The Measurement of Depression

THE MEASUREMENT OF DEPRESSION

Edited by
ANTHONY J. MARSELLA
University of Hawaii
The Queen's Medical Center, Honolulu

ROBERT M. A. HIRSCHFELD
National Institute of Mental Health

MARTIN M. KATZ
Albert Einstein College of Medicine-Montefiore Medical Center

THE GUILFORD PRESS
New York London

The opinions expressed herein are the views of the individual authors and do not necessarily reflect the official position of the National Institute of Mental Health or any other part of the U.S. Department of Health and Human Services.

Published 1987 by The Guilford Press
A Division of Guilford Publications, Inc.
72 Spring Street, New York, N.Y. 10012

Printed in the United States of America

Last digit is print number: 9 8 7 6 5 4 3 2 1

Library of Congress Cataloging-in-Publication Data

The measurement of depression.

Bibliography: p.
Includes index.
1. Depression, Mental—Diagnosis—Congresses.
I. Marsella, Anthony J. II. Hirschfeld, Robert M. A.
III. Katz, Martin M.
RC537.M43 1987 616.85′27075 86-29552
ISBN 0-89862-694-3

To our wives, partners, and friends:

Joy Marsella

Ellen Hirschfeld

Barbara Katz

Contributors

Nancy C. Andreasen, MD, PhD, Department of Psychiatry, School of Medicine, University of Iowa, Iowa City, Iowa

Christine K. Cross, MA, Group Operations, Inc., Rockville, Maryland

Paul A. Gaist, Neurosciences Research Branch, National Institute of Mental Health, Rockville, Maryland

Robert M. A. Hirschfeld, MD, Center for Studies of Affective Disorders, Clinical Research Branch, National Institute of Mental Health, Rockville, Maryland

Karen John, PhD, Department of Psychiatry, Yale University, New Haven, Connecticut

Martin M. Katz, PhD, Division of Psychology, Department of Psychiatry, Albert Einstein College of Medicine – Montefiore Medical Center, New York, New York

Donald F. Klein, MD, New York State Psychiatric Institute, New York, New York; Department of Psychiatry, College of Physicians and Surgeons, Columbia University, New York, New York

Gerald L. Klerman, MD, Department of Psychiatry, Cornell University Medical Center, New York, New York

Stephen H. Koslow, PhD, Neurosciences Research Branch, National Institute of Mental Health, Rockville, Maryland

Peter M. Lewinsohn, PhD, Department of Psychology, University of Oregon, Eugene, Oregon

Anthony J. Marsella, PhD, Department of Psychology, University of Hawaii, Honolulu, Hawaii; World Health Organization Field Psychiatric Research Center, The Queen's Medical Center, Honolulu, Hawaii

Judith G. Rabkin, PhD, MPH, New York State Psychiatric Institute, New York, New York; Department of Psychiatry, College of Physicians and Surgeons, Columbia University, New York, New York

Lynn P. Rehm, PhD, Department of Psychology, University of Houston, Houston, Texas

Paul Rohde, MA, Department of Psychology, University of Oregon, Eugene, Oregon

A. John Rush, MD, Department of Psychiatry, University of Texas Health Science Center at Dallas, Dallas, Texas

Peter E. Stokes, MD, Division of Psychobiology, Payne Whitney Psychiatric Clinic, New York Hospital – Cornell University Medical Center, New York, New York

Myrna M. Weissman, PhD, New York State Psychiatric Institute, New York, New York; Department of Psychiatry, College of Physicians and Surgeons, Columbia University, New York, New York

Preface

It has been suggested that our present age be called an "age of melancholy." Given the fact that as many as 10% of Americans presently suffer from depressive disorders and that one of every four Americans will suffer from a significant depressive experience in the course of his or her lifetime, it is clear that this comment may be an accurate description of our times. Indeed, officials from the World Health Organization estimate that there are more than 100 million people in the world who are suffering from clinical levels of depression. And they suggest that there is every indication that the incidence of depressive disorders around the world is likely to grow, because of increases in (1) life expectancy, (2) rates of chronic diseases associated with secondary depression, (3) rapid psychosocial changes associated with the onset and maintenance of depression, and (4) the use of medications that have depression as a side effect.

Depressive disorders include a spectrum of biological, psychological, and behavioral dysfunctions that vary in severity and duration. At one end of the spectrum, there is the experience of normal depression, in which an individual may feel a transient period of sadness, generally in response to clearly identifiable stressors. The depressed mood associated with normal depression varies in duration but normally does not last more than a week. If the depressed mood continues for a longer period of time, and if sleep difficulties, eating problems, mental and physical exhaustion, and feelings of hopelessness and despair develop, the problem exceeds the boundaries of normal depression and approaches the status of a clinical depression. A clinical depression represents a more severe problem and may require professional care. At the most severe end of the spectrum, the experience and manifestation of depression reach psychotic levels. In this instance, an individual suffers extreme sadness and despair, and may lose contact with reality and develop delusions, hallucinations, and severe motor and psychological retardation. When depression assumes these proportions, professional care is almost always necessary.

The tremendous individual and cultural variability in depressive experience and disorder has made research and professional care difficult. As a result, in recent years, much effort has been expended on developing valid measures of the problem. It is now recognized that the successful diagnosis, treatment, and prevention of depression may require the measurement of all dimensions of a person's functioning — biological, psychological, and social. The purpose of the present volume is to provide researchers, professionals, and students with a comprehensive and scholarly resource for identifying, understanding, and evaluating the many measures of depression presently in use.

The present volume consists of 13 chapters, each prepared by acknowledged research leaders in the field. The chapters were first presented as discussion papers at a workshop held in Honolulu, Hawaii, in 1984 under the sponsorship of the National Institute of Mental Health (NIMH) and The Queen's Medical Center of Honolulu. Following the workshop, each of the papers was revised and updated for publication in the present volume. The 13 chapters are divided into four main sections that cover the major perspectives in the measurement of depression: clinical, biological, psychological, and psychosocial.

The three chapters in Section I address the topic of clinical measurement. Chapter 1, written by Gerald L. Klerman, provides an overview of the field of depression and analyzes the use of the term "depression" to cover mood, symptom, and disorder. Chapter 2, also written by Gerald L. Klerman, summarizes medical, neurological, and substance abuse conditions that have depressive sequelae. The chapter notes that mental health professionals frequently fail to acknowledge these problems as sources of depression in cases they treat as primary depressions. In Chapter 3, the closing chapter in this section, Judith G. Rabkin and Donald F. Klein discuss the clinical instruments available for the measurement of depression, including structured interviews, clinician rating scales, and self-report scales.

The second section includes three chapters on biological measurement. Chapter 4, prepared by Nancy C. Andreasen, discusses major approaches to the measurement of genetic aspects of depression. In Chapter 5, Stephen H. Koslow and Paul A. Gaist review the measurement of neurotransmitters in depression, covering all the recent research hypotheses. Chapter 6, written by Peter E. Stokes, covers the measurement of neuroendocrines.

Section III includes four chapters on the psychological and behavioral measurement of depression. Chapter 7, prepared by Lynn P. Rehm, offers a review of recent developments in the behavioral assessment of depressive disorders and serves as a complement to Chapter 8, in which Peter M. Lewinsohn and Paul Rohde address the psychological measurement of depression. In Chapter 9, A. John Rush provides a discussion of the new developments in the measurement of cognitive aspects of depression. Chapter 10, the final contribution in this section, has been prepared by Martin M. Katz; it suggests a unique conceptual approach to the measurement of depression, based on research efforts in the NIMH Collaborative Program on the Psychobiology of Depression.

The fourth and last section of the volume consists of three chapters on the psychosocial measurement of depression. Chapter 11, written by Robert M. A. Hirschfeld and Christine K. Cross, addresses both the historical and contemporary developments in the measurement of personality and depression.

Chapter 12, written by Karen John and Myrna M. Weissman, covers the familial and psychosocial measurement of depression; it summarizes the growing number of psychosocial measures and provides a complement to Chapter 11. And in Chapter 13, the final chapter in the volume, Anthony J. Marsella addresses the unique requirements involved in the cross-cultural measurement of depression.

We wish to express our gratitude to the many organizations and individuals who provided financial and personal assistance in the completion of this volume. NIMH, Rockville, Maryland; The Queen's Medical Center, Honolulu, Hawaii; the Upjohn Company, Kalamazoo, Michigan; and Dorsey Laboratories, Lincoln, Nebraska, all provided financial support for the Honolulu workshop in which the chapters were first presented and discussed. Our appreciation is extended to Dr. Robert Straw of the Upjohn Company and Charles Aono of Dorsey Laboratories for their interest and encouragement. We also extend our warm "aloha" to Susan Arkoff, Marie Aldover, Peter Campos, Thomas Leland, Paul Lister, Darryl Lum, and Carol Serota, of The Queen's Medical Center, for their contributions to the Honolulu workshop's success. Lastly, a sincere thank-you is extended to Seymour Weingarten, Editor-in-Chief of The Guilford Press, for his boundless patience and encouragement.

Contents

I. CLINICAL MEASUREMENT

1. **The Nature of Depression: Mood, Symptom, Disorder** 3
Gerald L. Klerman
Introduction, 3
Depression as a Normal Emotion in Humans and Animals, 4
Depression as a Symptom, 9
Depressive and Manic Syndromes and the Affective Disorders, 12
General Conclusions, 16
References, 18

2. **Depression Associated with Medical and Neurological Diseases, Drugs, and Alcohol** 20
Gerald L. Klerman
Introduction, 20
The Clinical Phenomena, 21
Nosological Considerations, 25
Pathogenic Mechanisms, 27
Conclusions, 28
References, 29

3. **The Clinical Measurement of Depressive Disorders** 30
Judith G. Rabkin and Donald F. Klein
Overview, 30
Introduction, 31
Some Measurement Considerations, 34
Structured Interview Schedules, 37
Clinician Rating Scales, 48
Global Illness Ratings, 59
Self-Rating Scales, 62
Conclusions, 78
References, 79

II. BIOLOGICAL MEASUREMENT

4. The Measurement of Genetic Aspects of Depression 87
Nancy C. Andreasen
Introduction, 87
Designing Family Studies, 88
Data Collection, 95
Analysis of Familial Data, 102
Summary, 106
References, 107

5. The Measurement of Neurotransmitters in Depression 109
Stephen H. Koslow and Paul A. Gaist
Introduction, 109
Measurement, 111
Neurotransmitter and Metabolite Levels in Biological Fluids, 113
Receptors, 116
Alternative Neurotransmitter Systems, 124
The NIMH Collaborative Program on the Psychobiology of Depression, 128
The New Biology, 139
References, 145

6. The Neuroendocrine Measurement of Depression 153
Peter E. Stokes
Introduction, 153
Growth Hormone, 154
Thyrotropin-Releasing Hormone Response, 161
Prolactin, 165
The HYPAC System, 167
Adrenocorticotropic Hormone, 181
Corticotropin-Releasing Factor, 182
Conclusion, 183
References, 185

III. BEHAVIORAL AND PSYCHOLOGICAL MEASUREMENT

7. The Measurement of Behavioral Aspects of Depression 199
Lynn P. Rehm
Introduction, 199
Behavioral Perspective on Assessment, 199
Assessment of Behavioral Aspects of Depression, 214
Conclusion, 232
References, 235

8. **Psychological Measurement of Depression: Overview and Conclusions** **240**
Peter M. Lewinsohn and Paul Rohde
Introduction, 240
Basic Issues, 241
Assessment of Affect: Dysphoria, 243
Assessment of Cognitive Functions, 245
Assessment of Social and Other Coping Skills, 251
Assessment of Subjective Quality of Experiences, 255
Discussion and Recommendations, 258
References, 260

9. **Measurement of the Cognitive Aspects of Depression** **267**
A. John Rush
Introduction, 267
Cognitive Measures Relevant to Beck's Theory of Depression, 271
Cognitive Measures Relevant to Seligman's Reformulated Learned Helplessness Theory of Depression, 281
Cognitive Measures Relevant to Rehm's Self-Control Model of Depression, 286
Other Measures of Depressive Cognitions, 288
Conclusions, 292
References, 292

10. **The Multivantaged Approach to the Measurement of Affect and Behavior in Depression** **297**
Martin M. Katz
Introduction, 297
Development and Characteristics of the Method, 299
The Timing and Specificity of the Action of Tricyclic Drugs, 305
Predicting Response in the Clinical Situation: The "Effect Size" of the Differences, 310
Conclusion, 315
References, 315

IV. PSYCHOSOCIAL MEASUREMENT

11. **The Measurement of Personality in Depression** **319**
Robert M. A. Hirschfeld and Christine K. Cross
Introduction, 319
Personality Traits, 322
Discussion, 339
References, 341

12. The Familial and Psychosocial Measurement of Depression **344**
Karen John and Myrna M. Weissman
Introduction, 344
The Measurement of Psychosocial Risk Factors in Depression, 346
The Measurement of Social Adjustment in Depression, 350
Comment on the Measurement of Social Adjustment, 370
References, 371

13. The Measurement of Depressive Experience and Disorder across Cultures **376**
Anthony J. Marsella
Introduction, 376
Culture and Psychopathology, 379
Culture and Depressive Experience and Disorder, 384
Cross-Cultural Measurement: Issues and Methods, 385
The Measurement of Depressive Experience and Disorder across Cultures, 389
References, 395

Index **399**

The Measurement of Depression

SECTION I

Clinical Measurement

CHAPTER 1

The Nature of Depression

Mood, Symptom, Disorder

GERALD L. KLERMAN
Cornell University Medical Center

INTRODUCTION

The term "depression" is applied to a range of emotional states, both normal and psychopathological. As a normal mood, depression is almost universal in human experience; for example, not to grieve after the loss of a loved one is somehow "less than human." Depressive mood, however, is not exclusively human; equivalent reactions occur in most mammals, especially primates. As a symptom, depression occurs as a component of reactions to stress and in patients with medical and psychiatric conditions. As a psychopathological state, the depressive syndromes are usually considered along with mania as belonging to the affective disorders.

"Mood" and "affect" are terms that are often used interchangeably with "emotion." "Emotion" usually refers to the total range of cognitive, bodily, and behavioral changes that fluctuate in psychic life. "Mood" usually refers to a sustained emotional state, and "affect" refers to the minute-to-minute fluctuations of emotion.

The terms "affective disorders" and "mood disorders" group together a number of clinical conditions whose common and essential feature is a disturbance of mood accompanied by related cognitive, psychomotor, psychophysiological, and interpersonal difficulties. Although human experience includes a variety of emotions, such as fear, anger, pleasure, and surprise, the clinical conditions considered within the affective disorders usually involve depression and mania. Some authorities have suggested that the term "mood disorders" would be the more precise designation, since, in the clinical disorders under consideration, the emotional changes are pervasive and sustained, meeting the definition of "mood." However, since historical continuity and clinical usage have preferred "affective disorders," that term is used in the third edition of the American Psychiatric Association's (1980) *Diagnostic and Statistical Manual of Mental Disorders* (DSM-III) and in this chapter.

DEPRESSION AS A NORMAL EMOTION IN HUMANS AND ANIMALS

Although this volume focuses on depression and affective disorders as clinical conditions, understanding their psychopathology is enhanced by viewing the depressed states within the range of normal experience and behavior in humans and animals.

The normality of depression poses problems for clinical practice and theory. For clinical practice, criteria are needed to specify the boundaries between the normal mood state and those abnormal states that merit clinical intervention. For theory, it is necessary to understand the nature of depression as a normal emotion and to elucidate which aspects of depression are common to both normal and psychopathological states in humans and animals, as distinguished from those features that are unique to the abnormal states.

Adaptation and Normal Depression

The most important insights concerning normal depressive emotion derive from Darwin's evolutionary theory. According to the criteria of evolutionary theory, a trait or behavior is adaptive from the phylogenetic viewpoint if it promotes the survival of the species; it is adaptive from the ontogenetic viewpoint if it promotes the growth and survival of an individual member of the species. Darwin applied his evolutionary approach to behavior, especially to emotional responses. Darwin (1882) postulated the evolution not only of morphological structures, but also of "mental and expressive capacities." He collected material to document the phylogenetic continuity of emotional expressions in animals, particularly among primates and human beings. However, his observations and theory lay dormant for many decades. Since World War II, there has been an upsurge of interest in the comparative biology of emotional states, and a significant convergence of findings from neurobiology, ethology, and comparative psychology has taken place.

At the same time, studies of human infant development, particularly those based on modified psychodynamic theory, have paralleled the work of these animal researchers. Bowlby (1969) and others have demonstrated that the genesis of emotion in the child is related to the vicissitudes of the child's attachment bond to mothering figures. Due to their prolonged state of dependency, human infants are highly vulnerable to the effects of separation and helplessness. The infant's depressive behaviors serve to alert the social group, usually the family, to his or her need for nurturing, assistance, and succor.

This pattern is true for the child, but what of the adult living in a modern industrial society? Is an urbanized man's or woman's depression only the perpetuation of previously developed evolutionary responses? If so, is the clinical depression of adults an adaptive response, or is it an earlier developmental state? Investigations into these questions involve clinical and biological research and theoretical analysis.

Although depression is a ubiquitous human experience, it is not a uniquely human condition. Most mammals, and especially primates, have the capacity to become depressed. This capacity is related to the biological helplessness of the mammalian infant, born into life incompletely developed and requiring a period of extrauterine nurturance and protection before becoming capable of independent biological survival. Naturalistic observations, particularly of dogs (Scott, Stewart, & DeGhett, 1970) and of primates (Goodall & Hamburg, 1971), have demonstrated the presence of depressive-like reactions to separation and loss — reactions with many similarities to human depression.

This biological fact of mammalian extrauterine dependence provides the substrate for the development of attachment bonds, particularly between the infant and the mother figure, and for powerful reinforcement of social learning and group behavior. Bowlby (1969) has expanded these animal observations to emphasize the importance of attachment bonding in human experience. The development of these attachment bonds and the associated social learning involve complex central nervous system CNS structures that have been inherited and modified through the evolutionary process.

In infants, a depressive response (e.g., crying, facial change, postural change) is almost universally precipitated by separation from the mothering figure. This has been documented in human infant studies of animal separation (Harlow, 1974; Kaufman & Rosenblum, 1967; McKinney & Bunney, 1969).

Although the child becomes biologically less helpless as he or she matures into adolescence, the capacity to respond to appropriate stimulation with depression persists and expands, and the range of stimuli also expands. In addition to actual separation through death or physical distance, other forms of environmental change serve as stimuli to the depressive response. With the development of perceptual and cognitive capacities, the child learns to anticipate the threat of separation from the parenting adults. The fear of abandonment is a prominent feature of the psychology of school-age children. Through social learning and stimulus generalization, other social situations involving disappointments, frustration of wishes, criticisms and reproaches, changes in interpersonal relations, and shifts in the dominant-submissive relationship come to act as precipitants of depressive symptoms.

The extent to which these normal reactions are related to the psychogenesis of clinical depressive syndromes has been a controversial area within psychiatry. The onsets of many episodes of clinical depressive symptoms and syndromes are temporally related to changes in life events, especially the occurrence of medical illness either for the individual or for a loved one. From these observations has evolved the concept of "reaction," "situational," or "psychogenic" depression.

The approach taken by Bowlby and other students of attachment behavior is in keeping with the psychobiological approach to mental illness first enunciated by Adolph Meyer (Klerman, 1979). Meyer attempted to apply Darwin's ideas about evolution and adaptation to psychiatric illness and viewed psychiatric illness within the context of the individual's attempt to adapt to his or her environment. In the history of thinking about affective disorders, there has been tension between the Meyerian approach, which has tended to view the range of depression (both normal and clinical) within the context of human experience and emphasizes the continuity of normal and clinical states, and the Kraepelinian approach, which has focused upon the pathological aspects of depression and the discontinuity between clinical disorders and normal experience.

The Adaptive Functions of Normal Depressive Mood

An adaptational approach based on evolutionary theory examines multiple functions of depression. It inquiries into the neuroanatomical structures and neurochemical mechanisms by which natural selection, genetic mutation, environmental conditioning, and social learning serve both to mediate the impact of environmental change and to organize, integrate, and terminate the emotional, metabolic, and goal-directed activities of the organism, in its normal depressive moods as well as in clinical depressive states. Four adaptive functions of emotions are relevant to clinical psychiatry: social communication, physiological arousal, subjective awareness, and psychodynamic defense.

Social Communication

The adaptive role of depressive emotion as social communication has been elucidated by animal studies, especially in primates, and by studies of human infancy.

Animal models of depression, based on the separation-loss paradigm, have behavioral validity. Not only have these animal experiments replicated the clinical syndrome of separation of depression observed in human infants, but they provide a means of testing hypotheses about behavioral, cognitive, and social consequences of early separations. The experiments thus have relevance for verifying many clinical theories relating the vulnerability of certain adults to affective disorders to their experiences in infancy and childhood.

Physiological Mechanisms

While clinical observation and animal experimentation have established the relationship of separation-loss to infant depressive affect and have clarified the role of depressive affect as a social signal, problems arise in specifying the neuroanatomical, electrophysiological, and neurochemical mechanisms by which these affective states are initiated, perpetuated, and terminated. Comparable mechanisms parallel problems that have been investigated for anxiety-fear, an emotion closely related clinically and developmentally to depression. Following upon the research of Cannon, it is accepted that anxiety-fear serves to arouse the organism in preparation for "fight or flight." This function is mediated by complex neuroendocrine systems, especially those involving hypothalamic and subcortical brain structures and the release of epinephrine from the adrenal medulla.

The comparable physiological mechanisms involved in depression are less well established. Research, mostly based on advances in psychopharmacology, implicates the CNS biogenic amines and neuroendocrine systems in these mechanisms. Although the evidence derives more from neuropharmacological studies than from direct observations in humans, the patterns and trends increasingly support a role for biogenic amines in the mediation of depressive responses.

Another hypothesis as to the mechanism of depression has been offered by Engel (1962) and Schmale (1973) and their associates. They proposed that the depressed state involves conservation-withdrawal, with reduced psychomotor and psychological activity. This is an intriguing hypothesis for which experimental verification is still required. Although the conservation-withdrawal formulation may be consistent with some behavioral features of infant and adult states, the clinical depressed state in adults is associated with increased adrenocortical activity and with anxiety and tension, presumably due to heightened adrenergic activity — changes inconsistent with the conservation-withdrawal formulation. One explanation for the apparent discrepancy is to hypothesize that the clinical depressions of adults involve a failure of mechanisms operative in normal and infantile states. Another explanation is in contrasting the initial protest response to separation with the later withdrawal.

Subjective Awareness

The subjective aspect of emotion has been emphasized by clinical research and theory. It is widely, if not universally accepted that the subjective components of human emotion, conscious or unconscious, play important functions in goal setting and the regulation of behavior, particularly in the judging of reality against personal values and goals.

Social-psychological studies have explored fluctuations in self-esteem, self-image, interpersonal relations, and behavioral approaches that search for sources of reinforcement in the social world of subjects as related to their mood fluctuations. Beck (1969) has described cognitive dysfunctions in depressed patients, particularly their impaired capacity to judge themselves and their performances realistically, and from these observations he has developed his cognitive-behavioral psychotherapy of depression. The capacity of human beings to relate affective awareness to associated ideas and cognitive representations serves important self-regulating functions in maintaining self-esteem and in setting and modifying goals. This capacity depends on the species' achievement of language and rational thought — evolutionary attainments of great significance.

Intrapsychic Processes

The fourth function of depression, intrapsychic defense, is frequently discussed in clinical settings, especially those influenced by psychoanalytic approaches; nevertheless, it represents an area of continuing debate.

Freud maintained a strong biological view that derived human emotional capacities from instinctual drives. He also emphasized the continuity between adult behavior and infant behavior. Thus, psychodynamic theory stimulated interest in the developmental aspects of emotions, particularly in the possible role of early childhood experiences as determinants of adult psychopathology. Psychodynamic thinking also stressed the important and perhaps crucial role of emotional experience that is not directly within the conscious awareness of the self but is potentially recoverable by reconstruction, free association, dreams, projective tests, or hypnosis.

Originally, Freud viewed emotions as derivatives of drive discharge. Later, psychodynamic theory of emotion included the initiation of defense mechanisms. After Freud's writing about anxiety in the mid-1920s, psychodynamic theorists emphasized the defensive functions of affects in ego psychology.

Bibring (1953), Rapaport (1967), and Chodoff (1974), and other analysts, have criticized the classic psychoanalytic theory of depression as being exclusively based on drive and instinctual forces and as offering insufficient attention to ego functioning. The classic theory of depression does not regard depression as a primary affective state, but rather as the result of transformation of another drive affect, aggression. Recent research and clinical experience do not support this view. Although psychodynamic theory has reinterpreted its formulation regarding anxiety to incorporate Cannon's discovery of adrenergic mechanisms into Freud's concept that anxiety serves as a signal to initiate ego defenses, similar formulations of depression have been slow to appear. If we extend this single theory of anxiety to a single theory of depression, depression can be regarded as deriving from multiple sources, not only from intrapsychic conflict. Regardless of its origins, once it arises into consciousness or unconsciousness, it can serve like anxiety as a signal for danger to the self, albeit of a different sort than anxiety. The nature of the responses, including defense, that would result within such a single concept of depression has not been fully elucidated.

Conclusions on Depression as a Normal Emotion

Viewed in the framework of biological adaptation, the capacity of human beings to react to environmental changes, especially separation and loss, is the outcome of mammalian and primate evolutionary changes. As a consequence of millions of years of evolutionary development, this capacity has been adaptive for humans. In adult experience, however, the contingencies that initiate, perpetrate, and terminate depressive states are less specific than for the child, for whom separation is the major stimulus. Loss and separation constitute one category of larger groups of life event stimuli, which also include economic, social, and interpersonal changes. Many attempts have been made to develop a unified theory, and various theorists have focused on factors such as symbolic loss, life stress, self-esteem, helplessness and hopelessness, social role change, and reward and reinforcement. In my opinion, no comprehensive solution has yet emerged. The evidence of altered biological predisposition in persons liable to clinical states renders a simple environmental stress explanation unlikely.

DEPRESSION AS A SYMPTOM

Depression can occur as a symptom. These depressive symptom changes seldom occur alone; they are usually associated with bodily complaints or psychological and social impairment. Depressive symptoms may occur as reactions to personal experiences, such as grief and bereavement; in response to adverse social and economic circumstances, such as poverty or racial or ethnic discrimination; or as part of a reaction to medical and surgical illnesses. Patients with depressive symptoms are deserving of clinical attention even if these psychopathological features do not meet the diagnostic criteria for the full clinical syndromes. In these contexts, psychiatric intervention may be useful, although systematic clinical trials have not been undertaken.

Distinguishing Normal Depressed Mood from Symptom

Because clinicians and investigators do not fully agree as to the complete range of affective phenomena to be diagnosed as psychopathological, the boundary between normal mood and abnormal depression remains undefined. This situation has multiple consequences. In clinical practice, there are often inconsistencies in referrals and marked variations in decisions as to treatment, whether psychotherapeutic or psychopharmacological. Without valid diagnostic criteria, case findings are highly variable; epidemiological surveys are inconclusive or ungeneralizable; and it is difficult, if not impossible, to calculate accurate estimates of incidence, prevalence, and other basic rates.

Clinical Judgment

The occurrence of certain characteristic features (e.g., hallucinations, delusions, marked weight loss, and suicidal trends) indicates, according to almost all observers, that the boundary between normal and pathological depression has been crossed and that the patient has passed into the range of psychopathology. The presence of a recent overt stress (a precipitating life event) poses multiple dilemmas. Psychiatrists tend to think they understand emotional fluctuations as occurring in relation to the precipitating event. Often, they tend to minimize the severity of depressive reactions when the life stress seems apparent, and it is desirable for the classification of clinical states to be derived independently of environmental circumstances, whatever the duration, intensity, or presence of precipitating events.

Operational Criteria

The desirability of operational criteria is increasingly accepted. Clinical thinking usually implies a necessary-but-not-sufficient model of diagnosis, with emphasis on salient symptoms derived from the clinician's experience with ideal cases. Attempts to operationalize this model into standard criteria have been successfully developed in the past decade and are increasingly used in clinical and research settings. The development of operational criteria, such as the Research Diagnostic Criteria (RDC) and those of DSM-III, has led to the awareness of a large number of "subclinical affective states" (i.e., those clinical conditions in which depressive symptoms occur but are of insufficient number, intensity, and duration to meet criteria). These states are commonly detected in community surveys, as well as in primary care and other medical settings. The clinical and theoretical significance of such subclinical states has yet to be fully developed.

Psychometric Approaches

The necessary-but-not-sufficient approach, although appealing to the clinician because of its logical simplicity, has been criticized for its emphasis on pure forms of depression that may be relatively infrequent. An alternative approach has used multivariate statistical methods to generate scales. In recent years, much psychometric research has been conducted on rating scales used in diagnosing depression. Normative data have been collected for a number of standard scales, particularly the Beck Depression Inventory (BDI; Beck, 1969), the Zung Self-Rating Depression Scale (SDS; Zung, 1965), and the Hamilton Rating Scale for Depression (HRSD; Hamilton, 1960), so that it is now possible to identify cutoff points that distinguish normal mood from clinical states. However, while many persons in the comunity are distressed by depressive symptoms, only a minority meet the criteria for depressive conditions. A large number of studies have been undertaken using scales such as the BDI, the SDS, the Center for Epidemiologic Studies Depression Scale (CES-D), and the General Health Questionnaire (GHQ; Goldberg, 1979). These studies indicate that there are a large number of patients in the community and in many mental health and general health settings who score above the cutoff points established by psychometric validity studies. Only a percentage of these patients, as mentioned above, meet the criteria for a depressive disorder as defined by operational criteria. The significance of these scores is undetermined, and until this is fully established, the validity of this approach for screening and for research will be inconclusive. The risk factors related to high scores on psychometric tests are similar to those related to a nonbipolar major depression, but there are a number of serious difficulties, particularly for individuals undergoing periods of adversity or facing difficult long-term life circumstances.

Criteria Derived from Naturalistic Studies

Another approach derives from naturalistic studies of normal states. Prominent in this area are the excellent studies of normal mourning among widows. These studies offer criteria for delineating the duration and intensity of normal grief. In concert with the grief studies, systematic observations of subjects undergoing stressful events indicate that although mood complaints are common, clinical states are characterized not only by mood disturbance but by associated vegetative and bodily dysfunctions and by persistent and pervasive impairments in usual social performance.

Grief, Mourning, and Bereavement

The prototype for adult depression is grief, the almost universal depressive response to the loss of a loved one through death. The clinical symptomatology of grief has been widely recognized, and efforts are under way to explore the natural history of grief and to determine which grieving patients may be at risk for clinical depression. Relatively few psychobiological studies of grief have been conducted, and until we know more about neuroendocrine and other changes, important questions about continuity or discontinuity between normal grief and clinical depression must remain unanswered. There have been no systematic control trials, with the exception of the possible value of imipramine or other tricyclic antidepressants or monoamine oxidase inhibitors in grieving states. The conventional wisdom in most clinical circles is that the grieving process is normal and should not be interfered with lest adverse consequences occur. On the other hand, the intensity of affects generated in the grieving reaction may predispose the bereaved individual to higher risk for cardiovascular and other medical complications. A clinical trial of tricyclic antidepressants against placebo and/or against counseling would be of theoretical and practical value.

Depressive Symptoms as Reaction to Stress, Trauma, and Life Events

Stressful or traumatic events can cause a variety of emotional responses. Depressive and other mood symptoms often occur in this context, with mixtures of anxiety, disappointment, frustration, insomnia, and bodily complaints. The concept of "adjustment reaction" encompasses these responses. Studies of life events, such as unemployment, migration, and natural disasters, indicate that depressive symptoms occur quite frequently in these transitional adjustment states. Whether they are in conjunction with or subsequent to clinical disorders has been the subject of continuing controversy.

Depressive Symptoms as Reaction to Medical Illness

Depressive symptoms occur in a variety of medical states. Almost all chronic mental illness and acute states that are life-threatening or seriously disabling are accompanied by some measure of depressive symptoms. These may be transient and of relatively mild importance, or they may persist and reach the level of a syndrome.

The frequent occurrences of bodily complaints are of particular importance to psychiatrists working in medical settings, especially emergency rooms in general hospitals, consultation and liaison services of medical centers, and consultants to medical-surgical and related services. These may involve all organ systems, but pain, gastrointestinal complaints, headaches, and feelings of weakness and fatigue are particularly common. In fact, depressed patients may present without the depressed mood that is characteristic of the disorder, but may emphasize their bodily complaints, sleep disturbance, and feelings of apathy, lethargy, and weakness as their "tickets of admission" into the health care system. These conditions are referred to as "masked depressions," since they are based on a depressed syndrome, but without reported changes in mood and feeling state. The presence of persistent bodily complaints, particularly pain, should alert the psychiatrist to the possible occurrence of this condition.

DEPRESSIVE AND MANIC SYNDROMES AND THE AFFECTIVE DISORDERS

Having discussed the various aspects of depression as a normal emotion, let us turn to the various depressive syndromes and the affective disorders. These have had the attention of clinicians for many centuries and continue to be the source of increasing concern.

Some Historical Observations

Literary and clinical descriptions of depression — previously called "melancholia" and "mania" — date back to antiquity, as do speculations about the relationship of emotional states to health and illness. Scientific investigations of affective disorders, however, are only a century or two old.

The alternation of depressed and elated states was observed clinically through the 19th century, particularly by the French clinicians Falret and Ballenger. However, it was Kraepelin who brought together diverse states into the concept of "manic-depressive insanity."

The manic-depressive insanity classification was described initially by Kraepelin (1921) and subsequently modified by Bleuler (1951), with further contributions by various researchers over the past 75 years.

After Kraepelin's delineation of manic-depressive insanity as a diagnostic entity, debates arose over the breadth of the concept; additional diagnostic labels, such as "psychoneurotic depressive reaction" and "involutional melancholia," were included in textbooks, official governmental classifications, and semiofficial professional nosologies. The debates were partially resolved by the creation by Bleuler of the general grouping called "affective disorders." This particular grouping had many advantages, since it allowed for multiple subcategories, with possibly differing causes; offered more theoretical flexibility than the manic-depressive entity; and emphasized affect as a normal human faculty, thus not restricting the scope of psychiatrists' attention to insanity and other psychotic phenomena. However, many unresolved issues remain as to the scope of the affective disorders and the principles on which subcategories are to be delineated and validated.

Kraepelin's textbooks presented the basis for the modern classification of mental disorders. Based on the 19th-century medical illness model, disease entities were delineated by the methods of syndromal description and then correlated with pathology, histology, bacteriology, and natural history. Applied to mental illnesses, those approaches proved successful, especially for the infectious disorders (e.g., general paresis caused by CNS syphilis) and for nutritional diseases like pellagra.

Early in the 20th century, however, doubts arose over the adequacy of the approach for the group of functional disorders — those psychiatric syndromes for which no apparent structural or organic pathology could be demonstrated by the available methods. Among the functional disorders, the affective disorders in particular generated controversy. Kraepelin's concept of manic-depressive illness brought together a large number of clinical states — including mania, melancholia, and cyclic psychoses — and clarified many issues to create a brief period of unity. During the middle decades of the 20th century, however, the apparent unity achieved by Kraepelin's manic-depressive illness concept gave way to the proliferation of many new categories.

The "endogenous-reactive" and the "neurotic-psychotic" distinctions were proposed as new modifications of Kraepelin's concept of manic-depressive insanity. Debates arose over the validity of the DMS-III category of "psychotic depressive reaction." To add to the controversies, Kasanin's (1933) description of "schizoaffective psychoses" created a nosological bridge between schizophrenia and the manic-depressive disorders. In the 1940s and 1950s, borderline states and pseudoneurotic schizophrenia were described for patients in whom depression and other mood swings were prominent, creating yet another bridge between psychotic states and neurotic reactions — in that instance, between schizophrenia and depression.

The confusion was the consequence of multiple factors. As psychiatric services expanded outside the mental institutions and into general hospitals, outpatient clinics, social agencies, and private practice, increasing numbers of nonpsychotic and noninstitutionalized patients came to the attention of psychiatrists. Today, the preponderance of patients with affective disorders are neither hospitalized nor psychotic, and they manifest behaviors and symptom patterns differing in many respects from the classic syndromes formulated in the late 19th century.

Current Controversies in the Nosology of Affective Disorders

Although the second edition of the *Diagnostic and Statistical Manual* (DSM-II) and the *International Classification of Diseases* (ICD) do not have composite categories for the affecetive disorders (they are separated into psychotic and neurotic disorders in DMS-III), the affective disorders are grouped together as a general diagnostic class. This grouping has blurred, but not totally eliminated, the distinction between psychotic and neurotic forms. This trend is clearly seen in the research employing the RDC and also in the creation of a separate category for affective disorders in DSM-III. The creation of the category for affective disorders in DSM-III incorporates a large body of research on the psychopathological, biological, and therapeutic aspects of depression and mania.

The concept of bipolar depression has been widely accepted for its clinical utility in predicting positive response to lithium and adverse response to tricyclics. The bipolar diagnosis has proven a strong spur to research on genetic and biochemical correlates. The concept of unipolar depression is less well accepted. There is increasing awareness that all that is not bipolar is not unipolar. In DSM-III, there is no separate unipolar category.

The concept of neurotic depression has been radically revised. The DSM-III diagnosis of psychoneurotic depressive reaction was among the most common diagnoses in clinical practice. Research and clinical experience have increasingly questioned the utility and validity of this concept. "Neurotic depression" has multiple definitions, including (1) long-term personality difficulty, (2) precipitation by acute stress, and (3) underlying unconscious conflicts, as well as others. These criticisms (Akiskal *et al.*, 1979; Klerman, Endicott, & Hirschfeld, 1979) resulted in the deletion of this separate category in DMS-III.

Considerable research on the role of life events as possible precipitants of various forms of affective disorder has led to the question of whether there is a separate category of reactive or situational depression (Hirschfeld & Cross, 1982). Life events may increase the risk for a wide variety of disorders — not only affective disorders, but also schizophrenia and medical conditions. The specificity of life events for any clinical form of affective disorders is increasingly in question.

Since the 1950s, attention to endogenous depression has increased. Factor-analytic studies were initially undertaken by Kiloh and Garside (1963) and the Newcastle group. Numerous replications of the factor-analytic studies in the United States (Mendels & Cochrane, 1968) identified a cluster of symptoms, including early-morning wakening, loss of interest in activities and pleasure, loss of weight, and psychomotor change, either with agitation or retardation. Evidence has found that this symptom cluster, called "endogenomorphic" by Klein (1974), is independent of precipitating life events, but that it is highly predictive of response to electroconvulsive therapy (ECT) and to tricyclic antidepressants.

Another major advance in the affective disorders is the proposal by Robins and Guze (1972) to separate primary and secondary depressions based on the criterion of temporal coexistence of other psychiatric conditions, particularly schizophrenia and alcoholism. We (Klerman & Barrett, 1973) and others have proposed that the diagnosis of secondary depression be extended to include conditions associated with pre-existing medical disorder or drug reactions. The occurrence of mania secondary to medical conditions has led to a proposal for the category of "secondary mania" (Krauthammer & Klerman, 1978).

The large number of ambulatory patients with symptoms of both anxiety and depression causes nosological uncertainty. In clinical practice, these symptoms tend to be diagnosed as anxiety disorder and are most often treated with antianxiety drugs of the chlordiazepoxide series. However, a number of studies have questioned the therapeutic efficacy of this class of drugs in depressions. It is unlikely that a separate category for "anxiety-depression" will appear in future nomenclatures.

Although acceptance of the psychotic-neurotic separation of depression has diminished, the presence of delusions and other manifestations of psychoses, narrowly defined, is of clinical and therapeutic importance. Patients with delusions and hallucinations seem to respond poorly to tricyclic antidepressants. The nosological significance of this finding for the classification of affective disorders is still uncertain, although the practical significance for decisions as to treatment has gained increasing attention. There is uncertainty whether depressed patients with delusions are best treated with a combination of tricyclics and neuroleptics or with ECT.

The Contributions of DSM-III

Although a large number of patients have one or another of the depressed symptoms, only a proportion will have a combination of symptoms of intensity and duration that meet the criteria for a depressive disorder.

The DSM-III category of "affective disorders" groups all the affective disorders together, regardless of the presence or absence of psychotic features or association with precipitating life experiences. Within that group, the subcategory "major affective disorders" includes "bipolar disorder" (mixed, manic, or depressed) and "major depression" (single episode or recurrent). Under "affective disorders" there are two additional subcategories: "other specific affective disorders" (including cyclothymic disorder and dysthymic disorder) and "atypical affective disorders" (including atypical bipolar disorder and atypical depression).

The classification system for DSM-III has undergone successive modification and refinement, and some terms used previously have changed. "Involutional melancholia" is now classified within "major depression" (single episode), with "melancholia," or with "mood-congruent psychotic features." "Manic-depressive illness, manic type" is now classified as "bipolar disorder, manic type"; "manic-depressive illness, depressed type" is classified as "major depression" (single episode or recurrent); and "manic-depressive illness, circular type" is classified as "bipolar disorder" (manic, depressed, or mixed). "Depressive neurosis" is now classified as either "major depression" (single episode or recurrent, without melancholia), "dysthymic disorder," or "adjustment disorder with depressed mood." Furthermore, DSM-III accepts the evidence pointing to the importance of the distinction between unipolar and bipolar forms of affective disorders.

In my opinion, it must be emphasized that there is no one depressive syndrome. The DSM-III classification provides the reference point for a clinical subclassification.

GENERAL CONCLUSIONS

Grouping the affective disorders according to the patient's predominant symptoms represents less than the ideal basis for nosology. An ideal nosology would base classification on causes — genetic, psychodynamic, and/or biological. These and other factors have been proposed as causal for the affective disorders, and investigations are under way to establish their precise roles. It is probable that the conditions grouped together as "affective disorders" are heterogeneous as to cause, and that some or most are probably multifactorial in causation, involving complex interactions of genetic, biochemical, developmental, and environmental factors.

However, in view of the limited knowledge about the causes of most mental disorders, classification by type of psychological impairment has had great heuristic value. Since the late 19th century, mental disorders have been classified by the psychological faculty most impaired: intelligence (mental retardation), thinking and cognition (the dementias, the deliriums, the schizophrenias), social behavior (character and personality disorders), and mood (affective disorders). The approach based on mental faculties parallels the classification of medicinal disorders by organ (heart, kidney, etc.). The faculties of the mind assume the place of mental structures, equivalent to body organs in providing a basis for classification, when a causal classification is not yet sufficiently substantiated by research or clinical experience.

Within the past three decades, there has been an increase in the attention given to depression and other affective disorders. That attention has been increasing among mental health professionals and the public, especially in North America and Western Europe. These shifts in professional attention and public interest possibly reflect a historical trend, the emergence of a new "age of melancholia," in contrast to the "age of anxiety" that followed World War II. Precipitated in part by recent adverse global events and consequent doomsday prophecies concerning nuclear warfare, overpopulation, and ecological destruction, public attention to and acknowledgment of depressions and other affective states has increased during the 1970s. Coverage of mental illness by the mass media has reduced the stigma attached to depression, and a number of political leaders, astronauts, and figures in the arts and entertainment fields have publicly acknowledged that they have suffered from depression.

There have been other ages of melancholia in Western society. Robert Burton (1621/1927) described the widespread despair of 17th-century England in his classic, *The Anatomy of Melancholy*. The poets, novelists, and philosophers of the Romantic movement documented the *Weltschmerz* of the early 19th century. In the post-Civil War period, the American physician George M. Beard (1880/1980) described neurasthenia as prevalent in America, calling that malaise the "most frequent, most interesting and most neglected nervous disease" of modern times.

The current age of melancholia seems to be generated not so much by absolute levels of human misery as by the relative gap between rising hopes and the actual fulfillment of expectations. The earth's resources are limited; the population has grown rapidly, particularly after World War II; and recent sociopolitical movements have proved themselves incapable of creating the utopian futures promised by their ideologies. Those historical changes seem to be associated with an apparent increase in the incidence of affective disorders, particularly depression, as manifested by a rise in suicide attempts and by increased numbers of patients seeking medical and/or psychiatric help for symptoms of depression.

Those changes in the epidemiology of affective disorders have coincided with the development of new treatments, enhanced professional confidence, and new theoretical and research approaches. Impressive progress has been made in the quality and the quantity of research, both in clinical disciplines and in the laboratory sciences.

Acknowledgment

The writing of this chapter was supported by grants in aid from the National Institute of Mental Health (No. MH 25478-09); the Alcohol, Drug Abuse and Mental Health Administration; and the U.S. Public Health Service.

References

Akiskal, H. S., Rosenthal, R. H., Rosenthal, T. L., Kashgarian, M., Khani, M. K., & Puzantian, V. R. (1979). Differentiation of primary affective illness from situational, symptomatic and secondary depression. *Archives of General Psychiatry, 36*, 635-643.

American Psychiatric Association. (1980). *Diagnostic and statistical manual of mental disorders* (3rd ed). Washington, DC: Author.

Beard, G. M. (1980). *A practical treatise on nervous exhaustion (neurasthenia)*. New York: William Wood. (Original work published 1880)

Beck, A. (1969). Measuring depression: The Depression Inventory. In T. A. Williams, M. M. Katz, & J. A. Shield (Eds.), *Proceedings of the NIMH workshop on recent advances in the psychology of depressive illnesses*. Washington, DC: U.S. Government Printing Office.

Bibring, E. (1953). Mechanism of depression. In P. Greenacre (Ed.), *Affective disorders* (p. 13). New York: International Universities Press.

Bleuler, E. (1951). *Textbook of psychiatry*. New York: Dover.

Bowlby, J. (1969). *Attachment*. New York: Basic Books.

Burton, R. (1927). *The anatomy of melancholy*. New York: Tudor. (Original work published 1621)

Chodoff, P. (1974). The diagnosis of hysteria: An overview. *American Journal of Psychiatry, 131*, 1073-1078.

Darwin, C. (1882). *The expression of the emotions in man and animals*. London: John Murray.

Engel, G. L. (1962). Conversion symptoms. In C. M. MacBride & R. S. Blacklow (Eds.), *Signs and symptoms*. Philadelphia: J. B. Lippincott.

Goldberg, D. P. (1979). *Manual of the General Health Questionnaire*. Windsor, England: National Foundation for Educational Research.

Goodall, J., & Hamburg, D. (1971). *In the shadow of man*. Boston: Houghton Mifflin.

Hamilton, M. (1960). A rating scale for depression. *Journal of Neurology, Neurosurgery and Psychiatry, 23*, 56-61.

Harlow, H. (1974). *Learning to love*. New York: Jason Aronson.

Hirschfeld, R., & Cross, C. (1982). Epidemiology of affective disorders. *Archives of General Psychiatry, 39*, 35-46.

Kasanin, J. (1933). Acute schizo-affective psychoses. *American Journal of Psychiatry, 90*, 97-126.

Kaufman, I., & Rosenblum L. (1967). The reaction to separation in infant monkeys: Anaclitic depression and conservation-withdrawal. *Psychosomatic Medicine, 29*, 648.

Kiloh, L., & Garside, R. (1963). The independence of neurotic depression and endogenous depression. *British Journal of Psychiatry, 109*, 451-463.

Klein, D. F. (1974). Endogenomorphic depression. *Archives of General Psychiatry, 31*, 447-454.

Klerman, G. L. (1979). The psychobiology of affective states: The legacy of Adolph Meyer. In E. Meyer & J. V. Brady (Eds.), *Research in psychobiology of human behavior* (pp. 115-131). Baltimore: Johns Hopkins University Press.

Klerman, G. L., & Barrett, J. (1973). Clinical and epidemiological aspects of affective disorders. In S. Gershon & B. Shopsin (Eds.), *Lithium: Its role in psychiatric research and treatment* (pp. 201-236). New York: Plenum Press.

Klerman, G. L., Endicott, J., & Hirschfeld, R. (1979). Neurotic depressions. *American Journal of Psychiatry, 136*, 57-61.

Kraepelin, E. (1921). *Manic-depressive insanity and paranoia*. Edinburgh: E. & S. Livingstone.

Krauthammer, C., & Klerman, G. L. (1978). Secondary mania: Manic syndromes associated with antecedent physical illness. *Archives of General Psychiatry, 35*, 1333-1339.

McKinney, W., & Bunney, W. (1969). Animal model of depression. *Archives of General Psychiatry, 21*, 240.

Mendels, J., & Cochrane, C. (1968). The nosology of depression: The endogenous reactive concept. *American Journal of Psychiatry, 124*, 1-11.

Rapoport, D. (1967). Edward Bibring's theory of depression. In M. Gill (Ed.), *Collected papers of David Rapoport*. New York: Basic Books.

Robins, E., & Guze, S. (1972). Classification of affective disorders. In T. Williams, M. Katz, & J. Shield (Eds.), *Advances in the psychobiology of depressive illnesses* (pp. 283-293). Washington, DC: U.S. Government Printing Office.

Schmale, A. H. (1973). Normal grief is not a disease. In I. K. Goldberg, S. Maltiz, & A. H. Kutscher (Eds.), *Psychopharmacological agents for the terminally ill and bereaved*. New York: Columbia University Press.

Scott, J. P., Stewart, J. M., & DeGhett, V. S. (1970). Separation in infant dogs: Emotional response and motivational consequences. In J. P. Scott & E. C. Senay (Eds.), *Separation and depression: Clinical and research aspects* (Publication No. 94, pp. 3-32). Washington DC: American Association for the Advancement of Science.

Zung, W. (1965). A self-rating depression scale. *Archives of General Psychiatry, 12*, 63-70.

CHAPTER 2

Depression Associated with Medical and Neurological Diseases, Drugs, and Alcohol

GERALD L. KLERMAN
Cornell University Medical Center

INTRODUCTION

Depressive symptoms can occur in a variety of neurological and medical conditions, and in association with drug abuse and alcoholism. Sometimes the symptoms are of sufficient intensity, duration, and configuration to meet criteria for depressive syndromes in the third edition of the *Diagnostic and Statistical Manual of Mental Disorders* (DSM-III).

Similar considerations apply to symptoms of elation and euphoria, and to manic states, although these occur less frequently (Klerman, 1981; Krauthammer & Klerman, 1978, 1979).

There are four reasons why these phenomena are worthy of special attention:

1. For the clinician, careful differential diagnosis is crucial. Psychiatric clinicians should be alert to the possibility that depressive symptoms may be the clinical presentation of a life-threatening and/or treatable medical or neurological condition, such as brain tumor, carcinoma of the pancreas, or an adverse reaction to reserpine. Failure to identify these conditions can have serious clinical consequences.

2. For the clinician, careful diagnosis is also important for management and treatment decisions. The patient may have an associated medical condition that, while not causally related to the depressive symptoms, may influence the clinical course and the choice of treatments. This is particularly true where the patient's medical and neurological condition is being treated with a drug that may interact with the treatment chosen for depression, such as electroconvulsive therapy (ECT), lithium, tricyclic antidepressants, or monoamine oxidase inhibitors.

3. For the researcher concerned with homogeneity of samples for testing hypotheses, criteria are needed to exclude patients with associated medical

conditions, drug abuse, and alcoholism from studies of affective illness. This consideration, homogeneous sampling, was one of the motives leading to the proposal by Robins and Guze (1972) for the distinction between primary and secondary affective disorder.

4. For the theoretician, understanding the relationship between these associations can contribute to clarification of mechanisms of etiology and pathogenesis. The mechanisms may be either psychogenic or pathophysiological.

In this chapter, I review these phenomena with particular attention to their research and theoretical implications.

THE CLINICAL PHENOMENA

The following considerations are prompted by the clinical observations that depressive symptoms, often meeting the criteria for diagnosable disorder, occur in patients with a large number of medical and neurological conditions and in association with drugs and alcohol.

Medical Conditions

Table 2-1 lists the medical conditions frequently associated with high risk for affective disorder. These conditions include disorders of the thyroid, pituitary, and adrenal glands. Interest in the neuropeptides associated with these disorders, particularly adrenocorticotropic hormone (ACTH), endorphins, and others, has contributed to insight into the pathophysiology of depression. A large number of clinical affective conditions are characterized by hyperadrenal cortisolism. This seems to be true of various depressive states, as well as of bulimia and anorexia nervosa, and has many similarities to the phenomena in Cushing disease. However, recent research using the newly synthesized corticotropin-releasing factor (CRF) indicates that whereas in Cushing disease the impairment in regulatory activity lies in the pituitary, the impairment in psychiatric illnesses where hypercortisolemia is a major factor probably lies in the hypothalamus, with a failure of the feedback loop, reciprocal inhibition, and other regulatory activities.

Neurological Diseases

The correlation between anatomical brain damage by cerebral infarction and neuroanatomical regulation of affect has become the research interest for a number of colleagues in the Boston area, particularly Dr. Seth Finkelstein at McLean Hospital and Dr. David Bear at the New England Deaconess Hospital.

The euphoria associated with multiple sclerosis has often been described in

TABLE 2-1 Medical Conditions Frequently Associated with Higher Risk for Affective Disorder

1. Endocrine causes
   a. Acromegaly
   b. Hyperadrenalism
   c. Hypoadrenalism
   d. Hyperinsulinism secondary to insulinoma
   e. Hyperparathyroidism
   f. Hypoparathyroidism
   g. Hypopituitarism
   h. Hyperthyroidism
   i. Hypothyroidism
   j. Inappropriate antidiuretic hormone (ADH) secretion
2. Vitamin and mineral disorders
   a. Beri-beri (Vitamin B_1 deficiency)
   b. Hypervitaminosis A
   c. Hypomagnesemia
   d. Pellagra (nicotinic acid deficiency)
   e. Pernicious anemia (Vitamin B_{12} deficiency)
   f. Wernicke encephalopathy
3. Infections
   a. Encephalitis
   b. Hepatitis
   c. Influenza
   d. Malaria
   e. Mononucleosis
   f. Pneumonia
   g. Syphilis
   h. Tuberculosis
4. Neurological disorders
   a. Multiple sclerosis
   b. Tuberous sclerosis
   c. Wilson disease
5. Collagen disorders
   a. Systemic lupus erythematosus
   b. Polyarteritis nodosa
6. Cardiovascular disease
   a. Cardiomyopathy
   b. Cerebral ischemia
      i. Hypotension of cardiac origin
      ii. Cerebral arteriosclerosis
      iii. Cerebral embolization
   c. Congestive heart failure
   d. Myocardial infarction
7. Malignancy
   a. Carcinoid malignancy
   b. Pancreatic carcinoma
   c. Pheochromocytoma
8. Metabolic disorders
   a. Porphyria

Note. From *Antidepressant Treatment* by J. Griest and T. Griest, 1979, Baltimore: Williams & Wilkins. Reprinted by permission.

the literature, but recent evidence indicates that depressive symptoms are far more common.

Special attention should be given to the depressive reactions occurring in the elderly with senile dementia. In clinical practice, one of the important differential diagnostic distinctions is that of "pseudodementia." Impairment of thinking, concentration, and memory are frequently reported by elderly depressed patients. This syndrome was first described in England in the 1950s and led to case findings in nursing homes and other facilities. About 40% of patients over the age of 65 in British nursing homes who were diagnosed as having dementia were found to have reversible depressive conditions when treated with ECT and drugs (Kiloh, 1976; Post, 1975).

Recent evidence suggests that the depressive and dementia syndromes are not mutually exclusive. Dementia and depressive symptoms appear in the early stages of Alzheimer disease, multi-infarct dementia, and forms of subcortical dementia, particularly Binswanger disease. The subcortical dementias are particularly important because of neuropathological lesions in limbic areas.

Depressions Associated with Drugs Used in Medical Treatment

As shown in Table 2-2, a number of important interactions occur such that depression may be an adverse effect of a number of drugs. This has been most extensively studied with the drugs used in the treatment of hypertension,

TABLE 2-2 Drugs Frequently Associated with Depressive Reactions as Adverse Effects

Class name	Generic name	Trade name
Antihypertensives	Reserpine	Serpasil, Sandril
	Methyldopa	Aldomet
	Propranolol hydrochloride	Inderal
	Guanethidine sulfate	Ismelin Sulfate
	Hydralazine hydrochloride	Apesoline Hydrochloride
	Clonidine hydrochloride	Catapres
Antiparkinsonian agents	Levodopa	Dopar, Larodopa
	Levodopa, carbidopa	Sinemet
	Amantadine hydrochloride	Symmetrel
Hormones	Estrogen	Evex, Menrium, Femest
	Progesterone	Lipo-Lutin, Progestasert
Corticosteroids	Cortisone acetate	Cortone Acetate
Antituberculosis drugs	Cycloserine	Seromycin
Anticancer drugs	Vincristine sulfate	Oncovin
	Vinblastine sulfate	Velban

Note. From "Treatment of Depression in the Elderly" by G. L. Klerman and R. Hirschfeld, 1979, *Geriatrics, 34*, 51. Reprinted by permission.

particularly reserpine. Observations about reserpine-induced depression contributed to the formation of the early monoamine theories of depression.

Many animal models for screening possible antidepressant drugs used in pharmaceutical companies rely on the amine-depleted animal, where either reserpine or tetraquinonia are used to induce animal states of central nervous system (CNS) monoamine depletion. The behavioral validity of these states is still controversial.

There are complex reactions to corticosteroids, particularly cortisone and prednisone. While the majority of patients may show depressive reactions, a substantial porportion become elated and even manic or schizoaffective. The factors determining which patients react to steroids with depression and which with mania are worthy of investigation.

Depressions Associated with Recreational Drugs

In addition to depressive symptoms occurring as adverse effects of drugs used in treatment of medical conditions, depressive symptoms can also be associated with recreational drugs, most particularly amphetamines, cocaine, and the opiates.

Amphetamines and Cocaine

Among the various recreational drugs, the most significant reactions are those related to amphetamines and cocaine. These reactions are of interest pharmacologically and theoretically because of the known pharmacological effects of cocaine and amphetamine on release of the monoamines norepinephrine and dopamine, but not serotonin. Epidemics of amphetamine-related depression and suicide were reported after World War II in England and in Japan. We may be experiencing a similar epidemic of cocaine-induced affective disorders in the US. In addition to depression, both cocaine and amphetamines can produce a paranoid hallucinatory state indistinguishable from schizophrenia. This seems to occur during the period of ingestion of a high dose and is probably related to the dopaminergic actions. In contrast, the depressive reactions, including suicidal trends, are more likely to occur after cessation of the ingestion of the amphetamines and are hypothesized to be due to the noradrenergic actions. Rebound depression with amphetamines has been widely reported by students using amphetamines and also by street users.

Opiates

Depression also occurs in opiate addicts treated with methadone. It is unclear whether this is due to the consequences of the amphetamine action, to psychological reactions, or to some adverse affect of the methadone itself. A number of clinical trials have been used to treat methadone-maintained addicts, including those reported by Kleber *et al.* (1983) at Yale with imipramine and other tricyclics. Interestingly enough, brief psychotherapeutic efforts directed at mood disturbance have also been employed with this population, including the use of interpersonal psychotherapy by Rounsaville and colleagues (Rounsaville, Glazer, Wilber, Weissman, & Kleber, 1983; Rounsaville, Weissman, Crits-Cristoph, Wilber, & Kleber, 1982) in New Haven and two forms of psychotherapy, cognitive-behavioral and psychoanalytically oriented emotive expressive, reported by Luborsky, O'Brien, and Woody in Philadelphia (Woody *et al.*, 1983).

Depression and Mania Associated with Alcoholism

A major controversy concerning the significance of the association between depression and alcoholism exists, since depressive symptoms often precede the onset of heavy drinking. One hypothesis is that men in particular are predisposed to "treat" their dysphoric mood with alcohol. In this sense, depressive mood and dysphoria are antecedent and possibly prodromal components of the heavy use of alcohol.

At the same time, it is known that about 40% of alcohol-dependent individuals will experience a clinical depression within a year or two following delirium tremens or other withdrawal reactions.

In epidemiological and family studies, depression and alcohol are frequently associated. Winokur, Behar, Van Valkenburg, and Lowry (1978) used this association as the basis for one of Winokur's familial types of depression, depressive-spectrum disorder. However, recent epidemiological and family aggregation studies indicate that there is no genetic association, but that because these are two frequent disorders, a moderate percentage of families will have comorbidity of these two syndromes.

NOSOLOGICAL CONSIDERATIONS

As regards nosology, the situation is, in my opinion, unsatisfactory. Although almost all clinicians and diagnosticians acknowledge these phenomena, there is disagreement in how they should be regarded in relationship to other affective illnesses and how they must be classified. For example, Kielholz proposes the concept of "symptomatic depressions" for depressions occurring as part of the symptom picture of medical illnesses.

DSM-III

In DSM-III, these conditions may be classified in three ways. There is the category of "organic affective disorders," which is primarily intended for affective syndromes occurring in relationship to CNS disease. In addition, DSM-III has a category of "adjustment disorder with mood disturbance," if the clinician feels the depressive symptoms are a reaction to a medical illness. A third approach is to allow the clinician to use the multiaxial system, in which case the depressive or manic condition may be diagnosed as "bipolar affective disorder" or "major depression" or "dysthymic disorder." On Axis I and on Axis III, the medical or neurological condition is listed. The use of the multiaxial system allows the clinician to avoid any judgment as to the "chicken or egg" question (i.e., whether the mood disturbances were antecedent to or are independent of the medical condition).

The Distinction between Primary and Secondary Affective Disorders

Robins and Guze (1972) proposed a distinction between primary and secondary affective disorders. This is an initial separation based on two criteria: the chronology of onset in relation to the patient's psychiatric history, and the evidence of associated psychiatric illnesses. Within this classification, primary affective disorders occur in the group of patients who have previously been well or whose only previous psychiatric disease was mania or depression; secondary affective disorders occur in mentally ill persons with previous psychiatric illness. This diagnostic distinction is without reference to immediately apparent life stress or specific symptom patterns: The criteria for primary and secondary affective disorders do not include the presence or absence of a life event as a precipitant. The knotty etiological questions posed by the endogenous-reactive distinction can thus be postponed. This diagnosis is also independent of severity: Psychotic features are not important in the assessment of depressed patients, in decisions about treatment, or in prognosis and outcome. Etiological biases implicit in the older psychotic-neurotic diagnostic classification are therefore circumvented.

Exact data on the prevalence of affective disorders characterized as primary and secondary are not available. In a large sample of patients with depression seen in emergency rooms of general hospitals, 55% were found to have primary affective disorders and 33% secondary affective disorders; for approximately 10% of the patients, the diagnostic assignments could not be made.

Klerman and Barrett (1973) and others have noted that affective disorders are also often associated with general medical illness or drug reactions. Affective states, particularly depressions, often occur in patients with pneumonia, infectious hepatitis, or mononucleosis. Endocrine disorders, particularly those of the thyroid, adrenal, and pituitary glands, are often associated with mood dysfunction. Another important group of affective disorders is the consequence of drug effects, especially those of the rauwolfias, amphetamines, and steroids. The concept of secondary affective disorders, therefore, should be expanded to include affective states that are not only secondary in time to

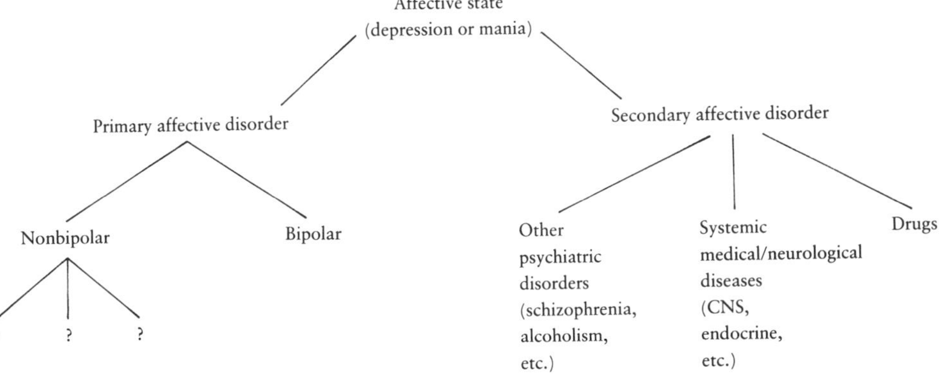

FIGURE 2-1 The primary-secondary distinction, and multiple diagnostic groups within the affective disorders.

other well-defined psychiatric syndromes, but also secondary to or associated with concomitant systemic medical diseases or drug reactions.

Secondary manic states also occur; elated mood and overactive behavior may be secondary to organized states or the effects of drugs. In patients with schizophrenic symptoms or with histories of a previous schizophrenic episode, an elated or manic episode would be considered part of the schizophrenic syndrome, according to the Robins and Guze criteria. For some psychiatric investigators, however, such an episode would be labeled schizoaffective.

The primary-secondary distinction is not a final diagnostic subclassification. Rather, it is valuable as an initial step toward classifying multiple diagnostic groups in a decision-tree approach, as shown in Figure 2-1.

PATHOGENIC MECHANISMS

Two mechanisms have been proposed in the depressive and manic syndromes associated with the conditions described above. One mechanism is psychogenic, regarding the depressive symptoms as "reactive to the illness"; the second mechanism is pathophysiological, looking toward the nature of the antecedent condition for clues as to the pathophysiology of depression.

Psychogenic Mechanisms: The "Reactive" Hypothesis

The conventional wisdom in clinical circles has been that these depressive symptoms are psychological reactions to the threat of illness and the stress of medical or neurological conditions. The crucial step in the sequence is the awareness by the individual, either consciously or unconsciously, that the medical illness involves some threat to his or her self-esteem, life circumstances, or survival. The related mechanism is that of a removal of denial, as is postulated to occur with alcoholics or drug addicts who become depressed after periods of withdrawal and abstinence. In the case of alcoholics, particularly according to the philosophy of Alcoholics Anonymous, the depressive symptoms are seen as a person's awareness of the adverse consequences of the drinking for his or her personal life as well as for friends and relatives, particularly family members.

The role of dysphoria in this sequence is complicated. Dysphoric mood is postulated to occur antecedent to the ingestion of alcohol and drugs and is postulated by many theoreticians to be the dynamic to motivate the future addict to use alcohol or some drug as a means of self-prescribed antidepressant treatment.

Pathophysiological Mechanisms

The other mechanism that may be involved is some pathophysiological mechanism, whereby the pathophysiology of the medical condition or the effects of the drugs alter those brain functions that subsume the regulation of affect. This is most evident in the case of drug reactions, such as the reserpine reaction, and also in the study of depressions and affective states related to brain lesions, such as stroke.

CONCLUSIONS

Separating depressive syndromes related to medical and neurological conditions follows a pattern widespread in other fields of medicine — for example, the distinction between central hypertension and symptomatic hypertension, or the distinction among anemia secondary to infection, to cancer, or to chronic ingestion of toxic substances such as benzene. Likewise, in diabetes, there is a distinction between secondary diabetes and primary diabetes; primary diabetes is further divided into early-onset and mature-onset forms.

The advantages of separating different syndromes are multiple. Clinically, it alerts the clinician to the need for careful differential diagnosis for treatment planning; for researchers, it ensures the homogeneity of samples for genetic and family studies and for treatment planning.

There is an additional research need — that is, to study intensively the clinical, psychopathological, and pathophysiological aspects of depressive disorders associated with specific disorders. Included in this group would be studies of depression in rheumatoid arthritis, multiple sclerosis, and pituitary tumors. These studies should include family studies to indicate whether or not a family history of affective disorder predisposes the individual patient to develop an affective illness in response to the drug or to the illness. This mechanism of familial predisposition has been proposed by Bunney (1978) and associates in understanding manic excitement as a response to tricyclics, and has also been suggested for patients with a depressive response to reserpine or to steroids.

Another research strategy would be to study intensively the pathophysiology of the disorder, particularly in instances of endocrine disorders.

Depression associated with viral conditions would be investigated as a site of action of the virus and might contribute to neuroanatomical understanding of brain centers involved in the regulation, perpetuation, and cessation of affective states. Pending the result of these investigations, the individual clinician will be confronted by the importance of diagnosing the associated medical condition and then determining whether or not it is antecedent to, consequent upon, or independent of the affective disturbance.

References

Bunney, W. E., Jr. (1978). Psychopharmacology of the switch process in affective illness. In E. Gershon (Ed.), *Psychopharmacology: A generation of progress* (pp. 1249-1259). New York: Raven Press.

Kiloh, L. G. (1976). Pseudodementia. *Acta Psychiatrica Scandinavica, 37*, 36-51.

Kleber, H. D., Weissman, M. M., Rounsaville, B. J., Wilber, C. H., Prusoff, B. A., & Riordan, C. E. (1983). Imipramine as treatment for depression in addicts. *Archives of General Psychiatry, 40*, 649-653.

Klerman, G. L. (1981). The spectrum of mania. *Comprehensive Psychiatry, 22*, 11-20.

Klerman, G. L., & Barrett, J. (1973). Clinical and epidemiological aspects of affective disorders. In S. Gershon & B. Shopsin (Eds.), *Lithium: Its role in psychiatric research and treatment* (pp. 201-236). New York: Plenum Press.

Krauthammer, C., & Klerman, G. L. (1978). Secondary mania: Manic syndromes associated with antecedent physical illness. *Archives of General Psychiatry, 35*, 1333-1339.

Krauthammer, C., & Klerman, G. L. (1979). The epidemiology of mania. In B. Shopsin (Ed.), *Manic illness*. New York: Raven Press.

Post, F. (1975). Dementia, depression, and pseudodementia. In D. F. Benson & D. Blumer (Eds.), *Psychiatric aspects of neurological disease*. New York: Grune and Stratton.

Robins, E., & Guze, S. (1972). Classification of affective disorders. In T. Williams, M. Katz, & J. Shield (Eds.), *Advances in the psychobiology of depressive illnesses* (pp. 283-293). Washington, DC: U.S. Government Printing Office.

Rounsaville, B. J., Glazer, W., Wilber, C. H., Weissman, M. M., & Kleber, H. D. (1983). Short-term interpersonal psychotherapy in methadone-maintained opiate addicts. *Archives of General Psychiatry, 40*, 629-636.

Rounsaville, B. J., Weissman, M. M., Crits-Christoph, K., Wilber, C., & Kleber, H. (1982). Diagnosis and symptoms of depression in opiate addicts. *Archives of General Psychiatry, 39*, 151-156.

Winokur, G., Behar, D., VanValkenburg, C., & Lowry, M. (1978). Is a familial definition of depression both feasible and valid? *Journal of Nervous and Mental Disease, 166*, 764-768.

Woody, G. E., Luborsky, L. McLellan, T., O'Brien, C. P., Beck, A. T., Blaine, J., Herman, I., & Hole, A. (1983). Psychotherapy for opiate addicts: Does it help? *Archives of General Psychiatry, 40*, 639-645.

CHAPTER 3

The Clinical Measurement of Depressive Disorders

JUDITH G. RABKIN
DONALD F. KLEIN
New York State Psychiatric Institute
College of Physicians and Surgeons, Columbia University

OVERVIEW

Improving diagnostic reliability is still a major challenge in American psychiatry. Advances in differentiated therapeutic techniques and biological procedures for studies of pathophysiology both require reliable diagnoses to allow generalizability. As Helzer and Coryell (1983) have observed, "After all the attention that has been given to diagnostic precision in psychiatry in the past few years, it is frustrating to think that differences in results across studies may still be partially attributable to criterion variance" (p. 1202). Furthermore, even though the specific criteria of the *Diagnostic and Statistical Manual of Mental Disorders*, third edition (DSM-III), may provide the basis for a descriptively homogeneous classification, their application may be inconsistent. Reliability is not determined solely through the use of criteria, but also through their application by interviewers who are sufficiently knowledgeable to elicit the relevant data in a clinically meaningful way across the range of psychopathology that will be encountered.

Even if criterion variance were not an issue, DSM-III does not offer full coverage with regard to salient illness variables such as severity and chronicity, nor does it include some subtypes that may prove useful to study. As the authors of DSM-III well recognized, this manual was not intended to solve all of the scientists' problems with regard to diagnostic reliability and validity. It has the more limited goal of moving the psychiatric profession toward reliable clinical communication.

In this chapter, we offer an overview of measures of depression. We have restricted our review (with rare exceptions) to published instruments designed either for diagnosis of depressive syndromes and subtypes or for assessment of severity. We consider only those instruments designed for adults, where the patient is the principal informant, and for which at least some psychometric data are available. We have included the most widely used and useful measures, but have made no effort to describe every published instrument. We have also excluded personality measures and scales for assessing specific areas of functioning (e.g., social adjustment, cognitive style), since they are addressed in other chapters of this volume.

After introductory observations, we review four categories of measures: structured diagnostic interviews, clinician rating scales, global illness ratings, and self-rating scales. We describe various measures of reliability and validity reported for individual scales. Excellent discussions of psychometric issues in the measurement of psychiatric disorders are provided by Endicott and Spitzer (1980), by Wittenborn (1972), and in the collection of papers edited by Pichot (1974).

INTRODUCTION

Bertrand Russell has reminded us that "a difference that makes no difference is no difference." We take this gnomic remark to indicate that by erecting a categorical distinction or arriving at a measurement dimension, we hope to make a difference. What is commonly called "validity" simply means that such a distinction or dimension allows us to make a difference. If we can assert something, arrived at through some measurement process, that then enables us to assert more or less correctly something else that was not tautologically implicit in the measurement, then our initial measurement has proven useful and presumably reflects some aspect of reality. Therefore, ultimately, the test of our measures and our categories is that they advance our understanding and demonstrate this by proving their utility. Those that do not prove useful should be discarded as incorrect guesses.

The problem of specifying categories and dimensions in the diagnostic field of psychiatry can be reduced to stipulating more or less efficient ways of explicating expert judgments in a fashion that can withstand both incident reliability tests and consensus discussion. In other words, in a situation where we lack readily available valid criteria, there is no immediate choice but to appeal to authority. It is not surprising, therefore, that claims to divine revelation have played a large part in humankind's effort to understand and regulate its world.

However, we know that what is asserted without evidence can be denied without evidence. Historically, our psychiatric position is far from complete ignorance, but is still all too far from the hard knowledge of etiology and pathophysiology that is required as our ultimate validational criterion. Freud, in *The Future of an Illusion*, reminds us, "Ignorance is ignorance: no right to believe anything can be derived from it" (1927/1961, p. 32). Therefore, we must proceed on the basis of the limited knowledge that we have. If we have no knowledge, nothing is left but empty disputation. What knowledge do we have available?

Probably the simplest kind of diagnosis-relevant knowledge consists of the detection of symptomatic patterns. It is hypothesized that there exists a grouping of traits or measures that, in some sense, reflects an underlying unity rather than a chance collocation or congeries. This set of traits we refer to as a "syndrome."

The assertion of a syndrome is, in principle, questionable through the usual methods of probability analysis. If we know the marginal proportions of the consistent traits in a sample, we can readily estimate whether the postulated syndrome appears more often than might have been expected by chance assortment. If it in fact does so, then we can be assured that there is some intricate causal network interrelating these traits or making them manifestations of yet more deeply underlying causes. We wish to emphasize that we are not discussing the possibility of arriving at a syndrome via some statistical cluster analysis (a procedure we have criticized elsewhere), but rather the direct test of a hypothesized syndrome's existence as shown by a subgroup of improbable associations.

As far as we know, there has been no attempt in psychiatry to directly attack the problem of any given syndrome's existence via the method of adequate population sampling, measurement, and probalistic analysis. The problems are clearly enormous. Probability samples are hard to come by. Even if one were industrious enough to develop such a sample, the measurement of psychiatrically relevant characteristics is notoriously difficult and without arduous precautions will be quite unreliable. Furthermore, the relevant characteristics, such as hallucinations or delusions, are often rare and seldom common. Therefore, detection of the existence of a syndrome that affects perhaps less than 5% of the population may well be swamped by measurement error. The probability of a Type II error is great, even with very good measures. Not surprisingly, then, this frontal assault on testing syndrome hypotheses has been eschewed.

Psychiatrists are used to describing certain syndromes and often find others agreeing that they have observed the same pattern. Yet here skeptics can always raise the doubt that what has been observed reflects not an underlying unity, but a common prejudice or halo effect.

As stated earlier, we would like to go beyond expert consensus. Ideally, we would like to show that allocating a person to a certain syndromal category makes some difference to our understanding of that person; we can make a better prognosis, choose a more effective treatment, give more accurate genetic counseling, or the like. Indeed, we would like to be able to validate our categories against etiological and pathophysiological knowledge, but, barring that, we will accept validation against phenomena such as the response to treatment, long-term outcome, and familial patterns that are only loosely linked to the underlying realities.

However, even at this level, our scientific ambitions far outrun our abilities. Seldom can we put our categories to the test of even these relatively soft validational procedures. Therefore, it is common practice to beat a strategic retreat from concerns about validity to concerns about reliability.

Without reliability there can be no validity, and this is clearly true in the extreme. However, the usual statistical truisms about reliability may be actively misleading when applied to diagnosis. The reliability of a measurement procedure can be intuitively grasped as its ability to produce a similar ordering of the objects to which it is applied, across the range of measurement present in the sample.

Yet it should be immediately obvious that even procedures of quite doubtful reliability, which would lead to all sorts of mixups when repeatedly applied to the middle range within a sample, might still regularly allocate the extremes of the sample as being very close to the extremes. Since many of the traits used in the definition of psychiatric syndromes stipulate that the subjects lie at the extreme of some measurement distribution, the ability of a measure to make gradations reliably within the midrange is of little concern for the particular purpose of identifying the outlier. Therefore, although we can agree that when reliability is absent validity cannot be present, we do not have to agree that tests of apparently low reliability cannot be of substantial use in diagnostic categorization.

It is true that the use of such tests must frequently result in the decision to leave the subject uncategorized, but is this any substantial loss? It might even be a gain, in that it confronts us with the vivid evidence of our lack of comprehension even at such a primitive level of syndromal construction.

In the context of syndromal allocation, we probably cannot make the easy assumption that improvements in reliability necessarily will increase our validity correlations, especially since the magnitude of the correlations depends largely upon the behavior of those at the extremes of the distributions. It would seem that in any given sample, however, multiple measures can be independently applied. This would allow us to contrast the reliabilities of methods and assert their relative superiority even without expert diagnosis.

For any given binomial sample assessed with a binary measure, the reliability of the measure is a joint function of the sensitivity, specificity, and base rate. We are not simply interested in an overall index of reliability, because we distinguish two sorts of errors — false positives and false negatives. For purposes of diagnosis, we cannot simply equate these errors. Moreover, applying evaluative weights to these errors seems no simple business. In practice, there is probably no all-purpose set of evaluative weights; rather, we should retreat from the amalgamated reliability index and try to speak more directly about sensitivity and specificity.

The problem here is that we can estimate reliability by intercorrelating parallel measures (in classical test theory), but estimating sensitivity and specificity requires knowledge of the true prevalences, which is exactly what we do *not* know except as estimated by expert judgments. Therefore, even this simple discussion of reliability indicates how we are forced back upon the weak but necesary reed of expert judgment as a reference standard.

As long as we are in the realm of reliability, the most direct attack upon the relative utility of different diagnostic instruments would be a head-to-head comparison of these instruments in a sample that has been well defined by the consensus of several experienced senior investigators, who have also demonstrated good independent interrater reliability. (It is a reasonable question whether averaging is better than consensus. For instance, if a measure were clearly more sensitive and specific when measured against a consensus standard than an average standard, it seems clear that the consensus must be a better standard.)

The point of this introductory note is to help the reader realize that even when the question of reliability has been directly addressed through the usual procedures of internal consistency, interrater and test-retest reliability, or parallel-forms correlations, the diagnostically crucial issues of sensitivity and specificity still require assessment.

SOME MEASUREMENT CONSIDERATIONS

The use of scaling devices represents the hallmark of clinical psychiatric research. This is in large measure a reaction to the difficulty of using clinicians as references. Clinical judgment has been challenged. Why is this so? The main reasons are these:

1. Clinicians are not always thorough.
2. Clinicians are not always thoughtful.
3. Clinicians are not always learned about the possibilities with regard to differential diagnosis, and therefore may not systematically pursue appropriate lines of investigation.
4. Clinicians use idiosyncratic criterion sets; these idiosyncratic sets may be at the elementary level of feature description and label application. In fact, this is probably more of a problem historically than currently. Reasonably well-trained clinicians will apply descriptive labels reliably. The real problem comes with category assignment, since clinicians have not had standardized sets of inclusion, exclusion, and severity criteria available to them.

Therefore, talking very generally, scales force thoroughness of coverage, which provides the information to which explicit inclusion and exclusion criteria can be applied, thus yielding a category assignment. Clearly, scales do not make clinicians learned or thoughtful; it is a researchable question just how necessary this is.

Another way to look at diagnosis is that it has three stages: the elicitation of information, the evaluation of information, and the application of criteria.

The first two steps act in a complex feedback loop, in which the ongoing elicitation of information leads to a temporary evaluation that then prompts further investigation. The evaluation of the information takes many forms:

1. Did the patient understand the question?

2. Is the reply deceptive or honest? Face-saving? Sick-role-seeking? Socially desirable? Self-dramatizing?

3. Is the reply influenced by psychopathology to such an extent as to produce a less than veridical report?

4. Should the report be viewed in the context of the patient's medical status?

5. Should the report be viewed in the context of emotional and psychological reactions to particular life situations?

The evaluation of these questions and the new answers lead to new evaluations and new questions, until finally there is a stable perception and a recording of the expert's view of what is valid information. Conceivably, although it probably has not been done, the expert could also record the verbatim statements of the patients as well as his or her own formulations, and then apply syndromal criteria to both sets of data.

This description of the interview-evaluation process makes it clear that there is ample room for rater idiosyncrasy to distort the output. Accordingly, we require reliability checks to determine whether there is a problem or not. Understanding this process casts light upon the possibility of sources of unreliability and invalidity in the various diagnostic approaches.

Self-ratings leave us with only the bald statement of the patient's reply. It is likely that such replies are often invalid for schizophrenics, occasionally so for depressives, and somewhat less so for anxious patients. Another relevant dimension is the relative inaccuracy of inpatients as opposed to outpatients.

Structured interviews that allow minimum inference, such as the Diagnostic Interview Schedule, amount to an interpersonal questionnaire. Their advantage over a self-rating is the assurance that the patient actually understands the question, but other than this, the complex feedback loop of information elicitation and evaluation is purposely abrogated.

Structured interviews such as the Structured Clinical Interview for DSM-III address those aspects of symptomatology that are narrowly relevant to the diagnostic criteria. The problem here is that by narrowly focusing on symptomatically relevant criteria, the diagnostician relinquishes the opportunity to gain a broader view of the patient. Such nonsymptomatic data may allow for skepticism concerning the patient's statements, which may err either in the direction of social desirability and minimization or in the direction of self-dramatization and the like.

So far, we are emphasizing thoroughness in developing criteria-relevant information in the diagnostic setting, either clinical or epidemiological. Scales have other uses that may help us estimate severity within a category. This was the original use for which the Hamilton Rating Scale for Depression was developed. However, the term "severity" implies a unitary dimensionality that may not be present. Factor analysis frequently has been applied to rating scales, with the result that several more or less orthogonal dimensions may be shown. Clearly, one can have as many severities as one has dimensions. To complicate matters further, the method of factor analysis assumes that the sample is randomly selected from a multivariate, normally distributed population without sharp cleavage planes or internal mixtures. Therefore, what may appear to be a set of different dimensions may actually reflect a mixture of different categories.

Scales may also help in the measurement of change. A common procedure is to use factor-analytically derived scores, obtained both at baseline and at the end of treatment, as the dependent variables in treatment contrast analyses. The problem with this extremely widespread procedure is that factors that measure status are not necessarily particularly sensitive to change. Because items relate at one point in time does not imply that they are all going to change in a lockstep fashion. Although this problem was pointed out by Klein and Fink in 1963, only the Montgomery-Asberg Depression Rating Scale has paid specific attention to the issue of winnowing out items descriptive of depression that are particularly prone to change during psychopharmacological treatment.

Yet another use of rating scales is to select homogeneous samples to use in case control studies for the detection of biological and social mechanisms and correlates of psychopathology. It is generally not recognized that scales that have quite moderate correlations with validity criteria might still be able to generate very homogeneous samples if one is in the position of selecting a small minority of those measured. For instance, a score consisting of the sum of the standardized scores of a person's high school grade point average, IQ, and parents' social status might correlate .40 with the person's actual academic achievement in college. However, if a college is in the fortunate position of having 10,000 applicants and admission openings for only 100, then admitting the top 100 as measured by this seemingly poor predictive device will furnish an extraordinarily homogeneous sample of high achievers.

The fly in the ointment is that such a procedure is analogous to selecting diagnostic outliers by emphasizing severity. It is conceivable that studies of these outliers will be more influenced by those pathoplastic features that increase severity than by those causal features that bring a syndrome into existence. For instance, the dexamethasone suppression test (DST) is far more often positive in inpatient major depressives than in outpatient major depressives. Inpatient status has served as a hurdle for selection by severity. Conceivably, some epiphenomenon of severity such as weight loss might account partly for the increased DST nonsuppression in patients.

We raise these issues for consideration as the different types of measures are presented in the following review.

STRUCTURED INTERVIEW SCHEDULES

Introduction

Structured interviews were developed in order to standardize the inquiries made by raters as well as the response options for patients. More generally, they are intended to increase the reliability and reproducibility of the assessment process. They are research instruments, and each requires at least some interviewer selection and training procedures. Whether they should be regarded as necessary or desirable in any given clinical study depends on the study's design and goals, as Kendell (1975) has pointed out. In cross-cultural comparisons, for example, or multicenter studies with independent teams of investigators, they are clearly the preferred method for assessment. In long-term projects where patients are admitted to the study over a period of years, they guard effectively against "criterion drift." Otherwise, minor adjustments inadvertently may create a secular bias, with patients admitted earlier differing systematically from later admissions. By contrast, in a short-term study with only a small group of interviewers and one patient population, the need is less obvious. In the interests of diagnostic reproducibility, though, an unstructured clinical interview for research purposes certainly requires some justification, while a structured diagnostic interview has clear-cut attractions.

However, if the major value of structural interviews is to enforce thorough inquiry, then it is not clear that an unstructured interview that requires the eventual coverage of all pertinent data might not do as well. Superiority for the structured interview might come from the standardization of inquiry, but this requires demonstration.

At least 15 standardized diagnostic interview schedules in the English language have been developed over the past 25 years for assessment of adult psychiatric patients in research settings. Most, however, are no longer used, having been superseded by improved versions using the current diagnostic criteria. The earlier schedules did not yield psychiatric diagnoses, but rather scores on various symptom dimensions. Those developed in the 1970s provided diagnoses based on the Feighner criteria and the Research Diagnostic Criteria (RDC), and the newest, still in the development phase, will provide DSM-III–R diagnoses for most Axis I and several Axis II diagnoses, as well as scores on Axes III, IV, and V.

At present, there are three major options for current use, with a fourth being developed. These are the Present State Examination (PSE), constructed by Wing and colleagues in 1959 and modified in 9 subsequent editions; the Schedule for Affective Disorders and Schizophrenia (SADS), developed by Spitzer, Endicott, and colleagues in 1976 for use in the National Institute of Mental Health (NIMH) Collaborative Program on the Psychobiology of Depression; and the NIMH-sponsored Diagnostic Interview Schedule (DIS), developed by Robins and associates in 1980, originally for epidemiological population surveys but also applicable to patient samples. The Structured Clinical Interview for DSM-III (SCID) is now being field-tested by Spitzer and Williams.

Of the four structured interviews, the DIS is clearly different from the other three in significant ways, including degree of structure, extent of inference possible by rater, amount of rater training required, proportion of pathological cases expected, and anticipated sample sizes to be assessed. The DIS is the most structured, does not require or allow inferences or clinical judgments by the rater, and does not call for prior clinical training of raters. Because of its epidemiological focus, the expected sample size per study often exceeds 1,000, which is almost never true (alas) in clinical research. The attendant costs and need for economy are also far greater. Finally, in view of its use with community samples, the DIS will be used with many more respondents who have no psychiatric disorder; case finding is a specific goal with this interview in contrast to the others, which are typically used with people already identified as patients.

In reviewing the characteristics of each of the four interview schedules, a critical issue is whether anything substantial is lost by using the "economical" DIS in either community or clinical samples. Since reports of outcome research with the DIS are just beginning to appear in the journals and at professional meetings, it is too early to reach a firm answer, but the question warrants careful consideration.

In the United States at this time, the SADS is the diagnostic schedule of choice for investigators studying depressive disorders. For example, in the 13 months from January 1983 through January 1984, 38 papers with samples of depressed patients were published in the *Archives of General Psychiatry*. Of these, 13 studies included a structured interview schedule for diagnosis; 12 used the SADS; and 1 (published in January 1984) used the DIS. Such preferential selection may reflect either the particular utility of the SADS for depression research, or the absence of desirable alternatives 2—4 years ago when the studies published in 1983 were designed.

In this section of the chapter, we review each of the three currently available structured interview schedules, as well as the SCID, which at present exists only in draft form. We present for each its background, goals, format, scoring, advantages, and limitations, as well as the practical considerations of necessary rater qualifications, time required for the interview, format, data base, and subject suitability. (Table 3-1 presents these latter considerations in capsule form.) A brief concluding discussion addresses reliability and validity issues.

Present State Examination

The first edition of the PSE appeared in 1959, before the development of Feighner, RDC, or DSM-III diagnostic criteria. It was intended to provide a

TABLE 3-1 Characteristics of Structured Diagnostic Interviews

Schedule	Rater qualifications	Interview format and structure	Interview duration	Subject suitability	Data base	Time frame	How diagnosis is made	Diagnostic output
PSE	Clinically trained mental health professionals.	Close-ended; optional rater inquiries encouraged. 140 items.	15-60 minutes.	Medical and psychiatric patients; scoring system adapted for epidemiological studies.	Patient only	Last month.	By computer program.	Descriptive syndromes. *Depressive disorder*: irritability, lack of energy, delusions, simple depression, vegetative symptoms, loss of interest, miscellaneous.
SADS	Clinically trained mental health professionals.	Open- and closed-ended. Responses are rated on 6-point graded scales. RDC diagnoses are rated absent, probable, or present. 200 items (3rd edition).	90-120 minutes.	Medical or psychiatric patients; SADS-L for community and family studies.	All available sources of information.	Previous week; current episode at its worst; previous episode.	By interviewer after completion of interview.	RDC categories. *Depressive disorders*: major (plus 10 subtypes), minor, intermittent, bipolar I or II. Current plus past episodes; uses diagnostic hierarchies.
SCID	Clinically trained mental health professionals.	Open-ended questions followed by closed-ended; optional rater inquiries. Responses are rated true, false, uncertain. (22 pages of questions.)	45-60 minutes.	Medical or psychiatric patients aged 18+; SCID-NP for epidemiological or family studies.	All available sources of information including informants, charts, and referral notes.	Current episode at its worst.	By interviewer as interview progresses, pending supplemental data from other sources.	DSM-III diagnoses, Axes I, II, III, IV, V (planned). *Depressive disorders*: major, cyclothymic, dysthymic, bipolar. Current plus past episodes; uses diagnostic hierarchies.
DIS	Lay interviewers with 1 week of intensive training.	Closed-ended only. No probes. 263 items (Version 3).	45-75 minutes.	Designed for use with community respondents; also used with patients.	Respondent only.	Lifetime; past month; past 6 months; past year.	By computer program.	14 Feighner categories, 9 RDC categories, 32 DSM-III (Axis I) categories. *Depressive disorders*: No RDC subtypes except primary-secondary. Does not use diagnostic hierarchies.

reliable method for case identification and to differentiate among major classes of psychopathology. For its time this was innovative, especially in epidemiology research, where "caseness" was rated simply as presence or absence without regard for type of disorder (e.g., Srole's Midtown Manhattan Study; Srole & Fisher, 1978). The interview consists of a standardized series of questions accompanied by standardized definitions, and is intended for use by a skilled clinician. Basically, it is a cross-sectional symptomatic review that allocates symptoms in a syndromal scheme without considering illness course or history.

The PSE is based on, and retains the major features of, a routine clinical examination. In its current format (Wing, Cooper, & Sartorious, 1974), it consists of 107 questions addressed to the respondent, and an additional 33 observational ratings of behavior, affect, and speech. Among the 107 questions, only 54 are "obligatory" and must be asked in every interview. In the absence of any positive responses providing evidence of symptoms, and with a respondent who is judged to be a reliable reporter, these 54 obligatory questions constitute the entire interview. There are, in addition, 3 other categories of questions that are designed to clarify responses to the obligatory questions and to elicit additional information when symptoms are present. It is important to note that it is the clinician, not the respondent, who makes this determination.

Responses to the precoded interview are scored by a computer program known as CATEGO. It uses a logical decision-tree model in which all the PSE data are reduced to a specific set of symptoms; these symptoms, in turn, are analyzed to produce syndromes and then ultimately 6 descriptive categories that are not mutually exclusive. Neither the symptoms nor the syndromes themselves necessarily belong to a single diagnostic category, but may be part of several. The final output for each patient includes all the syndromes and descriptive categories that are present (Spitzer & Williams, 1980). The CATEGO program is available to other investigators by arrangement with Wing.

The PSE and CATEGO are able to generate some diagnoses from the 8th and 9th editions of the *International Classification of Diseases* (ICD-8 and ICD-9) — diagnoses that are seldom used in the United States. CATEGO also has been adapted to provide diagnoses based on the Feighner diagnostic criteria, although very few CATEGO-positive cases appear to meet these more restrictive research criteria (Wing, 1970).

Since the time frame of the PSE is the past month, its diagnostic utility is in some instances limited. It cannot, for example, be used to differentiate unipolar and bipolar disorder, or primary and secondary depressive disorder. In application, the PSE has been used predominantly in studies of schizophrenia, such as the International Pilot Study of Schizophrenia. Furthermore, it cannot generate either episode or lifetime diagnoses according to RDC or DSM-III criteria, and has restricted ability to provide some Feighner diagnoses. It is not commonly used in this country in studies of depression.

Basically, the PSE is a cross-sectional review that allocates symptoms in a syndromal fashion, but it takes little note of course or history. Because of this, it cannot be considered to produce a diagnosis, but, as its title affirms, only a present state measure.

Schedule for Affective Disorders and Schizophrenia

The SADS, as noted above, was constructed for use in the NIMH Collaborative Program on the Psychobiology of Depression. The SADS is designed to provide both current and lifetime RDC diagnoses, which were developed from the Feighner criteria at the same time. The purpose of the SADS is to enable research investigators to apply a consistent set of diagnostic criteria in a standard format in order to obtain homogeneous groups of subjects. The focus of the SADS is primarily "on those symptoms associated with and important to the differential diagnosis of affective disorders" (Endicott *et al.*, 1981, p. 98). Since it was designed as a research instrument, it is not intended either to cover all psychiatric disorders or to classify all psychiatric patients; those who fail to meet the specified criteria are placed in the residual category of "other psychiatric disorder."

There is actually a "family" of SADS interviews. The SADS itself is intended for use with psychiatric and medical patients. It consists of two parts; the first is an extensive inquiry about current symptoms and current episode, while the second focuses on previous history of psychiatric disorder. They can be administrated together or on separate occasions, with Part 2 deferred until a patient has begun to respond to treatment. The SADS-L is a "lifetime" version and emphasizes past history, thus resembling Part 2 of the SADS. It differs from Part 2 in that it does address the possibility of there being a current episode, which in the SADS is entirely covered in Part 1. SADS-L is used in studies in which there is no known current episode — for example, in assessment of relatives of patients, in the screening of normal controls, or in community studies.

The Family History — Research Diagnostic Criteria (FH-RDC) is an SADS adaptation meant for family history studies, where one member is interviewed about the psychiatric histories of each other family member. The SADS-C is intended for measuring change, as in clinical drug trials, and can be used either in conjunction with the SADS or as an independent rating scale (described in "Clinician Rating Scales," below). The SADS-C provides symptom factor scores, as well as a derived Hamilton Rating Scale for Depression score. In addition, special SADS supplements have been written by Jean Endicott and various collaborators for specific research programs. These include an SADS — Anxiety supplement, an interval SADS-L for longitudinal studies with repeated interviews, an SADS — Affective Disorders supplement for assessing atypical depression, a supplement for assessment of schizotypal and borderline features (the Schedule for Interviewing Borderlines; SIB), and a self-rating form (in preparation). In this section, we report only on characteristics of the SADS itself, which is the equivalent of the other structured interviews reviewed here. The edition currently in use is the third edition, dated October 1979.

Among the currently available research diagnostic interviews, the SADS is most "expensive" in terms of rater training requirements and interview duration. Raters are required to have preivous clinical experience, and the training takes several weeks. Detailed instructions, case vignettes, workbooks, and videotapes are available to facilitate training. The focus of the SADS is on the worst period of the current episode, but a subset of 45 scaled items is judged for level of severity during the past week. These weekly ratings lend themselves to assessment of change over time.

SADS ratings generally consist of scales of graded severity, usually with 6 points accompanied by brief descriptive statements to serve as anchors. These graded ratings permit differentiated assessments, but in fact are rarely reported in publications and for diagnostic purposes are converted into a dichotomous rating of symptom present or absent. For this reason, and because such scaled judgments increase the length of the interview, SCID authors Spitzer and Williams have chosen a simpler response format to expedite scoring. Interviewers, however, often prefer the use of graded scales, and they are in general of superior reliability.

Despite the costs of requiring trained clinicians as raters, SADS-L interviews have been conducted in community surveys. Weissman and Myers (1978) were the first to use the SADS in a community study of over 500 respondents, and Vernon and Roberts (1982) used the same schedule in their study of over 500 community residents. SADS interviews appear to be a viable alternative even in large-scale studies.

The SADS is particularly useful in depression research, because it provides criteria for identifying 10 subtypes of major depressive disorder, and the Affective Disorders supplement identifies an 11th subtype. Its widespread use allows investigators to compare their findings with those of other major research programs, facilitating incremental growth of knowledge about depressive disorders.

Diagnostic Interview Schedule

The DIS was commissioned by NIMH for use in its Epidemiological Catchment Area (ECA) studies, which entail estimation of the prevalence and incidence of specific psychiatric disorders in the general population. From the start, it was also intended for use with clinical samples, but the primary emphasis was on its utility with community respondents. Lee Robins and her associates at Washington University, in consultation with Spitzer and Williams at the New York State Psychiatric Institute, adapted the DIS from the Renard Diagnostic Interview, itself recently developed for diagnosis of patient samples according to Feighner criteria (Helzer, Robins, Croughan, & Weiner, 1981).

Distinctive features of the DIS include the following:

1. It is designed to be used by lay interviewers with 1 week of training.

2. It has a simplified format in which every question is read exactly as written to the respondent, who responds either "yes" or "no."

3. Decision making by the interviewer thus consists of only two components: Did the respondent understand the question, and did he or she say "yes" or "no"?

4. In contrast to other structured interview schedules, there are explicit rules about which questions are asked. There are no optional skip-outs or omissions, or opportunities for improvised questions.

5. Diagnoses are made on a lifetime basis. In addition, current diagnoses can be identified in 4 time periods: past 2 weeks, past month, past 6 months, and past year. Diagnoses for the current episode as such are not available.

6. The DIS provides diagnoses according to three sets of criteria: all Feighner; all RDC (but only one subtype of major depressive disorder, which is the primary-secondary distinction); and, in Version 3, 32 of 150 DSM-III Axis I diagnoses (Robins & Helzer, 1982). Its diagnostic coverage is thus potentially considerably more comprehensive than that of the PSE or SADS, and far fewer patients end up in residual categories.

The DIS has a set of computer programs that generate as many diagnoses as applicable. That is, it does not impose a hierarchical ranking of diagnoses and will provide as many diagnostic classifications for a given patient as are met. In contrast, the other research interviews skip "pre-empted diagnoses," which therefore cannot be recovered on a later occasion. For example, the SCID is designed specifically to generate DSM-III diagnoses. In the DSM-III hierarchical decision-tree system, the presence of a given diagnosis (e.g., agoraphobia) pre-empts another diagnosis (e.g., generalized anxiety disorder). That is, according to the nosological rules, if one diagnosis is given, the other cannot be assigned and is therefore not recorded. In the DIS, the data are nevertheless collected, and unless one is applying the DSM-III computer program to DIS data, the DIS will provide all diagnoses regardless of hierarchical rules. DIS computer programs can also provide a total symptom count and a count of the number of criteria met for each diagnosis, whether or not that diagnosis is positive (Helzer *et al.*, 1981, p. 393). For many research questions, this capacity is useful.

Preliminary reports on reliability and validity were based on comparisons of ratings for 216 patients assessed in separate sessions by lay interviewers and psychiatrists (Robins, Helzer, Croughan, & Ratcliff, 1981). The psychiatrists first completed the DIS and then were able to ask any further questions they thought were needed to clarify diagnostic assessment. In regard to the presence or absence of the diagnosis of depression, there was approximately 80% concordance for lay interviewers and psychiatrists for all 3 sets of diagnostic criteria. This is at best a crude index of interrater reliability, since it does not correct for chance agreement.

A preliminary report from the Baltimore center of the ECA collaborative project (Anthony *et al.*, 1985) provides some data regarding DIS correspondence to psychiatrists' assessments. At the John Hopkins site of the ECA project, four research psychiatrists reinterviewed 810 of the 3,481 community respondents who had been given DIS interviews. The purpose was to determine extent of diagnostic agreement between the DIS and a full clinical psychiatric examination which consisted of the PSE amplified by "additional items for DSM III diagnoses" and queries about clinical history. Unfortunately, the format of this "clinical reappraisal" (CR) interview is not described in this publication, so that it is unclear whether it more closely resembles another structured diagnostic interview or a clinical examination. Its average length was about 2 hours. No formal assessment of interrater reliability was conducted.

In the Anthony *et al.* (1985) paper, diagnostic findings are reported for four disorders: major depression, schizophrenia, alcohol use disorder, and antisocial personality. Across the 810 sets of interviews, concordance was not impressive. For major depression, the DIS found 40 cases, of which only 8 were also identified as such by the CR interview. The CR diagnosed as depressed another 14 respondents *not* diagnosed by the DIS. If the CR is used as a criterion of accuracy, this yields for the DIS a sensitivity of 36% and specificity of 93%. Overall, the DIS generated twice as many diagnoses of major depression as did the psychiatric examination. Agreement for other diagnostic categories was also limited: The DIS identified twice as many schizophrenics as the CR, while the CR found twice as many cases of alcohol use disorder and 55% more cases of antisocial personality. These findings certainly raise important questions about the correspondence of DIS diagnoses and psychiatrists' clinical diagnoses, which themselves may be substantially unreliable.

The major specific advantages of the DIS at this time include its relative brevity, use by lay interviewers, and computer-generated DSM-III diagnoses. Robins *et al.* (1981) report that it takes 45-70 minutes to administer, an estimate corroborated by Von Korff, Anthony, and Kramer (1982). It does seem likely that this will vary as a factor of respondent characteristics, including ethnicity and illness severity. For example, in a study being conducted in Puerto Rico, patients often do not accept the simple "yes-no" format of the DIS and talk at length, so that the average interview takes about 2 hours, not 1 (L. Jimenez, personal communication, 1986).

While the DIS was intended for community studies, it is also applicable to patient groups. One immediate advantage of using the DIS with patients is the availability of the community data to provide comparison groups and prevalence baselines. In the NIMH-sponsored ECA studies, the DIS has been given to over 10,000 community respondents, and the work is ongoing. This is a rich data bank indeed.

The main drawbacks of the DIS for depression research are its somewhat arbitrary time frames and inability to generate subtypes. As noted, most of the RDC subtypes are not included. Endicott (1981) also has questioned whether the DIS computer program "could accurately apply the RDC rules as they are written, since many of them require a careful consideration of the time sequence in the development of symptoms during a specific period of illness" (p. 1300). Another potential limitation is that all clinical information is provided by the respondent, without consideration of physicians' notes, observations of ward staff, relatives' accounts, or previous records. Finally, an equivocal feature of the DIS is that the computer makes the diagnosis, thus enhancing interrater reliability but perhaps not the validity of the diagnostic assessment.

Structured Clinical Interview for DSM-III

Spitzer and Williams are currently developing a new structured interview schedule under contract with NIMH, specifically designed to generatee DSM-III diagnoses (Spitzer & Williams, 1983a; Spitzer, Williams, & Gibbon, 1986). It is intended for use by clinically trained mental health professionals in making the major Axis I and selected Axis II diagnoses, and also will cover Axes IV and V.

The SCID is intended to generate diagnoses, not to provide the fullest possible description of psychopathology. The SCID has a large number of screening questions and cutoffs, so that if key components of a disorder are not met, associated features are not assessed. The sequence of questions follows DSM-III format, and the items rated are the DSM-III diagnostic criteria. The interview is organized by diagnostic category, with mandatory questions to establish the presence of essential diagnostic criteria, parenthetical questions to be asked when clarification is necessary, and requests for specific examples of a symptom the patient reports as present. In the absence of essential diagnostic criteria, the balance of items in this area are skipped. The interview follows hierarchical rules, so that the presence of a disorder (e.g., schizophrenia) that pre-empts another disorder (e.g., major depression) allows the interviewer to skip over the pre-empted disorder. In addition, the SCID is modular, to facilitate omission of diagnostic sections not relevant to a particular patient or study (Spitzer, 1983).

The SCID is designed to provide provisional or definite diagnoses for psychiatric or medical patients aged 18 or older. A modified version, known as SCID-NP, has been developed for interviews with people who are not identified patients (Spitzer & Williams, 1986).

Specific advantages of the SCID for depression research (presented in more detail in Table 3-1) include focus on current illness episode as defined by the patient; incorporation into the diagnostic assessment of reports from records and informants; and incorporation of revisions in diagnostic criteria based on field applications since the publication of DSM-III, particularly with regard to principles for diagnostic hierarchies. As of 1986, the SCID is the only structured interview schedule for adults to incorporate the changes included in DSM-III — R, the revised diagnostic criteria to be published in 1987.

The most obvious advantage of the SCID compared to the SADS or PSE for those who want DSM-III diagnoses is that the SCID is specifically intended to provide them. The advantages over the DIS, which is the only currently available interview providing DSM-III diagnoses, are the SCID's broader coverage of diagnoses and axes, possibly greater validity associated with its broader data base, more flexible system of inquiry, and incorporation of DSM-III revisions.

The major current limitation of the SCID for depression research is the lack of information about depressive subtypes not included in DSM-III, such as the primary-secondary distinction, the atypical syndrome described by investigators such as Liebowitz *et al.* (1984), bipolar II disorder, and other subtypes currently under active study. One solution would be development of supplements for specific research programs. Furthermore, the skip-out method precludes consideration of certain research questions and prevents reanalysis with alternative criteria.

The most recent version of the SCID (Spitzer *et al.*, 1986) includes sections on substance dependence and affective, psychotic, anxiety, eating, and adjustment disorders. The most extensive revisions in diagnostic classifiation are in the section on anxiety disorders. While the current version is available to all investigators who are willing to provide feedback to the authors, it is not yet a finished product. Sections for evaluating Axes IV and V are being planned.

Reliability and Validity Studies of Structured Diagnostic Interviews

A major impetus for the development of structured diagnostic interview schedules was to correct the lamentably poor level of diagnostic reliability that was the norm in psychiatric research. Together with the development of operational diagnostic criteria — the Feighner criteria in 1972, the RDC in 1978, the DSM-III in 1980 — the introduction of these structured interviews made it feasible to aspire to reproducibility in diagnostic classification, at least for the major disorders, for the first time.

Over the last decade, several types of reliability studies have been conducted in conjunction with the three major available interviews — the PSE, the SADS, and the DIS. The least expensive and least stringent method uses either written case vignettes or audiotapes or videotapes of patient interviews, which are then rated by others. When case vignettes are used, a large number of cases can be studied rather quickly to establish adequate interrater agreement.

Other measures of interrater agreement include joint interviews with an active rater and silent observer, and successive interviews of the same patient by different raters; the latter is the most demanding method and is also the most complex, since the patient's status may indeed change between occasions. All of these methods have been used in large-scale studies, each accompanied by the use of appropriate statistics, most commonly Cohen's kappa. Detailed review of statistical issues in assessing reliability of psychiatric diagnoses is provided by Grove, Andreasen, McDonald-Scott, Keller, and Shapiro (1981), and extensive reliability data for the PSE and SADS and one study of the DIS are summarized by Hedlund and Veiweg (1981). Additional data on reliability of the DIS are provided by Hesselbrock, Stabenau, Hesselbrock, Merkin, and Meyer (1982) and Robins *et al.* (1981). These data cumulatively suggest that trained raters can reproduce each other's diagnostic assessments with extremely satisfactory levels of reliability.

An important element in good interrater reliability is the rigorous training of raters prior to their study participation. Elaborate training materials, including videotapes, instruction booklets, and case vignettes, have been developed by the authors of the SADS and DIS to ascertain that raters are meticulously instructed in the methods and carefully supervised in their applications before actual interviewing is undertaken.

In sum, the overall levels of reliability with trained raters is acceptable for each of these instruments. As Grove *et al.* (1981) conclude, "Carefully constructed interview schedules and lists of diagnostic criteria, together with rigorous training of raters, have caused a quantum jump in the magnitude of psychiatric reliability in the last decade" (p. 412).

Establishment of validity is a far more difficult undertaking. We wish to reiterate Cohen's (in press) cautionary note that "an instrument can never be said to have 'been validated,'" but rather that there is evidence for "some degree of validity of a particular kind, for a particular use, when used in a particular use, when used in a particular way" in a given population.

The central problem in establishing criterion validity for diagnostic instruments is the lack of a "gold standard" against which to compare the results obtained with the various interview schedules. Since they are intended to constitute an improvement over "usual" clinical interviews, there is little point in comparing their diagnoses with those based on unstructured interviews. In some studies, diagnoses obtained by nonpsychiatrists were compared to those made by psychiatrists who used the same interview schedule, thus using psychiatrist status as the yardstick for validity (e.g., Robins, Helzer, Ratcliff, & Seyfried, 1982). This does not resolve the problem of finding a valid criterion for assessing the validity of diagnoses made by psychiatrists. It may also artificially inflate assessment of validity, as Endicott (1981) has suggested, since the person to be "validated" and the criterion rater, by using the same interview schedule, get the same input and use the same format for scoring; she sees this procedure as more useful in assessing reliability than validity.

In the absence of a gold standard, Spitzer (1983) has proposed a more modest "LEAD" standard. The acronym LEAD incorporates three elements: "Longitudinal," "Expert," and "All Data." "Longitudinal" refers to extended diagnostic evaluation beyond the initial evaluation customarily conducted when treatment is initiated. Observation of symptoms and illness course serves to confirm or disconfirm the validity of the initial diagnostic classification. "Expert" refers to the use of senior clinicians who have demonstrated their ability to make reliable diagnoses; these clinicians would make independent assessments and, together with other experts, generate a consensus diagnosis to constitute a criterion measure. "All Data" signifies the incorporation of information from all available records and informants. Together, these procedures can contribute to establishing what Spitzer (1983) refers to as the procedural validity of a particular diagnostic interviw schedule.

Comment

The three extant and one impending structured interview schedules are all effective in generating reliable psychiatric diagnoses for the major disorders. At present, given the improvements in diagnostic classification introduced since the PSE was developed, we think the preferred instruments are the DIS and the SADS. Between the two, the SADS may be preferable for depression research, since it provides criteria for 10 subtypes of major depressive disorder and has supplements available for even more extensive subtyping. It has practical drawbacks, since it requires the services of mental health professional rather than lay interviewers, and the interviews last about twice as long as those of the DIS; also, it generates only RDC diagnoses, while the DIS also provides the DSM-III distinctions of major, cyclothymic, and dysthymic diagnoses. The SCID, when available, promises to be the instrument of choice for those whose research only requires DSM-III diagnoses.

CLINICIAN RATING SCALES

Introduction

Clinician rating scales are probably the oldest techniques for formal assessment in psychiatry. In general, they require the interviewer to cover specific areas and they provide more or less specific response options, but the questions addressed to the patient are not specified. Even though interviewers are left to ask whatever question they choose, interrater reliability can be satisfactory when adequate definitions and anchor points are provided. Without such definitions and anchors, as Kendell (1975) has noted, "a rating scale is simply an unstructured interview covering a range of topics, and retains all the shortcomings of an ordinary interview beneath its veneer of respectability" (p. 147).

With rare exceptions, clinician ratings of severity of depressive disorder play a central role both in describing patient samples and in measuring change after treatment. Considering their central role in depression research, it is surprising how little attention, comparatively speaking, has been devoted in the literature to a critical appraisal of their relative merits, their interrelationships, and their individual advantages and limitations in different research contexts.

In our review, we discuss in some detail the handful of clinician rating scales that, singly or in combination, are employed as either inclusion criteria, outcome measures, or both in nearly all depression research conducted in the past decade.

Hamilton Rating Scale for Depression

The Hamilton Rating Scale for Depression (HRSD), introduced in 1960 (Hamilton, 1960), is the pre-eminent scale in its field — the standard clinician rating scale for assessing depressive severity, to which other rating scales are compared. Not only has it been used in the majority of all research studies of depressive disorders over the past 25 years, but its international popularity continues unabated (Cronholm & Daly, 1983). It is especially widespread in clinical psychopharmacology research, and its inclusion in NIMH's New Clinical Drug Evaluation Unit's (NCDEU's) standard assessment battery (Guy, 1976) has generated a large data base for comparative and analytic studies (Rhoades & Overall, 1983). Not only is the original scale still a cornerstone in the assessemnt of depression and its amelioration, but it has given rise to a number of spinoff measures, some of which are reviewed in turn.

The original HRSD was designed to quantify severity of illness only in patients already diagnosed as having "an affective disorder of depressive type" (Hamilton, 1960, p. 56), not as a diagnostic tool for identification of depression.

Although Hamilton identified 21 rating variables in his original paper, he specifically stated that the scale was intended to include only the first 17. The other four items — diurnal variation, derealization, paranoid symptoms, and obsessional symptoms — were excluded from the scale either because they do not measure depression or its intensity (diurnal variation) or because they "occur so infrequently that there is no point in including them" (Hamilton, 1960, p. 57; see also Hamilton, 1980).

Unfortunately, the scale has been used in several different versions, with Hamilton's 17 items, his 21 items, or his 24 items (the additional three are helplessness, hopelessness, and worthlessness). In actual use over the past decade, the 21-item scale seems to have been most often employed, perhaps because it is the form incorporated in the ECDEU assessment battery; it is to this format that our remarks apply, unless otherwise noted.

Hamilton designed his scale as a way of quantifying information from the patient elicited by an experienced clinician in an unstructured interview (without specified questions and probes). Hamilton expected the interview to take at least 30 minutes, and he also recommended consideration of ancillary data sources (charts; information from friends, relatives, and nurses) in making the final assessment.

Hamilton favored simultaneous interviewing by two clinicians to increase reliability of ratings. Ideally, one would conduct the interview and the other would ask supplementary questions at the end. The final HRSD should consist of the summed scores of these two raters. In practice, this recommendation is not routinely followed, largely because of problems of cost and logistics.

Scores on each item synthesize frequency and severity of symptoms. The rater is expected to give "due weight to both of them in making his judgment" (Hamilton, 1960, p. 57). The scores reported in the literature are the scale's total score, factor scores, or individual item scores.

As a rule, the HRSD score most often reported is the total score, which consists of the item totals assessed by a single interviewer. Used in this manner, the range for the 17-item scale is 0-50, and for the 21-item scale is 0-62. Total scale scores are particularly popular as inclusion criteria in psychopharmacology trials. Generally, baseline scores under 10 are considered too mild for such patients to be included in a drug treatment study. In the past, patients with scores over 17 were often excluded from placebo-controlled trials on ethical grounds, although this policy is now being modified.

While Hamilton himself did not provide standard cutoff points, in practice it is generally agreed that scores of 25 or more identify severely depressed patients; 18-24 represents the moderate range; and 7-17 signifies mild depression. A score of less than 7 is often used as the definition of "recovered" or "not depressed" (Endicott *et al.*, 1981).

The HRSD has been factored to generate a number of different solutions. The ECDEU handbook (Guy, 1976) presents a 6-factor solution, including "anxiety/somatization," "weight," "cognitive disturbance" (guilt, agitation, suicidal ideas, derealization, and paranoid and obsessional symptoms), "diurnal variation," "retardation," and "sleep disturbance." Hedlund and Vieweg (1979a) reviewed 6 other factor analyses. Across all, at least two stable factors emerge. The first to be extracted in most studies is described as a general factor of symptom severity. The second relatively stable factor is a bipolar variable with the anchors of anxious, agitated depression at one end and retarded depression at the other. In the ECDEU report, it corresponds to "anxiety/somatization." In general, factor scores have not been used widely in research analyses.

An elegant series of psychometric analyses recently was reported by Rhoades and Overall (1983). In their factor analysis, they used both orthogonal and oblique rotations to obtain 7 primary factors; factor scores for these factors were then intercorrelated to yield 2 higher-order factors — "vegetative depression" and "cognitive depression." Rhoades and Overall also developed 5 symptom profile patterns based on cluster analyses of 21-item

HRSD scores of 240 patients in drug trials. They identified 5 phenomenological types that seem to correspond to depressive subtypes more readily than most of the extracted factors seem to do. The 5 types are labeled "anxious," "suicidal," "somatizing," "vegetative," and "paranoid" depression. Discriminant-function weights were calculated for each type, and can be applied to a patient's HRSD raw item scores to obtain individual type scores in terms of which he or she can be classified as a particular phenomenological type. This method represents a novel, interesting, and as yet unvalidated application of the HRSD, which may extend the utility of its application.

At an item level, interrater reliability levels are far lower than those observed for either factor scores or total scores. Cicchetti and Prusoff (1983) studied the interrater reliability of each HRSD item both before and after 16 weeks of treatment in a sample of over 80 patients with primary depressive disorder according to RDC. As assessed before treatment, interrater reliability levels were found to be "excellent" for one item, "fair" for seven items (intraclass correlation coefficients of .40 to .60), and "poor" for all other items (intraclass coefficients below .40). At the end of treatment, interrater reliability was slightly better on most items, but still considerably less adequate than were factor or total scale scores. Therefore, the use of HRSD results at the item level requires justification.

Reliability and Validity

Hedlund and Vieweg (1979a) summarized information on reliability from 9 studies published before 1979. Internal-consistency reliability coefficients were reported for 4 studies; for 3 of these, they ranged from .83 to .94 (the other was lower). Interrater reliability was above .85 in seven of the eight studies in which it was reported in this review. In a more recent study of interrater reliability (Cicchetti & Prusoff, 1983), using intraclass correlation, the investigators found agreement to be far greater after treatment ($r = .82$) than at pretreatment baseline ($r = .46$). This probably reflects increased variance after treatment. While it seems generally true that good interrater agreement can be obtained with proper training on the scoring of individual items, there is enough variability of agreement levels cited in the literature to suggest that levels of interrater agreement should be assessed in all studies.

Validity of the HRSD is difficult to assess, in the sense tht the scale has become the standard against which other measures are compared. Consequently, if HRSD ratings disagree with other assessments, it may be difficult to determine which is "right." We can, however, describe the overlap of HRSD scores and others. Hedlund and Vieweg (1979a) reviewed 23 studies comparing HRSD total scores with scores on the self-rated Beck and Zung scales, as well as with global ratings made by clinicians. Based on these studies, they concluded that the HRSD "is consistently reported to reflect patient changes over the course of treatment" (p. 159) in psychopharmacological trials, and in general successfully quantifies severity of depression from a clinical interview.

Correspondence of HRSD and Clinical Global Impressions Severity and Improvement Scores

In order to study the relationships between the HRSD and the Clinical Global Impressions (CGI) instrument, we looked at their correlations at baseline and at week 6 for patients in five different drug trials with depressed patients conducted in our department. A total of 105 patients receiving placebo medication and 170 receiving an active antidepresant were included (although some data were missing in some comparisons). At baseline, the correlation between scores on the CGI Severity scale and the HRSD scores averaged about .50. At week 6, we found correlations of .81 or .82 between ratings on the CGI Improvement scale and HRSD total scores for active drug and placebo patients considered separately, and correlations of .80-.90 for the CGI Severity scale and the HRSD. Allowing for unreliability of measurement, these three instruments appear to have been essentially interchangeable at week 6. Although less highly intercorrelated at baseline, they were still strongly related. In general, we are confident that the HRSD is an accurate index of depressive severity for patients with diagnosed depressive disorder.

Hamilton Rating Scale Derivatives

Hamilton Endogenomorphy Subscale

The Hamilton Endogenomorphy Subscale (HES) was derived by Thase, Hersen, Bellack, Himmelhoch, and Kupfer (1983) for the specific purpose of providing an "expeditious and objective alternative" to chart review for retrospective diagnosis of endogenous depression. While studies designed since the publication of structured diagnostic interviews and objective diagnostic criteria can be compared with each other, it is often difficult "to place the findings of earlier studies into this current perspective," as Thase *et al.* noted (1983, p. 268). Because of the widespread use of the HRSD since its introduction in 1960, it provides a common data base across studies. By identifying a subset of HRSD items that together retrospectively identify the subtype of endogenous depression, older studies can be classified according to current terminology.

With this goal in view, Kovacs, Rush, Beck, and Hollon (1981) selected a subset of eight HRSD items intended to approximate Klein's (1974) concept of endogenomorphic depression. Thase *et al.* (1983) applied the same subset to another sample of depressed patients to validate the earlier study.

Format. The HES items include items 5-9, 16, 18, and 23 of the 24-item

HRSD. They are middle insomnia, late insomnia, work/activities, retardation, agitation, weight loss, diurnal variation (A.M.), and hopelessness. Their potential range is 0-22. For analysis of early studies using the HRSD 17-item scale, the first 7 items are used; this subset correlated almost perfectly (r = .94) with all 8 items.

Validity. High (≥8) and low scores on the HES were compared with RDC and DSM-III classifications made independently for the same sample of 147 patients. The HES high-low dichotomy yielded on overall concordance of 81% with the RDC subtype diagnosis of endogenous depression. Furthermore, 21 of the 23 definite endogenous depressives were identified. The HES correctly identified 93% of nonmelancholic but only 38% of melancholic patients diagnosed according to DSM-III. This lower level of sensitivity was largely attributable to a number of nonmelancholic patients who got HES scores of 8 or 9. Thase *et al.* (1983) suggest using a cutoff score of ≥10 to identify patients with the more restrictive diagnosis of melancholia.

Extension of the use of the HES to more severely depressed patients and replication of current findings with more heterogeneous outpatient samples are indicated before the HES is widely applied in retrospective diagnostic assessment. It seems, nevertheless, to be a promising research strategy that warrants further development and use.

Extracted Hamilton

As noted above, the SADS interview contains a subset of 45 items to be rated for the week prior to evaluation. The SADS-C incorporates items from this subset to constitute a change measure. Among these items are 20 that were written to correspond to HRSD items. One HRSD item (insight) has no SADS equivalent. Endicott *et al.* (1981) developed an algorithm for converting the SADS and SADS-C items to HRSD items (adding a constant value for the one missing item). They conducted a study to determine the level of agreement and comparative reliabilities of the HRSD and the equivalent SADS items, known as the Extracted Hamilton (EH). The sample consisted of 48 patients with an admission diagnosis of RDC depression. Five raters participated in different pair combinations; two at a time interviewed a patient and administered the SADS-C and then the HRSD. The Pearson correlation coefficient between the EH and real HRSD was .92. The variability in scores using the EH and real HRSD by the same rater was equivalent to the interrater agreement level for the HRDS. That is, "one would do at least as well in estimating an interviewer's real HR using his EH as one would using another observer's real HRSD" (Endicott *et al.*, 1981, p. 102).

These data support the use of the SADS-C as an alternative to the HRSD and indicate that the use of both scales on the same occasion constitutes an unnecessary redundancy.

Bech-Rafaelsen Melancholia Scale

The Bech-Rafaelsen Melancholia Scale, developed in Scandinavia, combines items from the HRSD and the Cronholm-Ottosson Depression Scale, which is another clinician rating scale used in Scandinavia. It is important to note that "melancholia" is here used as a synonym for "depression," and it is not equivalent to DSM-III melancholia. Like the HRSD, it is intended as a measure of severity, is based on clinician interview, and provides anchored 5-point scales for rating each of its 11 items (Bech, 1981). The authors provide standardized cutoff definitions of mild, moderate, and severe depression. They report interrater reliability coefficients of .82-.93 (Bech, Bolwig, Kramp, & Rafaelsen, 1979; Bech & Rafaelsen, 1980) and a correlation of .97 with the HRDS. It is not commonly included in American assessment batteries, but is used in Scandinavian studies.

Montgomery-Asberg Depression Rating Scale

A comparatively new clinician-rated scale, the Montgomery-Asberg Depression Rating Scale (MADRS), was designed for the specific purpose of measuring clinical change in drug trials. The authors (Montgomery & Asberg, 1979) administered the 65-item Comprehensive Psychopathological Rating Scale at treatment baseline to 106 patients with primary depressive illness, diagnosed according to Feighner criteria. Patients from both England and Sweden were included to broaden the scale's application. Sixty-four patients were retested after 4 weeks of treatment. The authors first selected the 17 items most commonly identified as present. Their sum, a measure of illness severity, was highly correlated both with HRSD scores (r = .94) and with global clinical ratings (r = .89) at week 4. From this set of 17 items, 10 were selected that showed most change after treatment and that also correlated highly with the total score of the remaining items. These 10 items constitute the final scale.

Each item is scored on a 7-point scale, with anchors provided for every other point. A score of 0 signifies absence of the symptom in question, while a score of 6 signifies the most extreme form. The graded points integrate both intensity and frequency of occurrence, and in some instances duration or degree of incapacitation as well. The time frame may be determined by each investigator as desired.

While no data about internal consistency reliability were reported, the reported interrater reliability coefficeints among pairs of trained raters are extremely high (.89-.97, with equivalent agreement on HRSD scoring). They are in fact extraordinary, since they included untrained as well as trained raters. The procedure for their computation was not described.

Change scores on the MADRS and HRSD were calculated for a sample of 64 patients participatng in medication trials, and were correlated with outcome (responder vs. nonresponder). The MADRS change score was slightly more highly correlated with outcome (point-biserial $r = .70$) than was the HRSD ($r = .59$), although these correlations are in the same range.

In general, the advantages of this new scale compared to the standard (HRSD) include its brevity and its apparent greater precision in measuring change (Cronholm & Daly, 1983). If the latter characteristics continues to be observable in subsequent studies, this will be a useful instrument to include in clinical trials.

Brief Psychiatric Rating Scale

Overall and Gorham (1962) designed the Brief Psychiatric Rating Scale (BPRS) to meet two needs: to provide a rapid method of assessing treatment change, and also to provide a comprehensive description of major symptoms in a variety of psychiatric disorders. At the time it was developed, its focus was on functionally psychotic inpatients, and it is still recommended primarily for inpatients (Guy, 1976). The instrument has been used in more than 200 treatment studies. Of these, about 70% were of schizophrenic patients. An excellent review of the literature regarding its psychometric properties and applications is provided by Hedlund and Vieweg (1980; 177 references).

The BPRS consists of scaled ratings on 18 "symptom constructs," which were derived from factor-analytic studies of change scores of earlier rating scales. This procedure was intended to identify groups of items representing relatively independent dimensions of symptom change.

For each of the 18 symptom constructs, brief scale definitions are provided on the rating forms, and a 7-point scale (0-6) is given. More detailed scale definitions and rating instructions are presented in the original article (Overall & Gorham, 1962), as are specific suggestions for training raters. The authors recommend a semistructured interview procedure beginning with an explanation about its purpose, general questions to obtain spontaneously volunteered information, and then direct questions as needed to complete the ratings. In general, there is less structure and more latitude for clinical inference in this scale then in the previously presented scales.

Of the 18 items, at least half are probably seldom seen in depressed patients (i.e., excitement, disorientation, unusual thought content, mannerisms, hallucinatory, conceptual disorganization, grandiosity, hostility, uncooperative). The consequence would be attenuation of score range and a weaker measure. In reporting findings from the BPRS, investigators use total scores, factor scores, and often item scores. While Hedlund and Vieweg (1980) located 22 reports of BPRS reliability in over 300 articles reviewed, none were based on homogenous samples of depressed patients. Most of the interrater reliability coefficients reported for samples of schizophrenic and other patients were .80 or higher — possibly greater in magnitude because of wider symptom range than would be found in a sample composed only of depressed patients.

In terms of validity, Hedlund and Vieweg (1980) found over 150 drug treatment studies in which BPRS was used along with other measures to assess treatment effect. With rare exceptions, the BPRS change scores were corroborated and supported by other clinical measures. Some data suggest, however, that "the BPRS may not be as sensitive to antidepressant drug effects" as the HRSD (Hedlund & Vieweg, 1980, p. 52). The BPRS has also been used to develop a system of typology (Overall, 1974). Six phenomenological types have been identified by cluster analyses of BPRS profiles. Three of these are depressive subtypes: anxious depression, hostile depression, and retarded depression. Computer programs are available for classifying patients according to this typology. Perhaps due to the subsequent development of the RDC and DSM-III, this typology does not appear to have been widely used in depression research.

In summary, the BPRS is a thoroughly documented research tool that is particularly relevant in treatment studies in schizophrenia. Quite a few of its items do not apply to depressive disorders. For this reason, and perhaps because there are other established scales used in studies of affective disorders, there is comparatively less information about its utility as a measure of change with depressed patients. The strongest argument for its use with depressed patients probably would be in multinational studies, since the BPRS is as widely known in Europe as in the United States. Aside from this application, it is probably not the scale of choice in measurement of depression.

The SADS—"Change" Form

The SADS-C is an abbreviated version of the regular SADS, described above (see "Structured Interview Schedules"). It includes 29 scaled items and several checklist items that are rated for the last week. If conducted as a separate interview, it takes 20-30 minutes to complete. It is intended either for follow-up evaluations when the SADS has been administered initially, or for use instead of the regular SADS when the goal is limited to a cross-sectional evaluation of severity of psyhcopathology.

The SADS-C uses the same 6-point ratings for responses that are used in the regular SADS, and requires the same level of clinical experience and training for the raters. Subsets of items can be combined to provide scale scores to assess anxiety, depression, endogenous features, manic features, and delusions/disorganization. In addition, the SADS-C includes the Global Assessment Scale (a global rating described below), and provides an EH score (see "Extracted Hamilton," above).

Newcastle Scales

The Newcastle Scales were devised to distinguish between endogenous and neurotic depressed patients in order to identify those most likely to respond favorably to somatic treatments. In the first step of scale development, Carney,

Roth, and Garside (1965) selected 35 items considered on clinical grounds to be valuable in discriminating between these depressive subtypes. The items included measures of illness history, family history, personality characteristics, and current symptomatology. These 35 items were rated before electroconvulsive therapy (ECT) and 3 and 6 months later for 129 depressed inpatients. The items were subjected to multiple-regression analyses where the outcome measure was either ECT response or clinical diagnosis.

The 10 items most highly correlated with diagnosis were selected to constitute the Newcastle Diagnostic Scale (also referred to as Newcastle Scale-I or N-I). The 10 items best predicting ECT response were selected to constitute the Newcastle ECT Prediction (or ECT Indices) Scale. Two items (weight loss and anxiety) appear on both scales, which together therefore have a total of 18 items.

On the scales, each item is assigned a weight, ranging from −3 to +3, derived from the multiple-regression analysis and converted into whole numbers. These weights reflect the independent discriminating power of each item. An item that is present is scored as indicated by its assigned weight. If it is absent, it is ignored. No consideration is given to severity or frequency. The total score for each patient is the sum of weights of items present in that case. On the Diagnostic Scale, eight items (adequate personality, no adequate psychogenesis, distinct quality, weight loss, previous episode, depressive psychomotor activity, nihilistic delusions, and guilt) each have a positive weight of 1 or 2; two items (anxiety and blames others) each have a negative weight of 1. The score range is thus −2 to +12, but if all 10 items are present and the negative weights are included, the patient would be given a score of 10. The scale is intended to provide a dichotomous classification of patients; a total score of 6 or more indicates "endogenous" and less than 6 "neurotic" depression (Carney & Sheffield, 1972).

The ECT Prediction Scale is similarly constructed: Five items have positive weights of +1 to +3 (weight loss, pyknic physique, early wakening, somatic delusions, paranoid delusions), and 5 items have negative weights (anxiety, worse P.M., self-pity, hypochondriacal, hysterical). Again, while the score range is −12 to +11, a patient with all symptoms present would receive a score of −1. A total score of 1 or higher is considered to predict good ECT outcome, and less than 1 a poor outcome.

A subsequent sample of 97 depressed patients was assessed before and 3 months after ECT (Carney & Sheffield, 1972). The Newcastle Scales again were found to be successful in differentiating between treatment responders and nonresponders, providing evidence for their validity. The Diagnostic Scale and ECT Prediction Scale correctly predicted outcome in 70% and 76% of the patients, respectively. Severity of illness as rated by the HRSD was found to be equal for patients classified as endogenous or neurotic.

In another study (Abou-Saleh & Coppen, 1983), 200 inpatients with primary depressive disorder and baseline HRSD scores over 15 were classified on the Newcastle Diagnostic Scale during their first week of admission. They were assigned either to ECT or to antidepressant medication and evaluated by the HRSD after 4 weeks of treatment. Patients with Newcastle scores in the middle range (4-8) showed a higher percentage of improvement on both treatments (41%) than those with lower (35%) or higher (29%) scores. In contrast, another 96 patients treated with lithium did not show this curvilinear effect; higher Newcastle scores (endogenous) were associated with greater improvement after 1 year of treatment. Abou-Saleh and Coppen comment that these findings are "intriguing" and not unexpected, since, they assert, "severely ill depressives" are known to have "less favorable responses to ECT and IMI than moderately ill depressives" (1983, p. 602). These data cast some doubt on the utility of the Newcastle Scales for predicting treatment response, however, which is what they were intended to do. While these scales continue to be used widely in England, their predictive properties remain to be clarified.

Atypical Depression Rating Scale

One depressive subtype that has received increasing attention in the last several years is that of "atypical" depression, also referred to as "neurotic" or "anxious" depression. This use is not the same as the DSM-III term "atypical depression," which constitutes a residual category for depressed patients who do not meet criteria for other DSM-III depressive disorders. The atypical depressed patient is often characterized by prominent character pathology, anxiety and/or somatization (Silberman & Post, 1982), reactive mood, oversleeping, overeating, extreme lethargy, and/or pathological rejection sensitivity (Liebowitz *et al.*, 1984).

The Atypical Depression Rating Scale was devised by Silberman and Post (1982) to provide a diagnostic index of atypical depression. It is designed to utilize all available data sources, including patient report. Part I, consisting of 14 items of varying specificity (e.g., manipulativeness, hysteroid phenomena), is rated for current or past depressive episode. Another 10 items in Part II, most of which are extremely general (e.g., stress or transference psychoses, disturbed sexuality), are rated for entire life history. One-sentence rating guides are provided for each item (e.g., "disturbed relationships — grossly pathological relationships such as severe dependency or lack of stable relationships"). The rating scale is broad in scope and, obviously, quite unstructured. Each item is scored 0 (absent), 1 (to some degree), or 2 (marked). Scores can range from 0 to 48.

The scale was used by its authors to assess 44 patients hospitalized at NIMH who met RDC for primary depressive disorder. Forty of them also met criteria for endogenous depression. Scores on the Atypical Depression Rating Scale were analyzed in relation to neuroendocrine and sleep measures as well as treatment response. In these analyses, patients were classified as atypical if they obtained scale scores of 6 or more (the median score).

The scale was found to discriminate a subtype of disorder that was associated with specific biological characteristics, including monoamine oxidase activity and slow-wave sleep. While the scale needs extensive further study in terms of reliability and validity, it is one of the few published measures of a significant diagnostic subtype, and as such may be useful for other investigative teams.

Atypical Depression Diagnostic Scale

Another scale for diagnosing atypical depression, the Atypical Depression Diagnostic Scale, has been developed at the New York State Psychiatric Institute. It is described by Liebowitz *et al.* (1984), but the scale itself has not been published and is being revised at this time. In format it resembles SADS items, with specified queries and 6-point response options with anchors. It covers the following areas: mood reactivity (the essential criterion) and weight gain or appetite increase, oversleeping, extreme lethargy, and rejection sensitivity of such proportions as to impair social functioning (associated criteria). In an ongoing clinical trial of phenelzine, imipramine, and placebo, over 200 patients identified by this scale as meeting full or partial criteria for atypical depression showed preferential treatment response to phenelzine. This pharmacological finding provides some evidence for the validity of the scale.

GLOBAL ILLNESS RATINGS

Introduction

Global ratings of illness severity and treatment-related improvement are widely used in clinical trials, and often serve as a key change measure. Such scales usually have between 5 and 11 points on a single continuum, although there are exceptions. Brief anchor points are indicated, such as "minimal improvement" or "much improved." Operational definitions are usually absent. While they are usually not used to describe samples, they can be useful as outcome measures.

Global ratings are usually regarded as "valid" virtually by definition. When they are correlated with clinician rating scales, this is almost always done to validate the latter. Discrepancies are assumed to reflect errors in the clinician rating scale, not flaws in the global ratings.

It is far from clear what considerations global ratings encompass, above and beyond assessments of symptom severity, or even the extent to which other factors influence them. Chipman and Paykel (1974) examined this issue in a study including clinician ratings of 30 symptoms plus global ratings for a sample of nearly 300 depressed women. The symptom scores were used as predictors and the global rating as the criterion variable in a multiple-regression analysis. A multiple R of .75 was obtained, indicating that assessment of symptoms accounted for only about half of the variance in the global judgment. As the authors note, "this leaves a good deal unaccounted for," which they regard as signifying a significant role for intuitive or "configural" synthesis of clinical data in this process (Chipman & Paykel, 1974, p. 674). Other contributions to global ratings may include individual opinions of the value or desirability of observed changes, or of what constitutes change.

Clinical Global Impressions

The CGI, mentioned above, consists of three iems or scales: Severity (of illness), (global) Improvement, and an Efficacy index. It is included in the ECDEU assessment battery for psychopharmacological trials (Guy, 1976), and routinely is used as an outcome measure in treatment studies.

The Severity and Improvement scales are 7-point measures. The scoring is similar to that found in most other scales, in the sense that lower is healthier. On the Severity measure, 1 means "normal," 2 means "borderline mentally ill," and 7 means "among the most extremely ill patients." On the Improvement scale, 1 means "very much improved," 2 means "much improved," 3 means "minimally improved," 4 means "no change," and 7 means "very much worse." The third item or scale, the Efficacy index, is a composite rating of therapeutic effect and drug side effects. This score, used far less often than the other two, calls for an estimation of therapeutic effect ("marked," "moderate," "minimal," "unchanged," or "worse") in relation to severity of side effects ("none," "do not interfere with functioning," "do interfere," "outweigh benefits").

The time frames can be variable for the Severity scale and the Efficacy index. The Improvement scale (for which there is no baseline) refers to change since admission to the study (Guy, 1976). The framework for ratings on the Severity scale is this: "Considering your total clinical experience with this particular population, how mentally ill is the patient at this time?"

Overall, the CGI Severity scale and Efficacy index are reported in drug trials less frequently than the CGI Improvement scale. When the latter is used as the basis for classifying patients as treatment responders or nonresponders, as is often the case, it is important to note the cutoff point used for this dichotomization. The more conservative use is to describe patients with CGI Improvement scores of 1 or 2 ("very much improved" or "much improved") as responders, while patients showing minimal improvement (a score of 3) are not considered responders.

A related problem of the CGI, apart from lack of a standard numerical cutoff for identifying treatment responders, is the terseness of scoring definitions. In our research group, we have tried to develop an operational criterion by agreeing to use the Improvement scores of 1 and 2 only for those patients who are considered to be responding satisfactorily to the current treatment, so that no alteration in treatment plan is indicated.

Global Assessment Scale

The Global Assessment Scale (GAS) is a single rating of overall functioning, assessed on a 100-point continuum. The GAS was derived from the Menninger Foundation Psychotherapy Research Project's Health-Sickness Rating Scale (HSRS; Waskow & Parloff, 1975). The HSRS was itself designed as an overall judgment of health status.

The GAS has 10 defined anchor points and ranges from 1 ("hypothetically sickest possible") to 100 ("hypothetically healthiest"). The anchors include considerations of degree of functional impairment, specific symptoms, quality of interpersonal relationships, and general severity of problems. Scores over 70 are considered to signify absence of disorder. Most outpatients will be given ratings in the 30-70 range, while scores below 30 signify a degree of severity usually found in inpatients.

The GAS authors have developed training materials and detailed instructions for raters. They have compiled a booklet of 23 case vignettes with a scoring key, to facilitate practice and to provide a basis for assessing acceptable levels of interjudge reliability in new studies. The test booklet itself includes not only the one-page rating scale with its 10 anchors, but six pages of instructions and examples. Interjudge reliability, concurrent validity, and predictive validity were assessed in five studies reviewed in the initial GAS publication (Endicott, Spitzer, Fleiss, & Cohen, 1976). Across samples, the precision of ratings was relatively high. The standard error of measurement was about 5 points for this 100-point scale, meaning that 95% of the time a rating given a patient will be within 10 points of his or her "true" rating. Validity was demonstrated by showing significant correlations between GAS scores and independently rated measures of overall severity, rehospitalization, and assessments of change in clinical status.

The GAS is applicable to patients with all forms of psychiatric illness, as well as to samples without known disorder. It has been incorporated into the SADS-C (see above), and can be used as a change measure as well as a method for describing cross-sectional severity of illness. It is distinctive in that it offers the opportunity to differentiate within a fairly broad range of well-being (scores of 71-100), which may be particularly useful in treatment follow-up studies. It also provides a greater scoring range and more numerous and more detailed anchor points than do most other global clinical assessments.

Raskin Three-Area Depression Scale

The Raskin Three-Area Depression Scale (RDS) is a cross between a clinician rating scale and a global assessment scale, consisting of three broad dimensions (or items), each of which is globally assessed. The three dimensions are behavioral signs, secondary symptoms of depression (e.g., sleep, appetite, or cognitive problems), and verbal expression of mood. Each is rated on a 1-5 scale of severity. Investigators usually report scores for the three individual items, and an overall depression score that is their sum and that has a range of 3 to 15. As Cicchetti and Prusoff (1983) showed, composite scores on the RDS, either at baseline or end of study, had considerably higher interrater reliability coefficients than did the individual items.

One problem with this scale is its constricted range in relation to its components. Since a score of 1 signifies "absence of impairment" and 2 is "minimal impairment," then it is easy to get scores of at least 7 even in the absence of significant psychopathology. The applied cutoffs — as exemplified in Weissman, Klerman, Prusoff, Sholomskas, and Padian's (1981) study, where an RDS score of ⩾7 was used as a study inclusion criterion — seem quite low.

SELF-RATING SCALES

Introduction

As a rule, investigators prefer to rely on clinician ratings rather then self-reports as dependent measures in efficacy studies. The limitations of self-reports are multiple. They are vulnerable to deliberate misrepresentation and to response biases (especially denial and exaggeration, but also social desirability, extremeness, and other systematic response sets). Response bias may actually pose less of a risk to the validity of report than is usually believed, according to recent rigorous studies in the related field of community psychiatric surveys. Gove, McCorkel, Fain, and Hughes (1976) found that the three response biases they studied — nay-saying, perceived trait desirability, and need for social approval — generally do not act as a "form of systematic bias that invalidates the pattern of relationships observed . . . but instead act as random noise" (p. 497). In other words, such biases may weaken but not necessarily distort self-reports on psychiatric measures.

Other concerns about self-reports include the possibility that the psychological terms they use may be differentially and perhaps idiosyncratically interpreted by respondents differing in level of education, social status, and ethnic background. Self-reports are also unsuited for elicitation of particular categories of psychopathology (e.g., inappropriate affect, reality testing, thought disorder), and for use by severely ill patients whose pathology disrupts their capacity for concentration or self-report. In such instances, an experienced clinician can gather useful information, and can integrate behavioral observations with material obtained from the patient to provide a comprehensive appraisal.

Another potential constraint on the utility of self-rating scales was articulated by Wittenborn (1972), who observed that they "tend to reveal relatively stable, characterological self-perceptions which do not change readily in response to fluctuations in the patient's affective state" (p. 86). Presumably as a result, self-report scales would be less sensitive measures of treatment-induced change. The available evidence does not support this assertion for outpatients, but it may be true for inpatients.

In view of the limitations of self-reports, few investigators would consider their exclusive use as outcome measures. They do, however, have striking assets, both practical and theoretical. The most apparent of their practical advantages is their conservation of professional time (and related expense). Furthermore, self-reports eliminate issues of inconsistencies and variations across interviews by the same clinician; problems of interrater reliability among team members; and, most important, systematic differences in ratings between research centers and over time. Indeed, the whole issue of reliability is simplified, becoming basically a matter of demonstrating stability of self-report and internal-consistency reliability among items (Hedlund & Vieweg, 1979b). Establishment of validity remains a challenge, but is no more of a theoretical problem with self-reports than with clinician ratings.

A major theoretical advantage of self-ratings is their ability to quantify subjective symptoms such as guilt. They also may be more suitable for detection and quantification of milder levels of depression (Hughes, O'Hara, & Rehm, 1982). Finally, when administered after treatment, they provide the best available index of consumer satisfaction. Nevertheless, for patients who rely heavily on denial, self-reports are of little value even for this purpose.

We wish to emphasize that the validity of the self-report scales reviewed in this section is restricted to those respondents independently diagnosed as having a primary depressive disorder. As Mendels and Weinstein (1972) convincingly demonstrated more than 10 years ago, self-report scales designed to assess anxiety and depression as separate conditions are clearly unable to differentiate them. Analyzing a battery of 6 depression self-report scales and 4 anxiety self-report scales administered to 76 patients with various diagnoses, they found only one general factor in the entire set. Furthermore, the anxiety scale scores did not correlate with each other any better than they did with depression scale scores, while depression scales were only marginally more highly intercorrelated. Overall, self-report scales as currently constituted cannot legitimately be used for differential diagnosis.

In this section, our review focuses largely on self-report scales designed to assess illness severity. We have also included one instrument, the Center for Epidemiologic Studies Depression Scale, designed to identify cases of depressive disorder in community samples.

Beck Depression Inventory

The Beck Depression Inventory (BDI) is analogous to the HRSD in the sense that it has come to serve as the standard in its class. Although there are more self-ratings than clinician ratings among depression scales, the BDI is almost always included when self-ratings are used.

The original BDI (Beck, Ward, Mendelson, Mock, & Erbaugh, 1961) has 21 items, each consisting of a graded series of statements ranging from 0 to 3 to signify severity. The respondent selects the single statement in each set that best represents his or her condition. This means that he or she has to consider and assess a total of 84 statements. The total score range is 0-63, and reflects both the number of symptoms and severity of each. The items were selected by Beck to represent "characteristic attitudes and symptoms that appeared to be specific for depressed patients and which were consistent with descriptions of depression contained in the psychiatric literature" (Beck, 1967, p. 189). Of the 21 items, 6 refer to vegetative symptoms, and the rest to mood and cognitive symptoms.

In a subsequent study (Beck, 1967), Beck performed item-total score correlations for 606 cases and selected the 13 items with the highest correlation coefficients to constitute a shorter form of the BDI. Beck and Beamesderfer (1974) reported a .96 correlation between scores on the short and standard forms for these patients. However, the 21-item form continues to be widely used, and is the one included in the assessment battery of the NIMH Collaborative Program on the Psychobiology of Depression.

Beck, Weissman, Lester, and Trexler (1974) have demonstrated high levels of internal-consistency reliability (using split-half reliability and item-total correlations). Concurrent validity was assessed by comparing BDI scores with global clinical assessments. Beck and Beamesderfer (1974) reported that in nine studies conducted in the United States and Europe, correlations in all cases were between .61 and .73. This has been corroborated more recently by Hamilton (1982). Several factor-analytic studies have identified physiological (insomnia, loss of libido, weight, appetite) and negative self-image (sense of failure, self-dislike, self-accusation, expectation of punishment) factors, as well as others not replicated by different investigators.

The selection of a cutoff score as a criterion for study inclusion has varied considerably for the BDI. As a screening device to detect depression among psychiatric patients, Beck recommends a cutoff score of 13. For identifying a relatively pure group of depressed patients for research purposes, he recommends a score over 21 (Beck & Beamesderfer, 1974). These cutoffs are arbitrary, but may serve as rough guides for assessing equivalence of samples when BDI scores are listed as inclusion criteria.

Comparison of the BDI and HRSD

In commenting on the comparative utility of these two scales, standards in their respective classes, some observers refer to the BDI as primarily a measure of cognitive function and the HRSD as primarily a measure of somatic symptoms (Hughes *et al.*, 1982). In fact, about half of their items overlap, and the remainder of each scale either concerns attitudes and beliefs about self and future (BDI) or describes additional somatic symptoms (HRSD). On either scale, patients who meet criteria for major depression will obtain scores of at least moderate severity.

Several investigators have studied the correspondence of BDI and HRSD scores by administering both to a series of depressed patients. Bailey and Coppen (1976) found, for a sample of 42 patients tested weekly over time, that a total of 425 pairs of scores generated a correlation coefficient of .68. Overall, a high concordance of ratings was found for two-thirds of their sample, with significant discrepancies observed for the others. The authors were unable to identify characteristics of patients associated with high or low concordance.

Bech *et al.* (1975) conducted a similar study, using clinical global assessments as well. Their observed correlation between the BDI and HRSD was comparable to that of Bailey and Coppen ($r = .72$), while either scale was also highly correlated with global clinical ratings (BDI and global rating, $r = .77$; HRSD and global rating, $r = .84$). Equivalent relationships were reported by Hamilton (1982), and by Hedlund and Vieweg (1979a).

Investigators who have compared the utility of the two scales with patients of various severity levels report that they are about equal in their ability to distinguish between more and less severely depressed patients (Hedlund & Vieweg, 1979a). Studies of their intercorrelation have found greater agreement between measures made after treatment than before it, probably due to the greater variability of scores on each scale obtained at that occasion.

In summary, the HRSD remains the preferred measure of the two for assessing depressive severity, if the means are available to use either. In the absence of sufficient clinical resources, or for some specific practical or research question, the BDI may serve as an acceptable approximation of the HRSD.

Symptom Checklist — 90

The Symptom Checklist — 90 (SCL-90) was developed from the 58-item Hopkins Symptom Checklist, itself originally derived from the Cornell Medical Index. As its name indicates, it is a self-administered 90-item symptom checklist on which the respondent indicates presence and severity of distress of symptoms associated with a broad range of psychiatric disorders.

Unlike scores for other instruments we have described, the SCL-90 scores are not based on the total scale. Instead, nine separate factor scores and three global scores are generated. The factors were derived from many factor-analytic studies including over 2,500 patients. These statistically derived factors have been reproduced by "clinical-rational" clustering by experienced raters working with 1,000 cases (Derogatis & Cleary, 1977).

The depression factor of the SCL-90 is its longest and has 13 items. The factor score reflects both number of symptoms reported and their severity (rated on a 5-point scale). The individual items focus on mood and loss of interest, with 2 items concerning somatic symptoms and one each about self-blame, suicidal thoughts, hopelessness, and worthlessness. Other relevant SCL-90 factors include somatization, interpersonal sensitivity, phobic anxiety, and general (free-floating) anxiety.

The three global scores describe overall distress, and do not specifically apply to depressive severity. They are probably most useful when study samples include patients with different disorders, for whom comparative assessments of illness severity are desired.

The psychometric properties of the SCL-90 have been assessed in numerous studies. Summarizing the earlier (pre-1974) literature, Derogatis, Lipman, Rickels, Uhlenhuth, and Covi (1974) reported internal-consistency coefficients of .86 and a pretreatment test-retest coefficint of .81 for depression factor scores. Like others (see Guy, 1976), we have found these scores to be sensitive to treatment-induced changes (although changes of similar magnitude were also found on most of the other SCL-90 factors as well, which may indicate that improvement induces an overriding halo effect).

Zung Self-Rating Depression Scale

Zung originally developed the Zung Self-Rating Depression Scale (SDS) to provide a quantitative, self-administered, brief assessment of depression in patients with a primary diagnosis of depressive disorder. The 20 items are intended to represent three domains: affect (2 items), somatic concomitants (8 items), and psychological concomitants (10 items) (Zung, 1965, 1974). The respondent is asked to rate each item on a 4-point scale in terms of the frequency ("a little," "some," "a good part," "most of the time") that it applies to him or her. Sometimes the response options are ambiguous or awkward — as applied, for example, to the item "I notice that I am losing weight." The total score is derived by dividing the sum of the item raw sscores by the maximum possible score of 80, multiplied by 100 (ranging from 25 to 100). Zung has provided cutoff scores as follows: below 50, within normal range; 50-59, minimal to mild depression; 60-69, moderate depression; 70-99, severe depression.

Several factor-analytic studies have been conducted both with patients and normal samples, with anywhere from one to seven factors identified (Hedlund

& Vieweg, 1979b). No investigator has found factor scores to be more useful than the total score in differentiating between depressed and other samples, or between levels of severity. Consequently, their utility has not been established.

In contrast to Hamilton and Beck, Zung has not restricted his scale to differentiating levels of severity in diagnosed cases of depressive disorder; he also has used it to investigate baseline levels of depression in the general population (Zung, 1974). He found that a cutoff score of 50 or more identified 88% of depressed patients, and also correctly identified 88% of normals as such. That is, both sensitivity and specificity were .88. Considering, however, how highly SDS scores are correlated with self-reports of anxiety (Mendels & Weinstein, 1972), it seems unlikely that the SDS can serve as a diagnostic index specifically for depressive disorder in a population where both anxiety and depression are likely to occur.

Carroll, Fielding, and Blashki (1973) compared scores obtained on the HRSD and the SDS for a total of 67 depressed patients. Some were severely ill inpatients, others were moderately ill day hospital patients, and the rest were mildly ill patients seen in office practice. The HRSD successfully discriminated between mean scores for all three groups, but the SDS did not. In fact, the SDS did not differentiate between the psychotic and mildly ill patients, which, as Carroll and colleagues noted acerbically, is the least one ought to be able to expect from a rating scale. Correlation coefficients between scores of the 3 patient groups were .40 for inpatients, .37 for day hospital patients, and .61 for outpatients. At the item level, corresponding items were found to have correlations from .11 to .67. In addition to its weak showing as an index of depressive severity, the SDS was difficult for the inpatients to complete without help. Their retardation, indecisiveness, and difficulty in concentrating interfered with their ability to respond on ther own.

Hedlund and Vieweg (1979b) reviewed the cumulative evidence published up to 1979 concerning the correspondence of SDS scores with those of other rating scales. They concluded that "except for studies by Zung and associates, trained observer ratings such as those associated with the HRSD are consistently reported to discriminate more reliably between diagnosed depression and other diagnostic groups . . . , [and] between various levels or degrees of clinical judgements," as well as to reflect treatment-related changes more consistently (1979, p. 54). We agree with their conclusion that the SDS is not the instrument of choice in estimating depressive severity or its change after treatment, although it may have a role as an adjunctive clinical or screening scale.

Zung's Depression Status Inventory

Zung's Depression Status Inventory was developed as a clinician-administered version of the self-report SDS. It covers the same items and is also intended to provide a global measure of the intensity of depressive symptoms. It is reported to have a Pearson correlation coefficient of .87 with the self-rated form (Guy, 1976). The Inventory as well as the SDS is included in the ECDEU assessment manual as one of the instruments suggested for standard assessment batteries for use in clinical trials. It is not, however, widely used.

Wakefield Self-Assessment Depression Inventory

Snaith and his colleagues wanted a short, simple, clear self-rating scale of depressive severity. Among available scales, they regarded Zung's SDS as the simplest to complete, but felt that not all items were equally useful. Accordingly, they selected the 10 SDS items that occurred most frequently and added 2 items concerning anxiety to constitute the Wakefield Inventory. They also modified the response format to give these options: "yes, definitely"; "yes, sometimes"; "no, not much"; "no, not at all."

The cutoff score for classification as depressed was studied by administering the scale to 100 patients diagnosed as having primary depressive disorder, and to 200 normal controls. Using a cutoff between 14 and 15, only 3% of patients and 7.5% of normals were misclassified. Forty-six patients at various stages of treatment were administered the HRSD and filled out the Wakefield Inventory. The correlation between scores was .87. Snaith, Ahmed, Metha, and Hamilton (1971) also correlated scores after deleting the somatic items from the HRSD and obtained a correlation of .89. They concluded that evidently little is lost by excluding somatic symptoms from their inventory.

The authors recommended that this scale is indicated when a major consideration is simplicity and brevity in assessing severity of illness. It has been superseded, however, by the Leeds Scales, which they now prefer.

Leeds Scales

Just as the Wakefield Inventory is a modified version of Zung's SDS, the Leeds Scales for Self-Assessment of Depression constitute a revised form of the 12-item Wakefield Inventory. The purpose of revision was to "more nearly cover the range of common symptoms of depressive illness and anxiety states" (Snaith, Bridge, & Hamilton, 1976, p. 151). Response format was modified to give the respondent a choice of these four options: "not at all;" "not much;" "sometimes;" and "definitely." The 10 new items cover somatic symptoms (daytime sleepiness, appetite, palpitations, dizzy attacks), self-blame, fear, tension, and suicidal thoughts.

The authors developed subscales to provide separate measures of severity of depression and anxiety ("general scales") and overlapping subscales to measure severity of endogenous depression and anxiety neurosis ("specific scales"). Each subscale contains six items.

Snaith and colleagues compared the Specific Depression subscale (6 items) from the Leeds Scales with other rating scales to assess their relative ability to discriminate between levels of severity in patients with depressive disorder (Kearns *et al.*, 1982). They used abbreviated versions of the HRSD and the BDI, and standard forms of the MADRS and their own Wakefield Inventory in this study. Severity, the dependent measure, was determined by clinical interview. Ratings for 62 occasions were included. The analysis consisted of sorting scores generated by each rating scale according to five levels of severity, and comparing them to clinical judgments. All scales were found effective in distinguishing between "very severe" vs. "severe" at one end and "mild" versus "recovered" at the other. The MADRS did best in distinguishing among intermediate levels, followed by the HRSD. The BDI (administered by a clinician) and the self-rating scales (Wakefield and Leeds) were all weaker. The authors concluded that the Wakefield Inventory and the BDI "should now be discarded" as research instruments (Kearns *et al.*, 1982, p. 48). Although their own scale, the Leeds, did just as poorly, they did not recommend that it be discarded, for reasons not presented.

In our opinion, the advantages of the Leeds Scales over Zung's SDS (or, for that matter, any other self-rating scale) remain to be demonstrated. We present it here to acquaint the reader with its composition, should it be cited in the literature.

The Pleasure Scale

The Pleasure Scale of Fawcett, Clark, Scheftner, and Gibbons (1983) is a new self-report instrument intended to provide a quantitative assessment of anhedonia. In recent years, this concept has come to be seen as having central importance in the differentiation of depressive subtypes (Klein, 1974), and has been incorporated as an essential criterion in the DSM-III diagnostic category of melancholia.

"Anhedonia" is defined as impairment or loss of the capacity to experience pleasure in normally enjoyable situations. It is not an exclusive characteristic of depressive disorders; Kraeplin and Bleuler identified it as a schizophrenic symptom, and Freud associated it with neurotic conflict. Klein, Gittelman, Quitkin, and Rifkin (1980) have emphasized the importance of distinguishing between anhedonia and demoralization, which commonly accompanies all forms of depressive disorder and which also may occur in the absence of other diagnosable disorders. Demoralization refers to "belief in one's ineffectiveness, engendered by severe life and defeat. It is a change in self image . . . in the direction of helplessness" (Klein *et al.*, 1980, p. 230). While the anhedonic person can neither anticipate nor actually experience pleasure, the demoralized person's ability to anticipate pleasure is diminished, but his or her ability to enjoy pleasures associated with drive reduction (i.e., consummatory activities) is unimpaired.

The Fawcett Pleasure Scale consists of 36 sentences, each meant to portray a situation that virtually anyone would regard as gratifying. These "items" were selected from a larger pool developed by a panel of clinicians. The respondent is asked to imagine how much pleasure he or she could experience in each situation, and to rate each item on a 5-point scale of magnitude of pleasure. High scores signify greater capacity for pleasure.

Fawcett *et al.* (1983) have conducted two studies with the Pleasure Scale, both to assess its reliability and to compare its scores with those of comparable rating scales administered at the same time. Internal consistency was measured by split-half reliability (.89, .94), Cronbach's alpha (.96, .94), and item-total correlation coefficients (ranging from .50 to .80). Results of a unidimensional latent trait analysis suggest that the scale items do represent a single dimension, implying that loss of pleasure capacity affects "all itemized experiences . . . in a relatively uniform way" (Fawcett *et al.*, 1983, p. 81).

Pleasure Scale scores were found to be significantly but not highly correlated with such related instruments as the BDI ($r = -.46$), the Chapman Anhedonia Scale ($r = -.42$), and Weissman's Social Impairment Scale ($r = -.44$). They were unrelated to age (which may be a significant improvement over the Chapman scale) or measures of global impairment or neuroticism. Most (88%) of depressed patients had scores that did not differ from those of normal respondents; only a small minority showed extreme anhedonia, which corresponds to clinical impressions. While further work with this scale is indicated, it is an interesting addition to measures available for assessment of depressive subtypes.

Carroll Rating Scale for Depression

The Carroll Rating Scale for Depression (CRS) is an adaptation of the 17-item HRSD in a self-rating format. Items of the HRSD that are scored 0-4 are here represented by 4 separate items, while those that are scored 0-2 are represented by two. (It is assumed, although not demonstrated, that patients who endorse the more severe version of an HRSD item will also endorse the less severe version, thus giving a higher total score to that symptom area in a manner equivalent to a higher weight assigned by a clinician.) There are altogether 52 items, presented in scrambled order. The response format is "yes-no" and the maximum score is 52, as on the HRSD.

The concurrent validity of the CRS has been assessed in several studies by correlating CRS total scores with those derived from the HRSD and other scales. The diagnostic constitution of the patient samples is related to the strength of the observed relationships between the scales, which are higher for more homogeneously depressed samples and lower for diagnostically mixed samples. Carroll *et al.* (1973) found a correlation of .85 between the CRS and HRSD for 46 endogenously depressed inpatients. More recently (Carroll, Feinberg, Smouse, Rawson, & Greden, 1981), the scores of 97 endogenous patients on both scales on several occasions were compared, and a correlation coefficient of .80 between measures was obtained. Assessment of internal-consistency reliability for both scales was done in this study; the median item-total correlation coefficient for the CRS was .55 and for the HRSD was .54.

Inpatients with a range of psychiatric diagnoses were given the CRS, HRSD, and BDI on a total of 279 occasions. The two self-rating scales were more highly intercorrelated ($r = .86$) than either was with the HRSD (CRS and HRSD, $r = .71$; BDI and HRSD, $r = .60$). In another series of inpatients with various diagnoses, the CRS and HRSD were administered on the same day for 865 occasions; their correlation was .75 (Feinberg, Carroll, Smouse, & Rawson, 1981). For a subset of patients with unipolar endogenous depression, the correlation was .83, compared to .66 for patients with nonendogenous depression. The lower concordance between self-report and clinician ratings for the latter group was due to the patients' reporting more symptoms than the clinicians rated.

In the same study, global ratings of depression were made by patients (using the Visual Analogue Scale; see below) and clinicians (using a 4-point global rating scale). Two structured scales (CRS and HRSD) correlated more highly with each other than with either global rating, whether made by patient or physician. It would seem that "global ratings by *either* clinician or patient traded the advantages of ease, speed and repeatability for a loss of precision" (Feinberg *et al.*, 1981, p. 208).

Another group of investigators (Nasr, Altman, Rodin, Jobe, & Burg, 1984) administered the CRS and the 24-item HRSD to 64 depressed outpatients. The mean HRSD score for all patients was 23 ± 8, and the mean CRS score was 22 ± 11. The overall correlation was .84. In contrast to the findings of Feinberg *et al.* (1981), no differences were found between the interscale correlations for endogenous vs nonendogenous patients in this much smaller sample.

The CRS was also administered to 119 employees of a medical center who presumably were representative of the general population (Carroll *et al.*, 1981). The mean score was 4.6 ($SD = 0.4$). The authors propose a cutoff score of 10 if the CRS is used as a screening instrument, with higher scores signifying the presence of significant depressive symptoms.

Overall, the CRS shows both statistically and clinically significant correlations with the HRSD. While it is not proposed as a substitute in research protocols, it appears to be a convenient and economical alternative in particular situations. It may be useful for weekly monitoring or for assessing concordance between doctor and patient assessments of clinical progress. It may also be useful in routine clinical practice, either to monitor change or to serve as a screen to identify patients who need more extensive evaluation of depressive symptoms. Its use as a community screening test requires considerably more study.

Hopelessness Scale

Hopelessness is not necessarily a component of depressive disorders, nor is it directly correlated with depressive severity. It is, however, believed to be related to suicidal intent, and as such may be regarded as a defining characteristic of a subset of depressed patients.

Beck *et al.* (1974) developed a 20-item true-false scale to assess hopelessness, which they defined as negative expectancies concerning oneself and one's future. Of the items on the Hopelessness Scale (HS), 9 are keyed false and 11 true; the total score has a range of 0-20. Beck *et al.* reported an internal-consistency reliability coefficient of .93 in their initial study of 294 inpatients who recently had attempted suicide. Item-total correlation coefficeints ranged from .39 to .76; these were all statistically significant, but they suggest that the total score is much more reliable than any single item.

Concurrent validity was assessed by comparing HS scores with clinician ratings of hopelessness, with total BDI scores, and with the score on the BDI item of pessimism. All of these measures were significantly and moderately intercorrelated.

Since its introduction in 1974, the HS has been used in a number of studies exploring the relationships among hopelessness, depression, and suicidal intent. Dyer and Kreitman (1984) summarized eight such studies and reported the results of their own. In all, HS scores were significantly correlated with measures of suicidal intent, even when severity of depression was controlled. The scale appears effective as a measure of hopelessness, which may be an important dimension to assess both in selecting patients for research participation, and for describing the nature of study samples.

HRSD Microcomputer Self-Rating Format

Carr, Ancill, Ghosh, and Margo (1981) developed a self-rating microcomputer version of the HRSD. Items were rephrased as simple questions, with four response options. Some response options (e.g., for items concerning mood, guilt, anxiety, tension) are differentiated in terms of severity. Others (e.g., for items concerning insomnia, somatic complaints) refer to frequency. Four items concerning suicidal thoughts have only two response options (yes-no).

The scale is programmed so that 21 frames are presented consecutively on the microcomputer monitor, including 3 of instructions and then 18 of questions, one at a time. Each frame remains on the screen until an appropriate response is entered, so that respondents are obliged to answer every question. The procedure takes about 10 minutes for a patient to complete.

Carr *et al.* (1981) administered the HRSD microcomputer scale to 125 depressed patients (including 50 inpatients), of whom 75 were also given global ratings of depressive severity by their treating psychiatrists. The mode of test administration was accepted by all patients, and the scale scores correlated as highly with the global ratings in this study (r = .78 for outpatients and .72 for inpatients) as reported elsewhere between clinician ratings and pencil-and-paper self-report scales.

A normal control sample of 43 also responded to this computer-administered scale. An "arbitrary" (probably *ex post facto*) cutoff score of 10 (out of a possible total score of 46) was used; only 4 patients and no controls were misclassified.

Overall, microcomputer scale administration is an extremely promising assessment method. Both patients and staff like it, and there is some evidence that the method facilitates candor, especially in potentially stressful areas such as acknowledgment of suicidal ideation. We look forward to an expansion of this technique in the assessment field.

Depression Adjective Check List

The Depression Adjective Check List (DACL) was designed to measure "transient depressive mood, feeling or emotion" (Lubin, 1965, p. 57). There are four forms for male respondents and four for females, each consisting of 32 adjectives (22 positive and 10 negative), which the respondent rates as "applies to me" or "does not apply to me." The checklist format was selected because of ease of administration, face validity, and acceptance by patients. Average length of time needed to complete a checklist is about 2½ minutes.

Lubin, in his initial (1965) publication, reported acceptable levels of split-half reliability (.82-.93 for normal as well as patient samples), and high levels of intercorrelation between the various lists, indicating their equivalence. The checklists successfully discriminated between normal and patient samples in terms of mean scores, and were significantly (but not highly) correlated with BDI scores.

Commenting on the utility of the DACL, Tasto (1977) described the scales as reliable, sensitive to change as a function of treatment, and effective in differentiating between depression and other psychiatric disorders. He noted that their major limitation is inadequacy in distinguishing severe from moderate levels of depression.

The DACL seems potentially useful when multiple mood ratings are desired within short time periods. The availability of several equivalent forms promotes the feasibility of frequent ratings, as does their brevity.

Visual Analogue Scale

In the Visual Analogue Scale procedure, a straight line, usually 100 mm in length, is presented to the respondent (Aitken, 1969). Anchors are provided only for the endpoints. In rating depressed mood, for example, the anchors might be "depression absent" on the left and "extreme depression" on the right. The depression score is the distance in millimeters between the patient's response and the left-hand end of the line. Although clinician or patient may be asked to respond, the scale is usually administered to the patient. The scoring may be made using a 100-point scale, or any other classification of responses (e.g., deciles, quartiles) that the investigator prefers.

The advantages of this method include ease and speed of administration, face validity, and the absence of any demand to choose between specified alternatives. Despite the apparent crudeness of this measure, it has been used with success in several treatment studies. Hamilton (1982) reports that "it provides extremely useful information" (p. 10). It appears to be most useful when repeated mood self-assessments are required within a short time frame.

General Health Questionnaire

The General Health Questionnaire (GHQ) was developed by Goldberg (1972) in London to serve as a self-administered screening test for detection of psychopathology among community respondents. Goldberg was particulaly interested in its application with general medical patients, although it also has been used in community surveys. Vieweg and Hedlung (1983) have written another of their excellent reviews about this scale, and the interested reader is referred to this publication, whose highlights we summarize.

Goldberg intended to include 4 domains in the scale: depression/unhappiness; anxiety and psychological disturbance; social impairment; and hypochondriasis. He consulted earlier questionnaires such as the Cornell Medical Index and Maudsley Personality Inventory in developing items. An initial item pool was tested with patients and normals, and those discriminating best were factor-analyzed. Sixty items were then selected to represent a general "severity of illness" factor and specific symptom clusters. Subsequently, shorter versions have been constructed, with 30, 28, 20, and 12 items. The standard used is the GHQ-28.

GHQ items are scored by the respondent on a 4-point scale according to his or her recent experience, and then the item is scored dichotomously as present or absent. For example, in response to a question such as "Have you recently been feeling sad or gloomy?" the response options are "less so than usual," "no more than usual," "rather more than usual," and "much more than usual." The first two are scored as absent (0) and the others as present (1). The total score consists of the sum of items scored as present. In some forms, Likert scoring based on severity has been used, and subscale scores can be computed if the 28-item version is used. No cutoff scores for case identification are standard. Vieweg and Hedlund quote Tornopolsky's advice that "it is necessary to recalibrate the GHQ every time on representative samples from the population it is intended to be used on" (Vieweg & Hedlund, 1983, p. 79).

The instrument is satisfactory in terms of item-total, split-half, and test-retest reliability analyses. Its validity, however, remains unclear. While total scores show substantial correlations with other psychiatric rating scales, its misclassification rate of "cases" in the general population is too high to warrant its use as a screening instrument in that context. Cleary, Goldberg, Kessler, and Nycz (1982) compared GHQ responses with SADS-L diagnoses for a sample of American medical patients. They did not find the GHQ subscale scores useful for identification of specific psychiatric syndromes.

Overall, the GHQ seems to work best as a general indicator of psychological distress and/or demoralization for medical patients who may benefit from a psychiatric referral. It has not been shown effective as a diagnostic instrument for depression, and we do not recommend its use for that purpose either in clinical or research settings.

Center for Epidemiologic Studies Depression Scale

Assessment of disorder in the general population poses specific challenges, including the need to determine what level of impairment constitutes a "case" and what cluster of symptoms conforms to the definition of a syndrome. Since the base rates of disorder in community studies are, relatively speaking, very low, issues of false positives and false negatives become central in assessing the utility of assessment procedures designed to generate population prevalence rates. Even a small lack of specificity may grossly inflate the estimate of population prevalence.

All of the clinician rating scales and self-rating scales described above are intended for use with patients already diagnosed as depressed, with the exception of global ratings suitable for patients with any psychiatric diagnosis. While these scales are sometimes used in community studies, such use is not their intended use, and the results are often misleading in the direction of overestimating illness rates.

Probably the most rigorous method for establishing illness prevalence rates in the general population is the use of structured diagnostic interviews such as those described earlier in this chapter, or the Psychiatric Epidemiology Research Interview (PERI) developed by Dohrenwend and associates (Dohrenwend & Shrout, 1981). The PSE has been adapted for use in community surveys (Wing, Mann, Leff, & Nixon, 1978); the DIS was specifically designed for them; and the SADS has been used successfully with general population samples. The PERI, which is an intricate, sophisticated, and lengthy structured interview, includes components designed to assess dimensions of psychopathology using symptom scales, measures of social functioning, and a detailed assessment of stressful life events. The PERI does not yield diagnoses. All of these procedures require time and trained staff, so that their expense often prevents their application in any but the most ambitious and generously supported programs.

The Center for Epidemiologic Studies Depression Scale (CES-D) was developed by the Center for Epidemiologic Studies at NIMH specifically to meet the need for a brief, inexpensive measure of depression suitable for use in community surveys. Such an instrument could serve either as the initial screen in a two-stage assessment procedure such as that advocated by Dohrenwend and his associates, or, more ambitiously, as a basis for generating prevalence rates in its own right.

The CES-D consists of 20 items that were selected from other depression scales, including the BDI, the SDS, and the Minnesota Multiphasic Personality Inventory (MMPI). Six major symptom areas were identified, and a few items were selected to assess each. The areas are depressed mood, guilt/worthlessness, helplessness/hopelessness, psychomotor retardation, loss of appetite, and sleep disturbance. Each item is rated on a scale from 0 to 3 in terms of frequency of occurrence during the past week; the total score may range from 0 to 60. Although it can be used as an interview questionnaire, it is more often used as a self-rating scale.

A major question is the choice of the cutoff point used for classification of a respondent as "depressed." Most investigators have used a cutoff score of 16. Boyd, Weissman, Thompson, and Myers (1982) showed that over 99% of a sample of depressed outpatients with RDS scores over 6 scored 16 or higher on the CES-D. A score of 16 is equivalent to 6 symptoms reported as occurring for most of the previous week, or to more than half of the symptoms for fewer days.

As summarized by Roberts and Vernon (1983), the internal-consistency reliability and test-retest reliability of the CES-D are both good. What remains to be determined is its criterion validity. To date, the scale's correspondence to diagnosis of clinical depression in community respondents has been assessed in three samples.

In the second wave of a longitudinal community survey, Myers and Weissman (1980; Weissman & Myers, 1978) administered both the SADS and CES-D to 515 community residents. In the third wave of interviews 6 years later, 482 respondents were given both instruments. These investigators found in both data sets that the CES-D generated consistently much higher point-prevalence rates(15% to 25%) of depressive disorders than those based on SADS diagnoses (about 5%). Furthermore, the correlation between RDC diagnoses derived from the SADS and case identification by the CES-D was rather modest (r = .43). As Boyd *et al.* (1982) reported in a subsequent publication, the predictive value of the CES-D in the data set of 482 subjects was found to be 33%. The sensitivity of the CES-D was 64% (i.e., the scale correctly identified as depressed two-thirds of the subjects with RDC diagnoses of depression), and its specificity was 94% (i.e., 94 out of 100 people identified as depressed by the CES-D were in fact depressed according to RDC). Translated into survey terms, of 1,000 respondents given the CES-D, assuming a true point prevalence of 5%, 33 cases would be correctly identified, 17 cases would be missed, and 60 respondents would be identified incorrectly as cases. This yields an estimated point prevalence of 9.3%, which is an 86% overestimate.

Another recent study using both the CES-D and SADS was conducted by Roberts and Vernon (1983). In the first stage of their community survey, 528 people were asked to respond to the CES-D and other self-report measures. In Stage 2, shortly afterwards, clinical interviewers administered the SADS. The CES-D was found to identify correctly 60% of those identified as depressed by the SADS (sensitivity), and to identify correctly 86% of the noncases (specificity). These results are slightly less favorable than, but generally similar to, those reported in the New Haven samples of Weissman and colleagues. In the latter, Myers and Weissman (1980) concluded that symptom scales such as the CES-D are "only rough indicators of clinical depression in the community" (p. 1081). Roberts and Vernon, looking at the cumulative evidence, concluded that "it may be unrealistic to expect such instruments to generate differential diagnoses" and that "the CES-D should be used with considerable caution as first-stage screening instrument" (1983, p. 45) because of its lack of sensitivity.

Breslau (1985) examined the utility of the CES-D in differentiating between major depression and generalized anxiety, using NIMH-DIS diagnoses as the criterion. The 310 respondents were mothers of chronically medically ill children. Of the sample, 30% obtained scores over 16 on the CES-D, while 5% met criteria for major depression and 6% for generalized anxiety according to the DIS-generated DSM-III diagnoses. The predictive value of the CES-D for major depression was 15%, and for generalized anxiety it was 17%, reflecting a failure to discriminate between major depression and generalized anxiety. In addition, a low specificity rate (73% for both current major depression and generalized anxiety) was found, due to the scale's inability to distinguish current from past disorders of either kind. Breslau concluded that the CES-D was not a specific measure of depression in this sample of women at high risk for psychiatric disorder (or at least demoralization), exposed as they were to continuous life stress.

There seem to be at least three major considerations contributing to the limitations of the CES-D as a measure of population prevalence of depression. First, many CES-D items are not essential symptoms of major depressive disorder, and serve equally well as symptoms of other syndromes or even of nonspecific demoralization. Second, the essential criteria for an RDC diagnosis of major depression are either inadequately covered or are missing entirely. Third, as Zimmerman (1983) pointed out, there is a problem in case identification associated with any scale involving score summation for the purpose of case identification. Application of diagnostic criteria entails "counting" only those symptoms that reach a specified level of severity; if the symptoms are there but below threshold levels, they are disregarded for diagnostic purposes. In symptom scales, many symptoms may be present at a low level of severity or frequency, but nevertheless contribute to the total score used for case identification. This characteristic probably contributes to the much higher prevalence rates of depression generated by self-reported screening scales compared to structured diagnostic interviews.

In summary, we agree with the conclusion of Weissman and colleagues and of Vernon and Roberts that the CES-D has not yet been shown to be a useful tool for determination of community prevalence rates of depressive disorder, either as a first-stage screening method or as an independent assessment of illness.

CONCLUSIONS

We have briefly described major measures used to assess clinical disorders in adults. Our compilation of measures is not exhaustive, nor have we included promising and innovative scales currently used by their authors but not yet published (e.g., Zimmerman's Inventory to Diagnose Depression, a self-rating scale for diagnosis of major depressive disorder). Nevertheless, our review does encompass the large majority of scales currently used in the clinical measurement of depression.

We offer several concluding observations. First, in the categories of clinician ratings and self-ratings, the most successful scales were introduced over a decade ago and have not been notably improved upon by subsequent efforts. This calls to mind the situation in psychopharmacology, where the first drug introduced in a class often remains the standard (e.g., imipramine among tricyclic antidepressants). It is our general belief that the most pressing unmet needs of the field are extensions of current available measures to include diagnostic subtypes not adequately assessed by available instruments. Other major measurement needs include considerably more evaluation of the specific contributions of existing scales; refinement of existing scales to improve their reliability and validity; and pursuit of measuring differential effects of treatment, assuming that they exist.

Further work to be done includes assessment of sensitivity and specificity of measures in carefully defined clinical populations (diagnosed with high inter-clinician reliability). While sensitivity is independent of the various diagnostic distinctions in a given sample, specificity requires certain contrasts. For instance, a scale may be specific for depression when administered to depressed patients and normal controls, but may fail to distinguish between depressed and anxious patients.

Finally, measures of depression should be augmented to include indices of anxiety symptoms such as spontaneous panic attacks and phobic avoidance, both historical and current. Accumulating evidence suggests differential treatment response for depressed patients with and without panic attacks (Liebowitz *et al.*, 1984). These data are also relevant to the primary-secondary distinction among depressive subtypes.

For hierarchical growth to take place, investigators have to use equivalent measures so that findings are comparable across studies. When different research centers use their own instruments, the results may be fascinating but difficult to evaluate in the broader context of accumulated experience. While the application of psychometrically sophisticated and well-validated but inappropriate instruments is useless, it is also true that newly produced measures are difficult to interpret in the absence of carefully designed studies of norms, psychometric properties, and outcomes in several samples. The proliferation of measuring instruments, as Reeder, Ramacher, and Gorelnik (1976) have observed, "not only fragments the field but inhibits the cumulative nature" of research knowledge (p. 1). Accordingly, we urge investigators to use existing measures whenever it is possible to do so, instead of inventing their own, in order to promote data comparability among sites, samples, and occasions.

References

Abou-Saleh, M. T., & Coppen, A. (1983). Classification of depression and response to antidepressive therapies. *British Journal of Psychiatry, 143*, 601-603.

Aitken, R. (1969). Measurement of feelings using visual analogue scales. *Proceedings of the Royal Society of Medicine, 62*, 989-996.

Anthony, J. C., Folstein, M., Romanoski, A., Von Korff, M., Nestadt, G., Chahal, R., Merchant, A., Brown, C., Shapiro, S., Kramer, M., & Gruenberg, E. (1985). Comparison of the lay Diagnostic Interview Schedule and a standardized psychiatric diagnosis. *Archives of General Psychiatry, 42*, 667-675.

Bailey, J., & Coppen, A. (1976). A comparison between the Hamilton Rating Scale and the Beck Inventory in the measurement of depression. *British Journal of Psychiatry, 128*, 486-489.

Bech, P. (1981). Rating scales for affective disorders: Their validity and consistency. *Acta Psychiatrica Scandinavica* (Suppl. 295), 1-101.

Bech, P., Bolwig, T. G., Kramp, P. & Rafaelsen, O. J. (1979). The Bech-Rafaelsen Melancholia Scale and the Hamilton Depression Scale. *Acta Psychiatrica Scandinavica, 59*, 420-430.

Bech, P., Gram, L., Dein, E., Jacobsen, O., Vitger, J., & Bolwig, T. (1975). Quantitative rating of depressive states. *Acta Psychiatrica Scandinavica, 51*, 161-170.

Bech, P., & Rafaelsen, O. J. (1980). The use of rating scales exemplified by a comparison of the Hamilton and the Bech-Rafaelsen Melancholia Scale. *Acta Psychiatrica Scandinavica, 62* (Suppl. 285), 128-132.

Beck, A. T. (1967). *Depression: Clinical, experimental and theoretical aspects*. Philadelphia: University of Pennsylvania Press.

Beck, A. T., & Beamesderfer, A. (1974). Assessment of depression: The Depression Inventory. In P. Pichot (Ed.), *Psychological measurements in psychopharmacology* (pp. 151-169), Basel: S. Karger.

Beck, A. T., Ward, C. H., Mendelson, M., Mock, J. E., & Erbaugh, J. K. (1961). An inventory for measuring depression. *Archives of General Psychiatry, 4*, 561-571.

Beck, A. T., Weissman, A., Lester, D., & Trexler, L. (1974). The measure of pessimism: The Hopelessness Scale. *Journal of Consulting and Clinical Psychology, 42*, 861-865.

Boyd, J. H., Weissman, M., Thompson, W., & Myers, J. K. (1982). Screening for depression in a community sample. *Archives of General Psychiatry, 39*, 1195-1200.

Breslau, N. (1985). Depressive symptoms, major depression and generalized anxiety: A comparison of self-reports on CES-D and results from diagnostic interviews. *Psychiatry Research, 15*, 219-229.

Carney, M. W., Roth, M., & Garside, R. (1965). The diagnosis of depressive syndromes and the prediction of E.C.T. response. *British Journal of Psychiatry, 111*, 659-674.

Carney, M. W., & Sheffield, P. B. (1972). Depression and the Newcastle Scales: Their relation to Hamilton's scale. *British Journal of Psychiatry, 121*, 35-40.

Carr, A. C., Ancill, R. J., Ghosh, A., & Margo, A. (1981). Direct assessment of depression by microcomputer: A feasibility study. *Acta Psychiatrica Scandinavica, 64*, 415-422.

Carroll, B. J., Feinberg, M., Smouse, P., Rawson, S., & Greden, J. (1981). The Carroll Rating Scale for Depression: I. Development, reliability and validation. *British Journal of Psychiatry, 138*, 194-200.

Caroll, B. J., Fielding, J., & Blashki, T. (1973). Depression rating scales: A critical review. *Archives of General Psychiatry, 28*, 361-366.

Chipman, A., & Paykel, E. (1974). How ill is the patient at this time?: Cues determining clinicians' global judgments. *Journal of Consulting and Clinical Psychology, 42*, 699-674.

Cicchetti, D., & Prusoff, B. (1983). Reliability of depression and associated clinical symptoms. *Archives of General Psychiatry, 40*, 987-990.

Cleary, P. D., Goldberg, I., Kessler, L., & Nycz, G. (1982). Screening for mental disorder among primary care patients. *Archives of General Psychiatry, 39*, 837-840.

Cohen, P. (in press). Psychometric issues in devising and assessing a psychiatric diagnostic interview schedule for children. *Journal of the American Academy of Child Psychiatry*.

Cronholm, B., & Daly, R. (1983). Evaluation of psychiatric treatment. In T. Helggson (Ed.), *Methodology in evaluation of psychiatric treatment* (pp. 3-32). Cambridge, England: Cambridge University Press.

Derogatis, L., & Cleary, P. (1977). Confirmation of the dimensional structure of the SCL-90: A study in construct validation. *Journal of Clinical Psychology, 33*, 981-989.

Derogatis, L., Lipman, R., Rickels, K., Uhlenhuth, E. H., & Covi, L. (1974). The Hopkins Symptom Checklist (HSCL). In P. Pichot (Ed.), *Psychological measurements in psychopharmacology* (pp. 79-110). Basel: S. Karger.

Dohrenwend, B. P., & Shrout, P. E. (1981). Toward the development of a two-stage procedure for case identification and classification in psychiatric epidemiology. In R. Simmons (Ed.), *Research in community and mental health* (Vol. 2, pp. 292-323). Greenwich, CT: JAI Press.

Dyer, J., & Kreitman, N. (1984). Hopelessness, depression and suicidal intent in parasuicide. *British Journal of Psychiatry, 144*, 127-133.

Endicott, J. (1981). Diagnostic Interview Schedule: Reliability and validity (letter). *Archives of General Psychiatry, 38*, 1300.

Endicott, J., Cohen, J., Nee, J., Fleiss, J., & Sarantakos, S. (1981). Hamilton Depression Rating Scale. *Archives of General Psychiatry, 38*, 98-103.

Endicott, J., & Spitzer, R. (1980). Psychiatric rating scales. In H. Kaplan, A. Freedman, & B. Sadock (Eds.), *Comprehensive textbook of psychiatry* (3rd ed., Vol. 3, pp. 2391-2409). Baltimore: Williams & Wilkins.

Endicott, J., Spitzer, R., Fleiss, J., & Cohen, J. (1976). The Global Assessment Scale. *Archives of General Psychiatry, 33*, 766-771.

Fawcett, J., Clark, D., Scheftner, W., & Gibbons, R. (1983). Assessing anhedonia in psychiatric patients. *Archives of General Psychiatry, 40*, 79-84.

Feinberg, M., Carroll, B., Smouse, P., & Rawson, S. (1981). The Carroll Rating Scale for Depression: III. Comparison with other rating instruments. *British Journal of Psychiatry, 138*, 205-209.

Freud, S. (1961). The Future of an illusion. In J. Strachey (Ed. and Trans.), *The standard edition of the complete psychological works of Sigmund Freud* (Vol. 21, pp. 5-56). London: Hogarth Press. (Original work published 1927)

Goldberg, D. P. (1972). The detection of psychiatric illness by questionnaire. London: Oxford University Press.

Gove, W., McCorkel, J., Fain, T., & Hughes, M. (1976). Response bias in community surveys of mental health. *Social Science and Medicine, 10*, 497-502.

Grove, W. M., Andreasen, N., McDonald-Scott, P., Keller, M., & Shapiro, R. (1981). Reliability studies of psychiatric diagnosis. *Archives of General Psychiatry, 38*, 408-413.

Guy, W. (1976). *ECDEU assessment manual for psychopharmacology, Revised* (DHEW Publication No. ADM 76-338). Washington, DC: U.S. Government Printing Office.

Hamilton, M. (1960). A rating scale for depression. *Journal of Neurology, Neurosurgery and Psychiatry, 23*, 56-62.

Hamilton, M. (1980). Rating depressive patients. *Journal of Clinical Psychiatry, 41*, 21-24.

Hamilton, M. (1982). Symptoms and assessment of depression. In E. S. Paykel (Ed.), *Handbook of affective disorders* (pp. 3-11). New York: Guilford Press.

Hedlund, J. L., & Vieweg, B. W. (1979a). The Hamilton Rating Scale for Depression: A comprehensive review. *Journal of Operational Psychiatry, 10*, 149-165.

Hedlund, J. L., & Vieweg, B. W. (1979b). The Zung Self-Rating Depression Scale: A comprehensive review. *Journal of Operational Psychiatry, 10*, 51-64.

Hedlund, J. L., & Vieweg, B. W. (1980). The Brief Psychiatric Rating Scale (BPRS): A comprehensive review. *Journal of Operational Psychiatry, 11*, 48-65.

Hedlund, J. L., & Vieweg, B. W. (1981). Structured psychiatric interviews: A comparative review. *Journal of Operational Psychiatry, 12*, 39-67.

Helzer, J., & Coryell, W. (1983). More on DSM-III: How consistent are precise criteria? *Biological Psychiatry, 18*, 1201-1202.

Helzer, J. E., Robins, L., Croughan, J. & Weiner, A. (1981). Renard Diagnostic Interview. *Archives of General Psychiatry, 38*, 393-398.

Hesselbrock, V., Stabenau, J., Hesselbrock, M., Mirkin, P., & Meyer, R. (1982). A comparison of two interview schedules. *Archives of General Psychiatry, 39*, 674-677.

Hughes, J., O'Hara, M., & Rehm, L. (1982). Measurement of depression in clinical trials: An overview. *Journal of Clinical Psychiatry, 43*, 85-88.

Kearns, N., Cruickshank, K., McGuigan, S., Riley, S., Shan, S., & Snaith, R. (1982). A comparison of depression rating scales. *British Journal of Psychiatry, 141*, 45-49.

Kendell, R. E. (1975). *The role of diagnosis in psychiatry*. Oxford: Blackwell.

Klein, D. F. (1974). Endogenomorphic depression. *Archives of General Psychiatry, 31*, 447-454.

Klein, D. F., & Fink, M. (1963). Multiple item factors as change measures in psychopharmacology. *Psychopharmacologia, 4*, 43-52.

Klein, D. F., Gittelman, R., Quitkin, F., & Rifkin, A. (1980). *Diagnosis and drug treatment of psychiatric disorders*. Baltimore: Williams & Wilkins.

Kovacs, M., Rush, A. J., Beck, A., & Hollon, S. D. (1981). Depressed outpatients treated with cogntive therapy or pharmacotherapy. *Archives of General Psychiatry, 38*, 33-41.

Liebowitz, M. L., Quitkin, F., Stewart, J., McGrath, P., Harrison, W., Rabkin, J., Tricamo, E., Markowitz, J., & Klein, D. (1984): Phenelzine vs. imipramine in atypical depression. *Archives of General Psychiatry, 41*, 669-677.

Lubin, B. (1965). Adjective checklists for the measurement of depression. *Archives of General Psychiatry, 12*, 57-62.

Lyerly, S. (1973). *Handbook of psychiatric rating scales* (2nd ed., DHEW Publication No. HSM 73-9061). Washington, DC: U.S. Government Printing Office.

Mendels, J., & Weinstein, N. (1972). The relationship between depression and anxiety. *Archives of General Psychiatry, 27*, 649-653.

Montgomery, S., & Asberg, M. (1979). A new depression scale designed to be sensitive to change. *British Journal of Psychiatry, 134*, 382-389.

Myers, J., & Weissman, M. (1980). Use of a self-report symptom scale to detect depression in a community sample. *American Journal of Psychiatry, 137*, 1081-1084.

Nasr, S., Altman, A., Rodin, M., Jobe, T., & Burg, B. (1984). Correlation of the Hamilton and Carroll Depression Rating Scales: A replication study among psychiatric outpatients. *Journal of Clinical Psychiatry, 45*, 167-168.

Overall, J. (1974). The Brief Psychiatric Rating Scale in psychopharmacology research. In P. Pichot (Ed.), *Psychological measurement in psychopharmacology* (pp. 67-78). Basel: S. Karger.

Overall, J., & Gorham, D. (1962). The Brief Psychiatric Rating Scale. *Psychological Reports, 10*, 799-812.

Pichot, P. (Ed.). (1974). *Psychological measurements in psychopharmacology*. Basel: S. Karger.

Reeder, L., Ramacher, L., & Gorelnik, S. (1976). *Handbook of scales and indices of health behavior*. Pacific Palisades, CA: Goodyear.

Rhoades, H. M., & Overall, J. E. (1983). The Hamilton Depression Scale: Factor scoring and profile classification. *Psychopharmacology Bulletin, 19*, 91-96.

Roberts, R. E., & Vernon, S. W. (1983). The Center for Epidemiologic Studies Depression Scale: Its use in a community sample. *American Journal of Psychiatry, 140*, 41-46.

Robins, L. N., & Helzer, J. E. (1982). Diagnostic Interview Schedule (letter). *Archives of General Psychiatry, 39*, 443-1445.

Robins, L. N., Helzer, J. E., Croughan, J., & Ratcliff, K. (1981). National Institute of Mental Health Diagnostic Interview Schedule. *Archives of General Psychiatry, 38*, 381-389.

Robins, L. N., Helzer, J. E., Ratcliff, K., & Seyfried, W. (1982). Validity of the Diagnostic Interview Schedule, Version II: DSM-III diagnoses. *Psychological Medicine, 12*, 855-870.

Silberman, E. K., & Post, R. M. (1982). Atypicality in primary depressive illness: A preliminary survey. *Biological Psychiatry, 17*, 285-304.

Snaith, R. P.. Ahmed, S. N., Metha, S., & Hamilton, M. (1971). The assessment of the severity of primary depressive illness: The Wakefield Self-assessment Depression Inventory. *Psychological Medicine, 1*, 143-149.

Snaith, R. P., Bridge, G., & Hamilton, M. (1976). The Leeds Scales for the self assessment of anxiety and depression. *British Journal of Psychiatry, 128*, 156-165.

Spitzer, R. L. (1983). Psychiatric diagnosis: Are clinicians still necessary? *Comprehensive Psychiatry, 24*, 399-411.

Spitzer, R. L., & Williams, J. B. (1980). Classification of mental disorders and DSM-III. In H. Kaplan, A. Freedman, & B. Sadock (Eds.), *Comprehensive textbook of psychiatry* (3rd ed., Vol. 1, pp. 1035-1072). Baltimore: Williams & Wilkins.

Spitzer, R. L., & Williams, J. B. (1983). *Development of a diagnostic clinical interview for psychiatric research* (Technical Proposal RFP NIMH DB-83-0007). Rockville, MD: National Institute of Mental Health.

Spitzer, R. L., & Williams, J. B. (1983b). *Instruction manual for the Structured Clinical Interview for DSM-III (SCID), 11/1/83 revision*. (Available from the Biometrics Research Department, New York State Psychiatric Institute, 722 West 168th Street, New York, NY 10032.)

Spitzer, R. L., & Williams, J. B. (1986). *Structured Clinical Interview for DSM-III — Nonpatient Version (SCID-NP 5/1/86)*. (Available from Biometrics Research Department, New York State Psychiatric Institute, 722 West 168 Street, New York, NY 10032.)

Spitzer, R. L., Williams, J. B., & Gibbon, M. (1986). *Structured Clinical Interview for DSM-III R-SCID, 8/1/86* (Available from Biometrics Research Department, New York State Psychiatric Institute, 722 West 168 Street, New York, NY 10032.)

Srole, L., & Fisher, A. (Eds.). (1978). *Mental health in the metropolis: The Midtown Manhattan Study* (rev. ed.). New York: New York University Press.

Tasto, D. L. (1977). Self-report schedules and inventories. In A. Ciminero, K. Calhoun, & H. Adams (Eds.), *Handbook of behavioral assessment* (pp. 153-193). New York: Wiley.

Thase, M. Hersen, M., Bellack, A., Himmelhoch, J., & Kupfer, D. (1983). Validation of a Hamilton subscale for endogenomorphic depression. *Journal of Affective Disorders, 5*, 267-276.

Vernon, S., & Roberts, R. (1982). Use of the SADS-RDC in a tri-ethnic community survey. *Archives of General Psychiatry, 39*, 47-52.

Vieweg, B. W., & Hedlund, J. L. (1983). The General Health Questionnaire (GHQ): A comprehensive review. *Journal of Operational Psychiatry, 14*, 74-81.

Von Korff, M., Anthony, J. C., & Kramer, M. (1982). Diagnostic Interview Schedule (letter). *Archives of General Psychiatry, 39*, 1443.

Waskow, I., & Parloff, M. (Eds.). (1975). *Psychotherapy change measures* (DHEW Publication No. ADM 74-120). Washington, DC: U.S. Government Printing Office.

Weissman, M., Klerman, G., Prusoff, B., Sholomskas, D., & Padian, N. (1981). Depressed outpatients. *Archives of General Psychiatry, 38*, 51-55.

Weissman, M., & Myers, J. (1978). Affective disorders in a U.S. urban community. *Archives of General Psychiatry, 35*, 1304-1311.

Wilson, P., Goldin, J., & Charbonneau-Powis, M. (1983). Comparative efficacy of behavioral and cognitive treatments of depression. *Cognitive Therapy and Research, 7*, 111-124.

Wing, J. K. (1970). A standard form of psychiatric present state examination. In E. H. Hare & J. K. Wing (Eds.), *Psychiatric epidemiology* (pp. 93-131). London: Oxford University Press.

Wing, J. K., Cooper, J. E., & Sartorious, N. (1974). *Measurement and classification of psychiatric symptoms: An instruction manual for the PSE and CATEGO program*. London: Cambridge University Press.

Wing, J. K., Mann, S. A., Leff, J. P., & Nixon, J. (1978). The concept of a "case" in psychiatric population surveys. *Psychological Medicine, 8*, 203-217.

Wittenborn, J. R. (1972). Reliability, validity, and objectivity of symptom rating scales. *Journal of Nervous and Mental Disease, 154*, 79-87.

Zimmerman, M. (1983). Self-report depression scales (letter). *Archives of General Psychiatry, 40*, 1035.

Zung, W. (1965). A self-rating depression scale. *Archives of General Psychiatry, 12*, 63-70.

Zung, W. (1974). The measurement of affects: Depression and anxiety. In P. Pichot (Ed.), *Psychological measurements in psychopharmacology* (pp. 170-188). Basel: S. Karger.

SECTION II

Biological Measurement

CHAPTER 4

The Measurement of Genetic Aspects of Depression

NANCY C. ANDREASEN
University of Iowa

INTRODUCTION

The study of genetic aspects of depression involves determining the extent to which disorders aggregate within families and attempting to determine the reasons for that aggregation. To call this study "genetic" is to some extent a misnomer, since it rarely succeeds in discovering purely genetic factors. Disorders aggregate within families for many different reasons. Members of the same family may develop tuberculosis because they are exposed to the same infectious agents. Children growing up in the same ghetto apartment may develop encephalopathy because they are eating the same lead-contaminated paint. The daughter of a depressed mother may develop depression herself because she has learned coping techniques of withdrawal and introjection through role modeling. Even if an investigator is searching for "purely genetic" factors in the transmission of illness, he or she must be alert to the possible influence of these nongenetic factors. Indeed, the days of searching for a single gene that causes mental illness may be as distant as King Arthur's Camelot. Most psychiatric illnesses will probably turn out to be polygenic and multifactorial in etiology.

The reasons for studying the extent to which disorders aggregate within families are multiple. First, of course, we may use this technique in order to determine the extent to which disorders are transmitted genetically and what type of transmission is occurring. Investigations of this type hope to increase our understanding of the etiology and pathogenesis of mental illness. Second, studies of familial aggregation are frequently used to help determine the validity of existing systems for classifying mental illness or to develop new ones. Most investigators believe that the affective disorders are heterogeneous and consist of several different subtypes. Genetic and family studies may be used in an attempt to identify more etiologically homogeneous subtypes. Finally, genetic and family studies may be used to explore the comparative phenomenology of mental disorders. When data are collected on the symptoms and course of illness among members of the same family, they can then be compared in order to determine the degree of similarity. If the disorders are very similar and tend to "breed true," this finding gives additional support both for the nosological validity of subtypes and for a more purely genetic cause.

DESIGNING FAMILY STUDIES

Most family studies begin with the "proband method." That is, a "proband" (an index case with a particular diagnosis such as depression) is "ascertained" identified, and family members are then studied. Beginning with this single tiny kernel, the study of families may then grow in a variety of different ways, depending on the questions being asked and the resources available.

Types of Studies

The Family History Method

The family history method is the simplest technique for collecting familial data. It involves simply interviewing the proband about illnesses that have occurred in other members of his or her family (Andreasen, Endicott, Spitzer, & Winokur, 1977). Usually this method is limited to collecting information on first-degree relatives (i.e., parents, siblings, and offspring), since the proband does not usually have very complete information about more distant second-degree relatives (grandparents, grandchildren, aunts, and uncles). The family history method is strengthened by adding information from another informant, such as the proband's mother or sibling. The proband's ability to give reliable and valid information is also affected by his or her own psychopathological condition. Patients suffering from schizophrenia tend to be relatively poor informants, while those with depression are usually relatively good informants.

The advantage of the family history method is that it is efficient and inexpensive, and provides some information about all available family members. Obtaining a complete psychiatric history of the proband's family requires only about half an hour, even when the information is collected in thorough detail. Often a relative visiting the proband can be used as a second informant. Thus this method requires little in the way of time or personnel. Most important, however, the family history method provides information about *all* relatives of interest. Thus it insures that the sampling of family members will not be biased. Unlike other methods, it permits the investigator to collect information on relatives who have died, committed suicide, migrated, become demented, or become lost to the family, and therefore are not available for interview. Thus even the most sophisticated designs, such as are described below, must in some cases rely on family history data to complete pedigrees in the cases of relatives who cannot be directly interviewed for some reason.

The major problem with the family history method is the quality of information obtained. Even the closest families usually do not have complete information on the psychiatric history of all first-degree relatives. For example, a family member who has had relatively mild untreated depression may not have described this fact to any other members of his or her family, and therefore this information can only be obtained through interviewing the relative in person.

Table 4-1 shows the extent to which information collected by family history agrees with information collected through direct interview of relatives. As this table indicates, the family history method provides a substantial underestimate. This underestimate is greater for milder disorders than it is for serious ones such as bipolar disorder. Particularly in the case of purely genetic studies, in which one is attempting to determine patterns of transmission within a given family, family history data will not be sufficiently accurate to answer the questions being asked.

The Family Study Method

The family study method involves direct interview of relatives. In the usual family study, interviewing is limited to first-degree relatives (Winokur, Clayton, & Reich, 1969). The family study method differs from the family history method in that all available relatives are interviewed in person concerning their past history of psychiatric illness. Thus the information obtained is more accurate, since it is based on firsthand experience. Usually the goal is to determine lifetime prevalence of illness in these relatives.

While information based on personal interviews is clearly more likely to be accurate in most cases, such data can be quite expensive to collect. Most patients have three or more first-degree relatives, and they do not always live nearby. Relatives must be located, contacted, and either brought to the

TABLE 4-1 Accuracy of Family History Method, as Validated by Direct Interview (n = 2,216)

	Sensitivity		Specificity		Predictive value	
Any illness	841/1,282	(66%)	738/934	(79%)	841/1,037	(81%)
Any affective illness	473/937	(50%)	1,100/1,279	(86%)	473/652	(73%)
Depression	397/713	(56%)	1,259/1,503	(84%)	397/641	(62%)
Mania	27/46	(59%)	2,139/2,170	(99%)	27/58	(47%)
Alcoholism	174/336	(52%)	1,797/1,880	(96%)	174/257	(68%)
Drug use disorder	45/118	(38%)	2,070/2,098	(99%)	45/73	(62%)
Antisocial personality	11/21	(52%)	2,146/2,195	(98%)	11/60	(18%)
Schizophrenia	4/13	(31%)	2,199/2,203	(99.8%)	4/8	(50%)

research medical center or visited in person. Sometimes they may be interviewed by telephone. Thus the improved information is obtained at considerable cost and effort.

Extended Pedigrees

The extended-pedigree study is a special case of the family study. In such studies, the investigator tries to identify very large informative families and to collect information on all members of such families (Ashby & Crowe, 1978). Usually these studies emphasize the use of the family study technique, but family history data will be collected on more distant relatives who have died or cannot be located, so that the pedigree can be as complete as possible.

An example of a large informative pedigree appears in Figure 4-1. Pedigrees are considered "informative" when they contain many family members who are affected with mental illness. When pedigrees are sufficiently large and many family members are affected, the pedigree can be analyzed in order to determine the mode of transmission. Various types of genetic models can be fit, and the goodness of fit can be assessed. In addition, biological markers (see below) can be added to the study in order to assist in exploring the mode of transmission.

Twin Studies

Family studies indicate the degree to which disorders run in families, but they permit separation of genetic from learned cultural factors only by inference (i.e., through the fitting of various types of models of transmission, including those that recognize the role of cultural factors). Therefore, other designs have also been developed in order to provide additional information. Twin studies exploit the fact that monozygotic twins have essentially the same genetic material, while dizygotic twins share only half their genetic material (Hrubek & Allen, 1975; Smith, 1974). Monozygotic and dizygotic twins can be evaluated to determine the degree to which they are "concordant," or share the same illnesses. The concordance rate in monozygotic and dizygotic twins can then be compared, and a monozygotic-dizygotic ratio can be generated. The higher the monozygotic-dizygotic ratio, the greater the likelihood that genetic factors are important. Thus twin studies give a somewhat purer estimate of the role of genetic factors. Nevertheless, even this technique is not totally pure, since it does not control for the psychological impact of being a twin, the fact that twins usually have low birth weight and are therefore prone to suffer from "environmental traumata," or the fact that there are different rates of perinatal complications in monozygotic versus dizygotic twins.

Adopted-Offspring Studies

Adopted-offspring studies provide the cleanest design for separating nature from nurture (Heston, 1970; Mendlewicz & Rainer, 1977; Rosenthal & Kety,

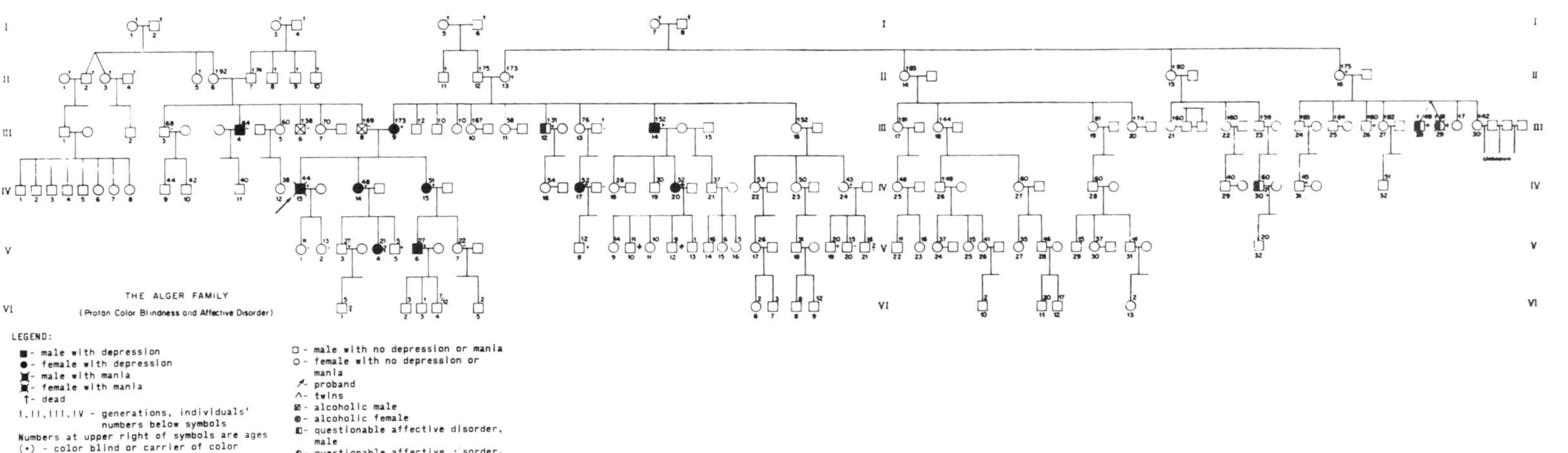

FIGURE 4-1 Example of extended pedigree. (From *Manic-Depressive Illness* by G. Winokur, P. J. Clayton, & T. Reich, 1969, St. Louis: C. V. Mosby. Reprinted by permission.)

1968). In these studies, the investigator identifies a cohort of mothers who have put their children up for adoption. Some of these mothers are identified because they are known to suffer from a particular type of mental illness, such as depression, while the other mothers are known to be well. In both instances, the adopted children are reared in normal families. Thus the tendency for an illness to pass from the mother to her child can be studied independently of maternal role modeling or other environmental influences. If the adopted child of a depressed mother develops depression, the familial cause is more likely to be purely genetic.

Even this relatively refined design is not without its inherent problems, however. Like twin studies, adoption studies require the ability to find a very special sample — mothers who have put their children up for adoption — and large amounts of time and effort to locate and interview the adopted children. In addition, most adoption studies have not thoroughly evaluated the extent to which the father might have mental illness. For example, a normal mother may have mated with a spouse suffering from some type of mental illness, such as antisocial personality. Information concerning the identity of the child's father, not to mention his psychiatric history, may be quite difficult to obtain, and yet such information is crucial in order to understand the results of these studies.

As this summary of methods indicates, the choice of any given method will always involve a series of compromises. There is no single ideal method for studying genetic or familial factors in affective illness or any other disorder. Rather, the best method to answer particular questions, and to meet one's budgetary constraints, must be selected. The results obtained must then be interpreted with a recognition of the limitations of the particular method selected.

Control Groups

The family history and family study methods require the collection of some type of control data, so that rates of illness in the probands' families can be compared with those in a control group in order to determine how familial the disorder may be. There are several potential pitfalls in the selection of a control group.

One approach to identifying a control group is to select a matched group. The first mistake that one might make — and it has been done, even though it is an obvious mistake — is to match the controls with the probands rather than the relatives. Rather clearly, there are potential differences between the probands and their relatives in some factors, such as age, sex, education, and socioeconomic status. If one is selecting a matched control group, then the next issue is how many variables will be required for matching. That decision will depend in part, of course, on the overall design of the study. Usually, the closer the match the better, but practical constraints tend to limit matching the sex, age, and some socioeconomic indicator.

Yet another problem is *how* to match. One design attempts to match each relative to a control. Several methods for obtaining matches are available. One has been called the "neighborhood method." The relative is asked to provide a list of approximately five people who live in his or her neighborhood but who are not close friends. A variant of the neighborhood method would involve using street guides and contacting households in order to find a match for the relative. Another type of method has been called the "acquaintance method." This involves asking a family member to list acquaintances (not friends) from places such as church, PTA, and the like, who match the relative in sex and age. The advantage of these techniques is that they provide relatively close matching on important variables that may affect the onset of an illness such as affective disorder. The disadvantage is that they may yield biased samples. In spite of trying hard to be objective, a relative may come up with a list of neighbors or acquaintances who share his or her tendency to have some type of psychopathology, thereby giving spuriously high estimates of illness in the control sample.

An alternate design for collecting controls involves the use of some other convenient group, such as medical controls. Again, the most obvious initial mistake is to match these medical controls to the proband. Ideally, a group of medical controls should be matched to the probands, and their relatives should then be subjected to family study in the same manner as those of the affectively ill proband. The advantage of this method is that it is relatively more random than the matching techniques just described and therefore less likely to yield a biased sample. The major disadvantages are that it is relatively difficult to apply and that the relatives may not provide a totally satisfactory match, particularly sociodemographically.

Yet a third technique for obtaining control data involves the use of epidemiological field surveys. In these surveys, a population may be sampled, or an attempt may be made to interview all people within a given area. Such surveys provide true population prevalence data, while the previous methods provide prevalence information concerning a subpopulation that may be more informative in a given study because of its matched characteristics. The mathematical models used for genetic analysis contain a term that requires an estimate of population prevalence. Therefore, such information is necessary to explore these models. On the other hand, good population data are extremely difficult to obtain, since they are usually obtained using instruments designed for epidemiological studies, while instruments used in family studies more closely approximate clinical interviews (even when they are structured). Thus there are always questions about the comparability of data.

Several problems may plague all attempts to collect control data — namely, refusal rate and response bias. Even when ascertainment attempts are extremely vigorous, some people will always refuse. It is impossible to know exactly how the refusers bias the sample. Some may refuse because they have been ill and do not wish to admit it, while others may refuse because they are very healthy and therefore too busy to participate. Of course, one attempts to describe the refusers as completely as possible and to show that they do not differ from those interviewed on important variables such as age, sex, and sociodemographic status, but this does not solve the problem completely. On the other hand, the accepters may also be a biased group. People who have enough free time to participate in a research study, particularly one with a relatively long battery, may be unusual in many different ways. They may be unemployed and may have depression either as a cause or a consequence of this. They may agree to participate because they suspect they may receive some help for problems they are having. Factors such as these can spuriously raise rates of illness among those who consent to participate.

Assortative Mating

A proband's spouse is not technically a first-degree relative, since the spouse shares no genetic material with the proband, but information on spouses is of course necessary in order to interpret information concerning children. It has been recognized for many years that people tend to be attracted to others who have characteristics in common with them, as expressed in the truisms that "like attracts like" or "birds of a feather flock together." Probands and spouses are likely to be similar in age, educational status, sociodemographic background, intelligence, and a variety of other factors — perhaps even the tendency to have mental illness or a familial predisposition to have it. Furthermore, since the proband is by definition ill, the spouse may himself or herself develop symptoms of illness in reaction to the stress of living with an ill mate.

Thus the spouses of probands are predisposed in several ways to have a higher illness rate than the general population. Spouses must, therefore, be included in family studies and evaluated in the same manner as the probands. Since it will be important to determine a spouse's own familial predisposition to illness, at a minimum family history data should be collected on the spouse. In cases where the children are an object of study, and in studies of those at high risk, then it may even be necessary to do family studies involving the relatives of the spouse.

Familial Markers

Genetic and family studies may be strengthened through the addition of various types of biological measures. Two types of familial markers are of interest: linkage markers and trait markers (Buchsbaum, Coursey, & Murphy, 1976; Gershon & Matthysse, 1977; Ott, 1976).

"Linkage markers" are markers that are known to have some association with a particular gene or chromosome. At present, molecular biologists are feverishly mapping the human genome; it is estimated that it may be successfully mapped *in toto* within the next 5-10 years. Even before this complete mapping occurs, it is possible to identify traits that are located on particular genes or chromosomes and that may be linked to some type of mental illness. On the basis of an association with color blindness, for example, an X-linked dominant mode of transmission has been proposed for bipolar illness. Although the finding has not been generally supported, more complex linkage studies continue, involving a variety of antigens and other markers.

A more indirect way of examining linkage is through the use of "trait markers" that may reflect a predisposition to the development of affective illness or be associated with its presence. Using this approach, one selects a trait or a characteristic that is presumed to be genetically determined and known to be associated with affective disorder, but that is not as yet genetically mapped. One example of this type of approach is the use of the ratio of red blood cells to plasma lithium. An elevated lithium ratio has been found to have a high monozygotic-dizygotic ratio in twin studies and to be associated with bipolar illness in family studies (Dorus *et al.*, 1983; Dorus, Pandey, Frazier, & Mendels, 1974; Mendlewicz & Verbank, 1981).

DATA COLLECTION

In the 1980s it is axiomatic that techniques for interviewing and evaluation must be made as reliable and as valid as possible. In addition, since it is never possible to collect a perfect data set, it is important to consider some of the factors that may impair data collection and decrease its reliability or validity.

Family History Data

At the moment, only one instrument is available for the collection of family history data, the Family History — Research Diagnostic Criteria (FH-RDC) (Andreasen *et al.*, 1977). This instrument consists of an interview guide, criteria for making diagnoses, and standardized forms for recording information concerning first-degree relatives (and second-degree relatives, if this is desired).

Because the data that can be collected through family history are limited in nature, criteria are provided only for major diagnoses: chronic schizophrenia, remitting schizoaffective disorder, chronic schizoaffective disorder, depressive disorder, manic disorder, organic mental disorder, unspecified functional psychosis, alcoholism, drug abuse, antisocial personality, other psychiatric disorder, and no known mental disorder. Some disorders of interest, such as bipolar II disorder, are not included on the FH-RDC because of the difficulty involved in obtaining sufficient information. This instrument also permits the reporting of data concerning hospitalization, treatment, attempted and completed suicides, social incapacity, and age of onset of illness.

The criteria in the FH-RDC are streamlined, because of the recognition that informants may not have sufficient information. For example, the criteria for depressive disorder are as follows:

A through E are required.

A. Evidence of a dysphoric mood change to either:
   1. A depressive mood (e.g., sad, down in the dumps, don't care, worthless, suicidal ideation, tearful); or
   2. Some other dysphoric mood (e.g., anxious, irritable, worried), and at least two of the following *associated* symptoms: loss of interest, appetite or weight change, sleep change, loss of energy, psychomotor agitation or retardation, guilt or self-reproach, impaired concentration.
B. At least one of the following is associated with symptoms in A:
   1. Electroconvulsive therapy or known antidepressant medication.
   2. Hospitalization.
   3. Suicidal behavior.
   4. Treated for either A1 or A2.
   5. Gross impairment in work, housework, or school, or social withdrawal.
   6. Had four *associated* symptoms listed in A.
C. No evidence suggestive of chronic nonaffective deteriorating course (but may have some residual symptoms).
D. No evidence that the period lasted less than two weeks.
E. Does not meet the criteria for schizoaffective disorder for the same period of illness. (Andreasen *et al.*, 1977)

These criteria permit the interviewer to make a diagnosis of depressive disorder if an informant reports that his or her relative had a depressed mood and either some form of treatment, or impairment in functioning, or four characteristic symptoms of depression. These criteria are considerably less stringent than, for example, those of the *Diagnostic and Statistical Manual of Mental Disorders*, third edition (DSM-III), or the Research Diagnostic Criteria (RDC).

The reliability of these criteria has been explored and found to be quite good. In addition, as has been shown in Table 4-1, they have relatively high sensitivity and specificity; on the other hand, they do clearly underestimate the rates of illness in relatives. The instrument permits the interviewer to make probable diagnoses as well. For example, if an informant reports that a relative was depressed but is unable to provide any additional information, the interviewer records this information as "other psychiatric disorder — probable depression." The sensitivity of the instrument is greater when these probable diagnoses are treated as definite, suggesting that any positive information on family history is likely to be fairly accurate.

Family history data are improved if the interviewer is encouraged to make detailed notes. Ideally, if sufficient time is available, the interviewer should even write up a short case history for each positive family member, providing as much detail concerning symptoms as possible. The data can later be reviewed clinically at the time that data analysis is being conducted.

Investigators who wish to provide estimates of prevalence or morbid risk in Families should be aware that even for the family history method, it is necessary to obtain a complete listing of all relatives and their ages, since these data will be required to calculate prevalence or morbid risk. A simple listing of relatives who are ill and their relationship to the proband is not sufficient.

Family Study Data

The collection of family study data requires an instrument suitable for making lifetime diagnoses. Several instruments of this type are currently available, although many widely used instruments (such as the Present State Examination) are not suitable for collecting family study data, since they only assess the current condition. The two instruments that are most widely used are the lifetime version of the Schedule for Affective Disorders and Schizophrenia (SADS-L; Endicott & Spitzer, 1978) and the Diagnostic Interview Schedule (DIS; Helzer, Robins, Croughan, & Welner, 1981).

The DIS was developed for epidemiological field studies. It covers a relatively broad range of diagnoses and is translatable into DSM-III diagnoses. Because it was designed for epidemiological field work, it does not require that the interviewer have extensive clinical experience. This is both a strength and a weakness of the instrument. It permits more flexibility in the recruiting of interviewers. On the other hand, interviewers who have not had firsthand experience with difficult forms of psychopathology, such as those occurring in schizophrenia or mania, may find it hard to interpret symptoms that are reported in the field. The DIS has been used in the Epidemiological Catchment Area (ECA) study of the National Institute of Mental Health (NIMH). Thus it is currently providing us with good population prevalence data concerning major mental illnesses.

The SADS-L is the lifetime version of a widely used clinical instrument, the SADS. It is designed for use by interviewers who have had some clinical experience, although they need not be physicians. In many studies, the SADS interviewer is a master's-level psychologist or social worker recruited from a clinical background. The SADS-L provides data concerning a slightly narrower range of disorders than the DIS. It is loosely translatable into DSM-III diagnoses, but not directly.

Whatever the instrument used, the collection of lifetime prevalence data has certain inherent problems that must be recognized by anyone who either collects them or tries to interpret them. When attempting to determine whether relatives have had a past episode of illness, the interviewer is often asking them to recall things that happened many years ago. The relatives must not only remember whether they were depressed, but also whether they had a wide constellation of symptoms, whether they were treated (and with what), when the symptoms began, how long they lasted, and so on. Again, recognizing that there are some constraints on memory, most diagnostic systems for estimating lifetime prevalence somewhat fewer criteria than would be necessary to make a diagnosis in a person who is currently ill.

In order to explore the extent to which relatives can recall past episodes of illness, we have done extensive reliability studies in the NIMH Collaborative Program on the Psychobiology of Depression (Andreasen *et al.*, 1981; Grove, Andreasen, McDonald-Scott, Keller, & Shapiro, 1981). These studies are ongoing, but some data have already been analyzed and reported.

In one study (Andreasen *et al.*, 1981), for example, we asked each of the five participating centers (Boston, Chicago, Iowa City, New York, and St. Louis) to send a single rater to two different "host" centers (Iowa City and Boston) to participate in two 1-week test-retest reliability studies. The raters participating in this study were senior experienced raters who had done a large number of SADS-L interviews. Each of the host centers was responsible for identifying 25 subjects from a pool of relatives and control subjects who were previously interviewed for the study. Each of these 25 subjects had been evaluated with the SADS-L by a rater in the host center 6 months previously. Subjects were selected to cover a wide spectrum of diagnoses, ranging from no mental illness to the more severe diagnoses such as bipolar disorder. Interviewers participating in the reliability study were kept blind as to the types of diagnoses involved.

The five raters representing the five participating centers traveled to Iowa City for 1 week and then to Boston 1 month later for 1 week to participate in the test-retest reliability study. Each subject was interviewed twice, once in the morning and once in the afternoon. Interviewer pairing was systematically rotated, with all possible rater pairs occurring at least four times. At the end of each day, the raters met with one another and reviewed their ratings and diagnoses. Sources of disagreement, such as variation in information provided by the subject on the two occasions, were noted. After reviewing their combined data, the raters completed a consensus SADS-L and RDC.

Thus four data sets were available for each subject: the original SADS-L and RDC completed by an Iowa City or Boston interviewer 6 months earlier; SADS-L and RDC completed in the morning by Rater 1; SADS-L and RDC completed in the afternoon by Rater 2; and a consensus SADS-L and RDC completed by both raters after conferring together.

Data concerning diagnostic reliability from this study appear in Table 4-2. The data concerning base rates are reported in addition to the intraclass *R*, since a low base rate provides a constraint on the estimate of reliability. With the exception of the diagnosis of incapacitating depression, the agreement between morning and afternoon evaluations was very high. On the other hand, when the initial diagnosis made 6 months earlier was compared with the consensus diagnosis agreed upon by the two reliability raters, the intraclass *R* for some diagnoses dropped markedly. This was particularly noticeable for bipolar II disorder. In this instance, the relatives were being asked to recall whether or not they had had mild hypomanic symptoms at any time in their

TABLE 4-2 SADS-L Test-Retest Study: Diagnostic Reliability ($n = 50$)

SADS-L/RDC lifetime diagnoses	Base rate (%)	Intraclass *R* Morning vs. afternoon	Initial vs. consensus
Bipolar I	10	1.00	.88
Bipolar II	6	.62	.06
Major depressive disorder	44	.87	.75
Primary	33	.70	.59
Secondary	6	.60	.51
Recurrent	15	.78	.21
Psychotic	9	.79	.24
Incapacitating	9	.19	.40
Alcoholism	25	.94	.72
Never mentally ill	33	.70	.63

lives. Clearly, some relatives reported this initially and failed to report it later on, or vice versa. In the case of mild disorders, it was often difficult to distinguish between normal variation and the presence of a disorder. Other diagnoses that showed some difficulty when initial versus consensus ratings were compared included recurrent major depressive disorder, psychotic major depressive disorder, and incapacitating major depressive disorder. Lowered reliability may have been due to a different problem in each instance. In the case of recurrent disorders, the relatives were being asked to remember the number of episodes, which may have been difficult to estimate. In the case of psychotic disorders, the relatives were being asked to recall the presence of psychotic symptoms when they may have been psychotic and therefore subject to confusion and perhaps disorientation. In the case of incapacitating disorders, there were problems with definition and determining an appropriate cutoff.

Diagnoses are based on the evaluation of symptoms, and therefore it is also useful to know whether symptoms can be recalled and rated reliably. Data from the same study concerning depressive symptoms appear in Table 4-3. With the exception of agitation-retardation, all the symptom items had excellent test-retest reliability in the morning versus afternoon situation. The raters attributed 80% of the disagreements on agitation-retardation to being given different information in the morning and in the afternoon. Reliability was also quite high in the initial versus consensus situation, although these values tended to be slightly lower, as would be expected. Only the variable of tiredness decreased to an unacceptable level of reliability: Interviewers found it difficult to achieve high levels of agreement when estimating the number of episodes that had occurred in the past. There was surprisingly good agreement in dating age of onset, with somewhat more difficulty in dating age at last

TABLE 4-3 SADS-L Depressive Syndrome Items

Item	Base rate[a] (%)	Intraclass R: Morning vs. afternoon	Intraclass R: Initial vs. consensus
Depressed mood	54	.71	.59
Impaired functioning	50	.80	.67
Appetite or weight change	44	.77	.79
Sleep disturbance	38	.70	.53
Tiredness	25	.72	.44
Loss of interest	33	.92	.60
Guilt	29	.71	.60
Trouble concentrating	31	.85	.50
Thoughts of death or suicide, suicide attempt	17	.80	.65
Agitation-retardation	19	.42	.38
Number of symptoms	—	.92	.74
Number of episodes of depressive syndrome	—	1.00	−.01
Number of episodes of major depressive disorder	—	.18	−.01
Age at onset	—	1.00	.64
Age at last episode	—	.30	.96
Hospitalized	10	.88	.78
Received medication	25	.95	.56
Preceded or followed by mania, hypomania	8	.88	.64
Incapacitated	8	.19	.19
Suicidal gesture	6	.91	.56
Associated with pregnancy	10	.73	.49

[a] Base rate is given if the rating was dichotomous.

episode. Information concerning treatment received was also collected with high levels of reliability.

This study used an extremely stringent design to explore the reliability of lifetime diagnoses in a nonpatient population. Test-retest reliability was evaluated using both short and long intervals. Raters from five different centers conducted the interviews, and subjects examined were drawn from two different centers. In spite of the stringent design, good to excellent reliability was found for rating symptoms and for making diagnoses. As a consequence, one can conclude that, when raters are carefully trained, lifetime diagnoses can be made reliably in nonpatient populations. Furthermore, relatives appear to recall past episodes well and to report them consistently. Thus, we can confront family study data with considerable confidence, in spite of a concern about difficulties in recalling episodes that have occurred in the past. The disclaimer must be added, of course, that the high degree of confidence pertains to relatively more severe disorders, such as major depressive disorder, and that reliability diminishes for milder disorders.

Techniques for Facilitating Analysis of Family Data

Investigators experienced in collecting family data have observed that several additional techniques are useful. Since most structured interviews yield only checked columns and keypunch forms, they typically do not reflect the richness of information that has actually been collected. Consequently, many studies now add a case narrative to supplement the computerized data. While these narratives cannot, of course, be used for computerized data analysis, they are frequently helpful as an aid in decisions about how to handle difficult cases. In addition, they are useful for training new raters, and they also serve as a check on quality control.

A second technique that has been found helpful is to summarize all the data concerning a single family on a "consensus pedigree." An example of such a pedigree appears in Figure 4-2. The consensus pedigree integrates family history and family study data. It requires that a relatively experienced clinician review all available materials, including the family history and family study data, and make a decision as to the most appropriate diagnosis or diagnoses for each relative. The usual rule is to place greater emphasis on data

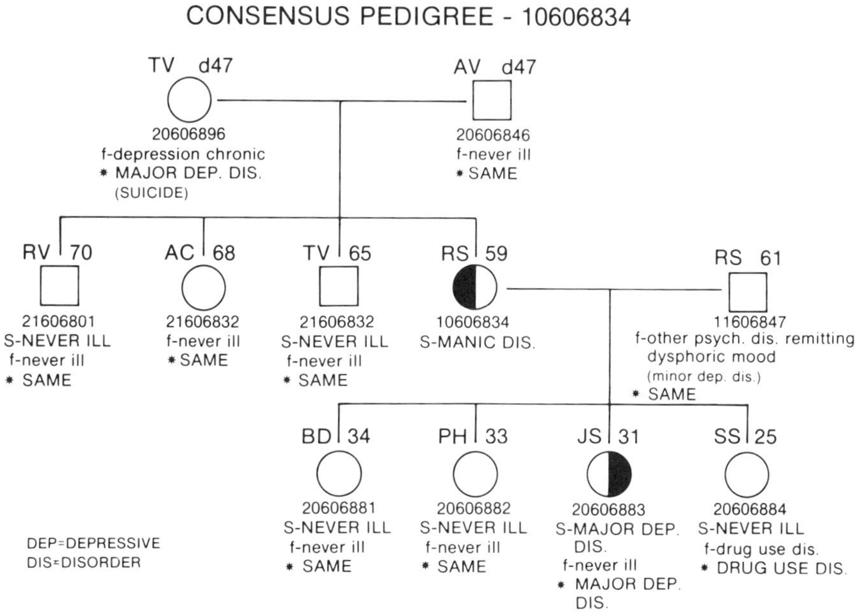

CONSENSUS PEDIGREE - 10606834

TV d47
20606896
f-depression chronic
* MAJOR DEP. DIS.
(SUICIDE)

AV d47
20606846
f-never ill
* SAME

RV 70
21606801
S-NEVER ILL
f-never ill
* SAME

AC 68
21606832
f-never ill
* SAME

TV 65
21606832
S-NEVER ILL
f-never ill
* SAME

RS 59
10606834
S-MANIC DIS.

RS 61
11606847
f-other psych. dis. remitting, dysphoric mood
(minor dep. dis.)
* SAME

BD 34
20606881
S-NEVER ILL
f-never ill
* SAME

PH 33
20606882
S-NEVER ILL
f-never ill
* SAME

JS 31
20606883
S-MAJOR DEP. DIS.
f-never ill
* MAJOR DEP. DIS.

SS 25
20606884
S-NEVER ILL
f-drug use dis.
* DRUG USE DIS.

DEP=DEPRESSIVE
DIS=DISORDER

FIGURE 4-2 Example of consensus pedigree.

collected by direct interview, but also to emphasize the most positive informative available, particularly in the case of some diagnoses (e.g., alcoholism or mania) where the interviewed informant may be prone to denial. Clearly, case narratives are useful to the person who must construct a consensus pedigree. Ideally, such pedigrees should also include information concerning age and age of onset. In many family studies, data analysis will proceed from the consensus pedigree rather than from family history or family study interviews, since the pedigree provides the most complete summary of information available.

ANALYSIS OF FAMILIAL DATA

Once familial data have been collected, they may be analyzed and presented in a variety of different ways, ranging from relatively simple to highly complex and technical. The selection of an appropriate technique will depend upon the question to be answered. In addition, the audience being addressed and the resources available to the investigator may be rate-limiting factors, since application of more technical genetic models requires special expertise.

Prevalence and Morbid Risk

The simplest way to analyze family data is to compare prevalence rates in two groups of interest, in order to determine whether one of the groups has higher familial rates of depression. For example, one might compare lifetime prevalence of affective diagnoses in the relatives of probands and the relatives of medical controls in order to show that depression runs more strongly in the families of the affected probands. Alternatively, one might compare two subtypes of affective disorder, such as bipolar versus unipolar or endogenous versus nonendogenous, to establish that one is more strongly familial than the other.

Many investigators prefer to report their data in terms of "morbid risk" rather than using simple prevalence figures, though. Relatives usually have a wide age range, and many of the younger relatives, particularly the children of probands, will be at risk of developing depression and may do so eventually; however, because of their young age they will not have developed the syndrome as yet, and therefore simple prevalence figures will provide an underestimate of the actual rate of illness in relatives. Consequently, familial data are frequently reported in terms of morbid risk, which includes an age-correction factor in order to provide a better estimate of rates in those relatives who have not yet passed through the age of risk. Several different techniques for calculating morbid risk are available, but they have in common the requirement that the investigator must have information about the usual age of onset of a particular disorder in order to calculate the age corrections. The data concerning age of onset can be drawn either from research literature, or they can be calculated using the known age of onset in the actual sample being studied. Age-of-onset figures for depression are available in the literature, although there is some suggestion that there may be an important cohort effect occurring, at least in the American population: The "baby boom" children are showing a much higher rate of depression than previous generations. If an investigator is interested in calculating morbid risk for diagnoses that have been less well studied and for nonaffective diagnoses, he or she may have some difficulty in finding literature norms. For example, good norms are not yet available for such diagnoses as substance abuse, cyclothmia, bipolar II, or antisocial personality. If the base rate in his or her own sample is sufficiently high, the investigator can develop age-of-onset data from this sample. In some instances, he or she may simply impute rational values. For example, by definition, the age of onset for antisocial personality is some time prior to age 20.

Table 4-4 shows some familial data presented in terms of morbid risk (Coryell *et al.*, 1983). These are data comparing rates of bipolar I, bipolar II, and unipolar affective disorder in the relatives of bipolar I, bipolar II, and unipolar probands, "BZ" in the third column stands for *Bezeugziffer*, meaning a number slightly smaller than the number of relatives actually interviewed. As this table indicates, the use of a morbid-risk calculation reduces the number of relatives estimated to be at risk, and therefore usually yields somewhat higher estimates of rates in relatives. This table also illustrates how familial data may be used to validate nosological categories. In this sample, the risk for bipolar I disorder was highest in the relatives of probands with bipolar I; that for bipolar II disorder was highest in the relatives of probands with bipolar II; and that for unipolar depression was highest in the relatives of unipolar probands.

Treating the Family as a Unit

Prevalence and morbid risk pool data from many probands and many relatives. Thereby they provide a rough index as to whether familial rates are

TABLE 4-4 Morbid Risks for Bipolar I, Bipolar II, and Unipolar Primary Major Depression among Interviewed Relatives

Proband diagnosis	Number of interviewed relatives	BZ	Number of relatives with lifetime diagnosis (morbid risk)		
			Bipolar I	Bipolar II	Unipolar
Bipolar I ($n = 82$)	328	278	8 (2.9)	7 (2.5)	63 (22.7)
Bipolar II ($n = 33$)	134	112	1 (0.9)	11 (9.8)	24 (21.4)
Unipolar ($n = 212$)	748	572	1 (0.2)	15 (2.6)	168 (29.4)

somewhat higher in some diagnoses than in others or than in a selected control group. Once one has established that a disorder is familial, however, one also wishes to know how *strongly* familial it is. Morbid-risk rates in a particular diagnostic group could be significantly increased because of the contribution of a subset of heavily loaded families, while some probands might come from families with a minimal number of family members affected or none at all. Thus pooling familial data may be misleading and may waste useful information. Consequently, investigators sometimes use a variety of other indices that indicate the degree to which a disorder is familial.

One approach is simply to determine how many probands come from families that are positive for a given disorder. An example of an analysis of this type, based on the same data set as that examined in Table 4-4, is shown in Table 4-5. This table divides the probands into bipolar I, bipolar II, and unipolar. It has then been determined how many in each diagnostic group came from families that were positive for that particular diagnostic group. As the table indicates, a familial background for bipolar I disorder tended to occur most strongly in bipolar I probands (8.5%), while families positive for bipolar II disorder were those associated with bipolar II probands (30.3%). On the other hand, a family history of unipolar disorder was relatively evenly spread throughout the three groups. These results suggest that, to some extent, bipolar disorders tend to sort differentially within families, and even that there may be some distinction between familial sorting of bipolar I and bipolar II disorder.

An alternate relatively simple way to determine the degree to which disorders sort within families is to calculate relative risk. The "relative risk" of having a positive family history for a specific disorder (i.e., of having at least one family member with the disorder) is the ratio of the proportion of positive families for probands with a particular disorder to the proportion of positive families for probands with all other disorders.

An example of this type of analysis is shown in Table 4-6 (Endicott *et al.*, 1983). The purpose of this analysis was to determine the extent to which psychoticism and bipolarity run in families. The sample for this study con-

TABLE 4-5 Numbers of Probands with Primary Major Depression with at Least One Interviewed Relative with Primary Major Depression

Proband diagnosis	*n*	Family history positive for: Bipolar I	Bipolar II	Unipolar
Bipolar I	82	7 (8.5)	5 (6.1)	50 (61.0)
Bipolar II	33	1 (3.0)	10 (30.3)	21 (63.6)
Unipolar	212	4 (1.9)	14 (6.6)	125 (59.0)

TABLE 4-6 Relative Risk for Hospitalized Subjects with a Major Depressive Syndrome of Having a Positive Family History for Selected Conditions

Family positive for:	Manic, hypomanic, schizoaffective manic (n = 103)[a]	Index episode psychotic major depressed (n = 40)[a]	Index episode schizoaffective depressed (n = 23)[a]	Ever delusions or hallucinations (n = 86)[a]
Major affective disorder (n = 188)[b]	1.00	1.08	0.96	0.97
Psychotic major depressive disorder (n = 11)[b]	0.71	3.69*	1.20	1.41
Manic, hypomanic, schizoaffective manic (n = 61)[b]	1.96*	1.26	1.07	1.03
Schizoaffective disorder (any type) (n = 6)[b]	1.89	3.23	2.39	2.47
Schizoaffective disorder, manic (n = 4)[b]	5.68	2.15	0.00	0.82
Schizophrenia (n = 6)[b]	1.89	0.00	5.98*	2.47
Unspecified psychosis (n = 2)[b]	∞	0.00	11.96*	∞
Ever delusions/ hallucinations (n = 23)[b]	1.46	2.82*	2.52	2.26*

[a] Number of probands with given disorder.
[b] Number of families positive for given disorder.
* $p < .05$ by Fisher's exact probability test.

sisted of probands who had evidence of bipolarity (manic, hypomanic, schizoaffective manic disorders), probands with psychotic major depressive disorder, and probands with schizoaffective depression. It was then determined how many had positive family histories of relevant disorders, such as major affective disorder, psychotic major depressive disorder, bipolar syndrome, schizophrenia, and unspecified psychosis. In addition, it was determined how many probands had ever had delusions or hallucinations and how many came from families in which these symptoms had occurred. Reading down the columns, one can observe that the relative risk for bipolarity was nearly doubled in the families of bipolar probands. The relative risk for schizoaffective mania was also increased. On the other hand, among the probands with psychotic major depression, the relative risk for psychotic major depression was quite high, as was the risk for schizoaffective disorder and for delusions and hallucinations. Probands with schizoaffective depression tended to come from families positive for schizophrenia or unspecified psychosis, and, finally, there was some suggestion that delusions and hallucinations even tended to sort within families. Thus, techniques such as these can give a preliminary indication of the extent to which disorders may be transmitted.

Segregation Analysis and Mathematical Models

If analyses of the type described above suggest a familial basis for disorders, as they have in most studies of affective disorder, then more complex and costly statistical analyses are justified. "Segregation analysis" involves looking at each family as a unit and determining the actual numbers of unaffected and affected members separately by relationship (e.g., parent, sibling, child) for each family. Correlation coefficients between the various types of relatives can be calculated.

Segregation analysis is often used to explore both purely genetic issues and nosological issues. Once segregation data are obtained and analyses are done, one can then try to determine the extent to which the data fit different types of genetic models. Some of these models assume simple Mendelian patterns of inheritance, such as the "single major locus" model, while some models are polygenic. In addition, there is a multifactorial model that assumes an interaction between environmental and purely genetic factors (Gershon, Baron, & Leckman, 1975; Reich, Cloninger, & Guze, 1975).

Recent refinements of these models have been used to examine nosological issues. For example, multiple-threshold models have been developed (Reich, James & Morris, 1972). These models can be used to determine whether, for example, unipolar and bipolar depressive disorders are mild and severe forms of the same inherited disorder. Threshold models assume that there is an underlying greater vulnerability, or liability to develop the disorder, which has a normal distribution. The point on this distribution beyond which people manifest the illness is called the "threshold."

One variant of this model that has been used frequently in recent nosological research is called the "two-threshold model." An illustration of this model appears in Figure 4-3. Mild illnesses, such as unipolar depression, are defined as having a wider (lower) threshold than more severe illnesses, such as bipolar disorder. Statistical techniques are available to determine the goodness of fit of a particular data set to this model. If the model fits well, then one can conclude that bipolar disorder and unipolar disorder are genetically homogeneous. Alternative, if the model does not fit well, they can be considered as possibly heterogeneous. As yet, this issue has not been resolved with the data sets currently available (Baron, Klotz, Mendlewicz, & Rainer, 1981; Gershon, Bunney, Leckman, Van Eeerdewegh, & De Bauche, 1976).

SUMMARY

There is no single "best" technique for studying the genetic aspects of affective disorder. Many designs are available, such as family history and family

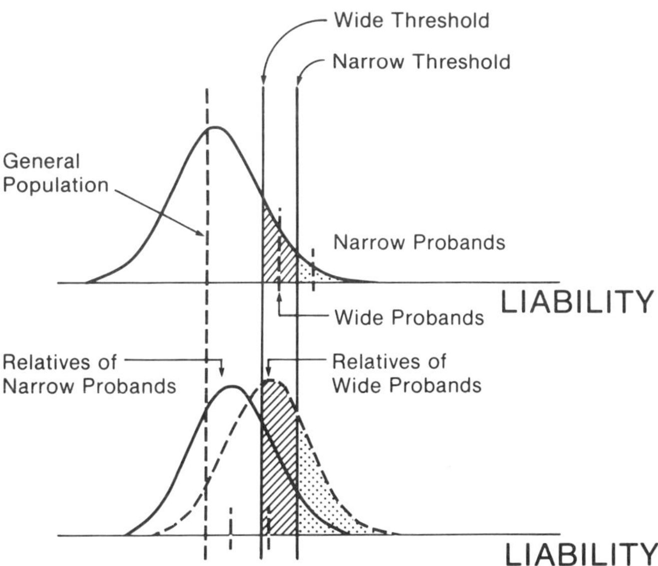

FIGURE 4-3 Example of a two-threshold model.

studies, twin studies, adoption studies, and extended-pedigree studies. Each of these designs illuminates a different aspect of the genetic issue. Each design involves a tradeoff in terms of the type of information obtained versus cost and efficiency. The same generalizations apply to techniques for analyzing familial data, which range from simple to highly complex. In spite of these caveats, however, some future directions seem clearly promising. For example, studies of high-density (multiplex) families and large multigenerational pedigrees are particularly powerful, especially when combined with the study of linkage markers and other biological markers.

Acknowledgment

The research reported in this chapter was supported in part by NIMH Grant No. MH31593.

References

Andreasen, N. C., Endicott, J., Spitzer, R. L., & Winokur, G. (1977). The family history method using diagnostic criteria: Reliability and validity. *Archives of General Psychiatry, 34*, 1229-1235.

Andreasen, N. C., Grove, W. M., Shapiro, R. W., Keller M. B., Hirschfeld, R. M. A., & McDonald-Scott, P. (1981). Reliability of lifetime diagnosis: A multicenter collaborative perspective. *Archives of General Psychiatry, 38*, 400-405.

Ashby, H. B., & Crowe, R. R. (1978). Unipolar depression: A family study of a large kindred. *Comprehensive Psychiatry, 19*, 415-417.

Baron, M., Klotz, J., Mendlewicz, J., & Rainer J. (1981). Multiple-threshold transmission of affective disorders. *Archives of General Psychiatry, 38*, 79-84.

Buchsbaum, M. S., Coursey, R. D., & Murphy, D. L. (1976). The biochemical high-risk paradigm: Behavioral and familial correlates of low platelet monamine oxidase activity. *Science, 194*, 339-341.

Coryell, W., Klerman, G., Hirschfeld, R. M. A., Keller, M. B., Fawcett, J., Endicott, N. C., Andreasen, N. C., & Reich, T. (1983). a family study of bipolar II disorder. *British Journal of Psychiatry, 145*, 495-498.

Dorus, E., Cox, N. J., Gibbons, R. D., Shaughnessy, R., Pandey, G. N., & Cloninger, C. R. (1983). Lithium ion transport and affective disorders within familiar of bipolar patients. *Archives of General Psychiatry, 40*, 545-556.

Dorus, E., Pandey, G. N., Frazier, A., & Mendels, J. (1974). Genetic determinants of lithium ion distribution: I. An *in vitro* monozygotic-dizygotic twin study. *Archives of General Psychiatry, 31*, 463-465.

Endicott, J., Nee, J., Coryell, W., Keller, M. B., Andreasen, N. C., & Croughan, J. (1983). *Major depressive syndrome with psychotic features: Evidence of differential familial association.* Unpublished manuscript.

Endicott, J., & Spitzer, R. L. (1978). A diagnostic interview: The Schedule for Affective Disorders and Schizophrenia. *Archives of General Psychiatry, 35*, 837-844.

Gershon, E. S., Baron, M., & Leckman, J. F. (1975). Genetic models of the transmission of affective disorders. *Journal of Psychiatric Research, 12*, 301-317.

Gershon, E. S., Bunney, W. E., Leckman, J. F., Van Eerdewegh, M., & DeBauche, B. A. (1976). The inheritance of affective disorders: A review of data and of hypotheses. *Behavior Genetics, 6*, 227-261.

Gershon, E. S., & Matthysse, S. (1977). X-linkage: Ascertainment through doubly ill probands. *Journal of Psychiatric Research, 13*, 161-168.

Grove, W. M., Andreasen, N. C., McDonald-Scott, P., Keller, M. B., & Shapiro, R. W. (1981). Reliability studies of psychiatric diagnosis: Theory and practice. *Archives of General Psychiatry, 38*, 408-413.

Helzer, J. E., Robins, L. N., Croughan, J. L., & Welner, A. (1981). Renard Diagnostic Interview: Its reliability and procedural validity with physicians and lay interviewers. *Archives of General Psychiatry, 38*, 393-398.

Heston, L. L. (1970). The genetics of schizophrenia and schizoid disease. *Science, 167*, 249-256.

Hrubec, Z., & Allen, G. (1975). Methods and interpretation of twin concordance data. *American Journal of Human Genetics, 27*, 808-809.

Mendlewicz, J., & Rainer, J. D. (1977). Adoption studies in manic-depressive illness. *Nature, 268*, 327-329.

Mendlewicz, J., & Verbank, P. (1981). Cell membrane anomaly as a genetic marker for manic-depressive illness. *American Journal of Psychiatry, 138*, 119.

Ott, J. (1976). A computer program for linkage analysis of general human pedigrees. *American Journal of Human Genetics, 28*, 528-529.

Reich, T., Cloninger, C. R., & Guze, S. B. (1975). The multifactorial model of disease transmission: I. Description of the model and its use in psychiatry. *British Journal of Psychiatry, 127*, 1-10.

Reich, T., James, J. W., & Morris, C. A. (1972). The use of multiple thresholds in determining the mode of transmission of semicontinuous traits. *Annals of Human Genetics, 36*, 163-184.

Rosenthal, D., & Kety, S. S. (Eds.). (1968). *The transmission of schizophrenia*. Oxford: Pergamon Press.

Smith, C. (1974). Concordance in twins: Methods and interpretation. *American Journal of Human Genetics, 26*, 454-466.

Winokur, G., Clayton, P. J., & Reich, T. (1969). *Manic-depressive illness*. St. Louis: C. V. Mosby.

CHAPTER 5

The Measurement of Neurotransmitters in Depression

STEPHEN H. KOSLOW
PAUL A. GAIST
National Institute of Mental Health

INTRODUCTION

Until the 1950s, the most common treatments for depression were psychotherapy and electroshock regimens. Pharmacologically, the treatment of depression was limited to stimulant drugs (i.e., amphetamines for hypoactivity and psychomotor retardation) or sedative drugs (i.e., barbiturates for agitation). During the 1950s several astute observations were made regarding the clinical effects of certain drugs being tested or used for medical conditions other than depression. These observations, supported by insights into the neurochemical effects of these drugs, provided the rational framework for research aimed at bridging the gap between the behavioral profile of depression and its underlying biochemical etiology.

Reserpinc, an alkaloid isolated from the *Rauwolfia serpentina* plant of India, was shown to produce in animals depression-like symptoms such as sedation and psychomotor retardation. Some patients receiving reserpine as a treatment for hypertension were also found to develop a depression-like syndrome. Specifically, 15% of a group of patients receiving reserpine as a treatment for hypertension experienced a mood alteration similar to that seen in patients with primary depressive disorder (Jensen, 1959). It was further noted that most patients who experienced an episode of depression while taking resperine had a prior history of depression not caused by the use of this drug (Ayd, 1958). In animal research, reserpine was found to impair the storage of serotonin (5-HT), dopamine (DA), and norepinephrine (NE) in nerve terminals, leading to the depletion of these central nervous system (CNS) neurotransmitters via the degradation of the neurotransmitters to inactive metabolites by the mitochondrial enzyme monoamine oxidase (MAO). This depletion, coupled with the clinical observations of the reserpine, suggested a possible connection between the amine systems and the behavioral effects.

Significant clinical observations were also made concerning iproniazid (Marsilid), a drug synthesized originally for the treatment of tuberculosis in the early 1950s. Iproniazid is a potent MAO inhibitor; therefore, its administration results in increased brain concentrations of the monoamine neurotransmitters NE and 5-HT. Clinically, iproniazid was shown to produce euphoric and hyperactive behavior in some patients. Reasoning that such properties would be valuable in the treatment of depression, Crane introduced iproniazid into psychiatry (Baldessarini, 1975). Shortly after its introduction, other investigations reported successful results when iproniazid was administered to depressed subjects (Berger & Barchas, 1977).

Based upon such observations, both Joseph J. Schildkraut, in the *American Journal of Psychiatry*, and William E. Bunney, with John M. Davis, in the *Archives of General Psychiatry*, formally postulated the "catecholamine hypothesis of affective disorders" in 1965. This milestone hypothesis, which addressed the possible link between the affective disorders and changes in CNS neurotransmitters (specifically the catecholamines), has been the guiding impetus for depression research for the last two decades. As originally stated in Schildkraut's paper, the hypothesis proposed that "some, if not all depressions are associated with an absolute or relative deficiency of catecholamines, particularly norepinephrine, at functionally important adrenergic sites in the brain" (1965, p. 509). Elation was conversely associated with an excess of the amines. Bunney and Davis, as well as several other researchers of the time, implicated 5-HT as well as the catecholamines in this hypothesis, since the available evidence could be equally applied to the serotonergic systems (Ashcroft *et al.*, 1966; Coppen, Shaw, Herzberg, & Maggs, 1967).

In addition to stating the hypothesis, both papers made the important observation that the ability to measure such an absolute or relative catecholamine deficiency (necessary for the direct testing of the hypothesis) would elude researchers of the day, due to the limitations of the experimental methodology available at that time. In citing the heuristic value of the hypothesis and the methodological limitations of the time, they set the stage for what has been one of the most intensive and extensive research endeavors of modern psychiatry. And, as was underscored by the original catecholamine theorists, progress toward an understanding of the pathogenesis of depression has been associated in large part with the development over the last 20 years of new methodologies by which to measure and test the implicated components of neurotransmission in the brain.

This chapter is devoted to outlining the major areas of research that have attempted to identify the biological components associated with affective disorders, emphasizing the role that the development of newer, more sensitive research methodology has played in these areas.

MEASUREMENT

Concurrent with the clinical observations of the effects of reserpine and iproniazid on behavior, basic researchers were beginning to unravel the mechanisms (neurotransmission) and the substances (neurotransmitters) that allow nerve cells to communicate with each other. Early studies used bioassays to identify and quantify neurotransmitters in whole brains. These early bioassay techniques were crude from the point of view of specificity (e.g., using the clam muscle for measuring 5-HT), but were exquisitely sensitive. Two technological advances — the use of fluorometric spectroscopy and the histofluorescence morphological technique — greatly facilitated research in the area of neurotransmission. The spectrometric technique, while not as sensitive as the bioassay technique, was more specific, since it was based on measuring the photofluor emitted by compounds at specific wave lengths of excitation and emission, thus allowing for the quantitation of neurotransmitters in gross brain regions. The histofluorescence procedure allowed for the visualization of the neurotransmitter in nerve cells and ultimately in terminal regions. These two approaches yielded quantitative data on the amounts of neurotransmitters contained in specific brain regions, as well as qualitative data on the anatomical distribution of the different neurotransmitter systems.

While the spectrometric and histofluorescence procedures produced important information about the chemical nature of the purported neurotransmitters DA, NE, and 5-HT, and provided the means to study the biosynthesis, storage, and metabolism of these important neurotransmitter systems, subsequent technological advances have resulted in analytic techniques with greatly increased sensitivity and specificity. Techniques such as gas chromatography-mass spectrometry (GC-MS), radioimmunoassay (RIA), radioreceptor assay (RRA), and high-pressure liquid chromatography (HPLC) coupled with specific chemical electrodes have provided researchers with previously unmatched investigative tools with which to study of field of neurotransmission, and, more specifically, the possible role of neurotransmitters in depression.

Combining the techniques of gas chromatography (GC) and mass spectrometry (MS) into one methodological approach — namely, GC-MS — has enabled researchers to reach previously unimaginable degrees of sensitivity, specificity, and flexibility in experimental design. GC separates the individual components from a mixture of compounds in a solution. MS allows for qualitative identification of the molecular structures of the separated compounds, and, by recording the ion density of specific fragments, the accurate measurement of even microquantities of the components contained alone or in a mixture in a solution. The limitation of this method is that the substance of interest must be volatile and stable at the elevated temperatures used in the GC process. Furthermore, the GC-MS procedure is technically complex and requires a high degree of expertise, as well as a high initial financial outlay for the instrumentation (though the cost of running the subsequent assays is small).

The RIA technique is an appealing method for the quantification of substances in biological fluids. RIA is based on the principle of competitive binding; that is, the amount of a radioactive substance specifically attached to a binding site is a function of the amount of unlabeled (endogenous) substance present. RIA is highly sensitive, allowing the quantification of substances in extremely small amounts (subnanograms to nanograms). Furthermore, RIA has good specificity, is relatively simple, and is versatile. RIA requires only routinely available laboratory equipment, and, once the assay is developed, it can be performed with relatively little expertise. Many samples can be processed quickly, and the costs of operation are comparatively low.

Major drawbacks to RIA are the considerable time and effort involved in developing a functioning system and validating its accuracy and specificity. In order to develop an RIA, it is necessary (1) to produce specific antiserum against the substance to be measured, making sure it has high affinity and specificity for that substance: (2) to have radioactively labeled antigen to compete with the unlabeled antigen for antibody binding sites; (3) to have a method to separate bound from free labeled antigen; and (4) to have unlabeled antigen for use as standards against which to measure the unknown concentrations. Another disadvantage of RIA, which should always be taken into consideration, is that almost inevitably there is a certain degree of nonspecific binding, as well as cross-reactivity with structurally related compounds. This necessitates a verification of the RIA procedure as to its specificity prior to its application.

The progress of cellular-level receptor research has been possible in large part because of the development of the RRA technique. This technique, like RIA, is based on the principle of competitive binding, and depends on the availability of radiolabeled compounds with highly specific activity. These compounds enable investigators to label and quantitatively assay receptor/recognition sites. Unlike RIA, RRA does not require specific antibodies to be developed and purified for the compound of interest. Instead, relatively specific brain membranes and high-specific-activity radioactive ligands are used to estimate unknown concentrations of the unlabeled ligand. A major concern in the use of this procedure is that it is an indirect assay and, as such, the specificity must be critically evaluated. Also to be remembered is the fact that radioligand binding can be easily influenced by unknown interfering substances.

Added to these powerful procedures is the newer HPLC technique. This technique has the resolving power to precisely separate substances with very similar chemical structures. HPLC utilizes a stationary phase (the column-packing particles) and a mobile phase (the elution solvent.) It is the unique interaction of the sample substance with these two phases that allows for the precise separation and distinction of molecules with very similar chemical structures. Another key element of the HPLC process is the continuous monitoring of the column effluent, which is the responsibility of the part of the HPLC instrumentation known as the detector. Detectors are of various types, and while they each have their respective range of sensitivity and mode of operation, their common qualities include (1) high sensitivity (2) predictable specificity for the compound of interest (3) a linear response to increasing amounts of the compound, and (4) an absence of response to the mobile phase. As compared to conventional column chromatography, HPLC is fast, versatile, and simple to operate. It has a sensitivity in the picomole-nanomole region, and gives excellent resolution. It can perform both qualitative and quantitative analyses, with the added advantage that the sample is not destroyed and fractions can be collected. Unlike GC, HPLC can be used to separate high-molecular-weight compounds and those that are unstable, polar, or nonvolatile, so long as the solute is soluble in the mobile solvent.

The development of these laboratory techniques has given the researcher ultrasensitive tools for studies in areas such as chemistry, biochemistry, biochemical pharmacology, neurobiology, and neurophysiology, all areas relevant to the study of the biological etiology of the affective disorders. With these techniques, analogous to the advent of the electron microscope, the presence, amounts, and distinctive qualities of substances and cellular components that were previously undetectable and unmeasurable have become accessible for study and scrutiny. These techniques and others like them have thrust the study of affective disorders into the new frontiers of receptor research, advanced neurotransmitter research, and cotransmitter (as well as neuromodulator) research. With these increasingly sophisticated techniques, and the resulting accumulation of information from these new research areas, there is a growing appreciation of the complexity of measurement.

NEUROTRANSMITTER AND METABOLITE LEVELS IN BIOLOGICAL FLUIDS

At the beginning of the 1970s, substantial knowledge of CNS neurotransmitter function had been accumulated, based on evidence gathered on the three important CNS neurotransmitters, NE, DA, and 5-HT. There was a basic understanding of their biosynthesis, storage, metabolism, and anatomical distribution in the CNS. The biogenic amine hypothesis, as cited earlier, proposed that a major biochemical abnormality in depression was that of insufficient levels of biogenic amines. Effective antidepressant pharmacological agents had been developed and were available for use in depression research. Armed with this increasing knowledge about the phenomemon of neurotransmission, the development of increasingly effective measurement techniques, a formal hypothesis to test, and the means with which to test it, the bioresearch of the affective disorders was well under way.

Prior to the introduction of the current brain-imaging techniques, the human brain did not lend itself to direct study. Researchers were therefore obligated to restrict themselves to the sampling of human fluids and tissues that could be obtained without undue harm to the subject. These procedures included the sampling of lumbar cerebrospinal fluid (CSF) and blood, and 24-hour urine collections. With these methods, samples could be collected from healthy subjects, patients with depression, and those who had been treated for depression with pharmacological agents. But even with these approaches, the analytical methods were for the most part not sensitive enough to measure the transmitters themselves, but were limited to the ability to measure some of their metabolites. In CSF, measurement was particularly difficult. The concentration of the metabolites was increased in many studies by blocking their transport out of CSF with a chemical agent, probenecid; however, the effects of probenecid itself may have confounded the measurement results obtained. Specifically, when one is using the probenecid technique, the proportion of transport block is uncertain; the ability to obtain a uniform level of transport block is uncertain: and the levels required for a total block of active transport are toxic in humans. Moreover, the probenecid agent is unsuitable for the metabolism of some neurotransmitters; the agent itself increases CSF and plasma NE; and it increases plasma free tryptophan. Obviously, then, using a CSF blocking agent to study brain function has many pitfalls, and results that have been derived from the use of such techniques must be interpreted with caution.

Research on CSF monoamine metabolite concentrations in depressed patients has emphasized the assessment of 3-methoxy-4-hydroxyphenylglycol (MHPG), 5-hydroxyindoleacetic acid (5-HIAA), and homovanillic acid (HVA), the principal metabolites of central NE, 5-HT, and DA, respectively. The data, however, do not provide consistent evidence regarding the direction of fluctuations in any of these metabolites, even when we consider only those studies that did not utilize the probenecid technique to obtain their results. Of nine such investigations of CSF MHPG concentrations in depressed patients, three reported decreased concentrations (Gordon & Oliver, 1971; Post, Gordon, Goodwin, & Bunney, 1973; Subrahmanyam, 1975), one reported increased concentrations (Vestergaard *et al.*, 1978), and five reported concentrations within the normal range of values (Berger *et al.*, 1980; Oreland *et al.*, 1981; Shaw *et al.*, 1973; Shopsin, Wilk, Sathananthan, Gershon, & Davis, 1974; Wilk, Shopsin, Gershon, & Suhl, 1972). Similarly, several studies reported decreased concentrations of CSF HVA in depressed patients (Goodwin, Post, Dunner, & Gordon, 1973; Mendels, Frazer, Fitzgerald, Ramsey, & Stokes, 1972; Papeschi & McClure, 1971; van Praag, Korf, & Schut, 1973), while others reported normal (Berger *et al.*, 1980; Sjostrom & Roos, 1972; van Praag & Korf, 1971) or increased (Bowers, 1974; Vestergaard *et al.*,

1978) concentrations. With regard to CSF 5-HIAA concentrations, decreased levels of the metabolite in depressed patients have been reported in several studies (Asberg, Thoren, Traskman, Bertilsson, & Ringberger, 1976; Ashcroft *et al.*, 1966; Coppen, Prange, Whybrow, & Noguera, 1972; Dencker, Malm, Roos, & Werdinius, 1966; Mendels *et al.*, 1972), whereas concentrations within the normal range of values have been reported in others (Berger *et al.*, 1980; Bowers, 1974; Goodwin *et al.*, 1973; Papeschi & McClure, 1971; Vestergaard *et al.*, 1978).

Studies of 24-hour urinary excretion products have focused on NE, epinephrine (E), and their metabolites normetanephrine (NM), metanephrine (M), vanillylmandellic acid (VMA), and MHPG. Here too, there have been conflicting results of decreased, increased, or normal excretion values for depressed populations and subpopulations (Beckmann & Goodwin, 1980; Edwards, Spiker, Neil, Kupfer, & Rizk, 1980; Hollister, 1981; Hollister, Davis, & Berger, 1980; Maas, Fawcett, & DeKirmenjian, 1968; Pickar, Sweeney, Maas, & Heninger, 1978; Roos & Sjostrom, 1969; Schildraut, 1973; Schildkraut, Orsulak, LaBris, *et al.*, 1978; Schildkraut, Orsulak, Schatzberg, *et al.*, 1978; Spiker, Edwards, Hanin, Neil, & Kupfer, 1980). One other approach that has been used in human studies with mixed results is the analysis of neurotransmitters in specific regions from postmortem material.

Though there has been a general lack of agreement in the research findings, there is still a general consensus that the biogenic amines play an important role in depression, and that this lack of agreement is, in part, more a function of problematic research design and measurement techniques than of biogenic amine neurophysiology (see Tables 5-1 and 5-2).

Early research with the first effective tricyclic antidepressant agents, imipramine and amitriptyline, suggested that these drugs worked by increasing the amount of active neurotransmitters in the synaptic cleft by preventing their reuptake. In a similar vein, treatment with MAO inhibitors appeared to

TABLE 5-1 Major Methodological Shortcomings in the Experimental Design of a Significant Number of Depression Studies

Subject characteristics

1. Heterogeneity in study samples:
   a. Diagnosis.
   b. Sex.
   c. Age.
2. Use of "neurological controls" as a comparison group.

Procedures

1. Small sample sizes.
2. Inadequate drug-free ("washout") period.
3. Lack of dietary control.
4. Level of physical activity not controlled.

TABLE 5-2 Major Methodological Shortcomings in the Measurement Techniques of a Significant Number of Depression Studies

General
1. Static, not dynamic measures.
2. Indirect measures used.
   a. In most cases metabolites, not neurotransmitters, measured.
   b. Usually no measures of receptors.
3. Peripheral and central neurotransmitter/metabolite contribution to measures not clearly differentiated (i.e., source of origin not clearly established).

Lumbar CSF measures
1. Gradient effects of the CSF not taken into account.
2. Measures do not indicate origin of metabolites/neurotransmitters within the brain.
3. Contribution of metabolites/neurotransmitters from spinal cord neurons or terminals not taken into account.
4. Diffusibility of some metabolites not taken into account.
5. CSF pressure effects not taken into account.

Urinary measures
1. Completeness of 24-hour collections difficult to assure.
2. Day-to-day concentration may vary (in multiple-day sampling).

Plasma measures
1. Plasma-CSF exchanges of metabolites and/or neurotransmitters not taken into account.
2. Free fatty acid influence on measurements (free and bound measurements) not taken into account.

Postmortem measures
1. Measures may be influenced by:
   a. Cause of death.
   b. Time of death.
   c. Time interval from death to analysis.
2. Uncertainty of diagnosis.

increase the concentration of neurotransmitters in the synaptic cleft by preventing intraneuronal metabolism of amines, making more available for release. Both of these treatments, then, appeared to result in more neurotransmitters being available to the postsynaptic neuron, thereby overcoming the proposed amine deficiency underlying the depressive symptomatology. Such synaptic mechanisms of antidepressant action appeared logicaly consistent with the depressant-like syndrome produced by reserpine treatment, which depletes the amine supply, and consistent with the biogenic amine hypothesis. A controversy regarding a role for the biogenic amines in human depression was precipitated by the development of new "atypical" antidepressant agents that did not alter the reuptake process of the biogenic amines. These "atypical" antidepressants fueled the growing belief that a neurotransmitter deficiency, as stated in the original biogenic amine hypothesis, was too simplistic a view to account entirely for the biochemical etiology of depression.

RECEPTORS

At about this same time, basic scientists working with rat brain tissue started to make inroads into the field of neurotransmitter receptors. Using techniques of "grind and bind" and specific radiolabeled agonists and antagonists, these scientists were able to characterize many of the neurotransmitter receptors — both on the presynaptic nerve terminal and on the postsynaptic neuron — with some degree of clarity, but not always with agreement. One major issue in neurotransmitter research is whether the binding of an agonist or antagonist to a "receptor" means it is a functional receptor site, or possibly just a nonspecific binding site. Thus, one goal in this field of research is to connect specific neurophysiological function to these sites.

Advances in this direction are being made. With the use of increasingly sophisticated radioligand assays it has been possible to quantify binding/ receptor sites within a specific region in order to characterize their appearance and to determine how physiological or pharmacological manipulation can regulate receptor density or receptivity. In addition, specific cellular responses that follow the activation of the particular binding/receptor sites have been studied electrophysiologically with the technique known as "microiontophoresis," which combines recordings from single cells and highly localized drug administration. The specific cellular responses that follow receptor activation have also been studied biochemically where the receptor is coupled to an enzymatic reaction such as the activation of a second messenger system (e.g., a cyclic nucleotide system). And finally, behavioral methods have been employed to study the behavioral consequences of receptor manipulation. Such research is making it increasingly evident that not only are there specific receptor moieties for specific transmitter substances, but there are also different molecular mechanisms by which these transmitters exert their effects.

Of particular interest to the study of depression is the activation of the adenyl cyclase system produced by the coupling of biogenic transmitters (and peptides) with their respective receptors. Adenyl cyclase is a membrane-bound enzyme that, when activated, catalyzes the transformation of cell adenosine triphosphate (ATP) to another molecule, cyclic adenosine monophosphate (cAMP). The generated cAMP then acts within the cell as a second messenger" which, by activating protein kinases, brings about altered cell function (see Figure 5-1). Thus, measuring changes in cAMP levels following receptor activation can be used as a means of evaluating receptor function and sensitivity (e.g., of beta-adrenergic receptors). Furthermore, the elucidation of second-messenger systems emphasizes the fact that potentially pertinent neuronal processes involved in the etiology of depression are not necessarily limited to neurotransmitters or receptors, but may also involve subsequent intracellular events. While these techniques for measuring receptors have their limitations (see Table 5-3), they have focused research attention on possible roles that presynaptic and postsynaptic receptors may play in depression, and have underscored the view of an increasingly complex etiology of depression.

It should be noted here that antidepressant drugs have been used extensively in conjunction with many of the aforementioned techniques. This is an

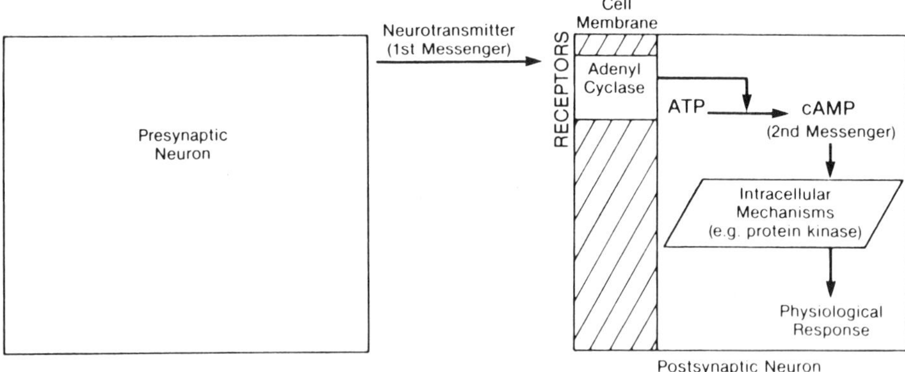

FIGURE 5-1 Second-messenger (cAMP) mechanism of neurotransmitter action. To be noted: (1) Second-messenger systems are an integral part of specific forms of neurotransmission and exist in the presence of other integral processes of neurotransmission (e.g., ionic processes). (2) cAMP is one example of a second-messenger system. There are other second-messenger systems (e.g., the guanine or cGMP system) that are activated by specific neurotransmitters. (3) Second-messenger systems exist presynaptically, as well as postsynaptically, and are activated by the stimulation of the presynaptic receptors. Adapted from Greengard (1978).

TABLE 5-3 Receptor Measurement Techniques

Technique	Receptor properties measured	Limitations
Biochemical		
Radiological binding	Identifies binding site(s).	Ligand may bind to sites other than receptors.
	Quantifies receptors (number and affinity).	No information regarding functional significance.
	Evaluates physiological or pharmacological regulation of receptor number.	Use of models of CNS receptors (e.g., lymphocytes) is of questionable significance.
Second-messenger activity	Characterizes mechanisms through which specific receptors operate. Serves as a functional measure of receptor responsivity.	Physiological significance of changes in second messenger not clear.
Electrophysiological	Characterizes integrated functional properties of receptor stimulation by ligand or neurotransmitter.	Net results are measured; such results may be influenced by events occurring beyond the cell or cell type being studied.
Behavioral	Provides information on overall behavioral consequences of receptor manipulation.	Gives overall effects and lacks precision; possibility of contributions from confounding factors is large.

obvious and practical approach, since determining the mechanism of action of effective antidepressant treatments not only helps in the further development of such agents, but also helps elucidate the biological substrates of depression. Acute antidepressant administration has been found to inhibit presynaptic reuptake of the neurotransmitter levels released, resulting in increases in neurotransmitters in the synaptic cleft. This is consistent with the biogenic amine hypothesis. It was theorized that this inhibition allowed the neurotransmitter to be present in the synaptic cleft for a longer period of time, thereby prolonging its effect and overcoming the neurotransmitter deficiency. But it was also noted that while the reuptake inhibition was an immediate effect of tricyclic antidepressant compounds, it took 2-4 weeks of treatment to induce the therapeutic effects in human subjects (Mandell, Segal, & Kuczenski, 1974). In addition (as mentioned previously), effective antidepressants that did not inhibit reuptake, such as iprindole, were discovered. Because they did not inhibit reuptake as the tricyclics did, they were termed "atypical" antidepressants. This "lag time" phenomenon, as well as these "atypical" antidepressants, emphasized our still incomplete understanding of the mechanisms by which antidepressants exert their effects. The attempt to find explanations for these "inconsistent" observations has led to the study of the effects of chronic antidepressant treatment upon presynaptic and postsynaptic receptors. In contrast to the effects of acute treatment with tricyclic antidepressants, it appears that the demonstrative effects of antidepressant treatments on receptors are seen only with semichronic or chronic antidepressant administration. For this reason, this discussion emphasizes results found with semichronic or chronic administration of antidepressant drugs.

Receptors for the adrenergic (NE) system have been designated "alpha-1" and "beta" for postsynaptic receptors, and "alpha-2" for presynaptic receptors. The postsynaptic beta-adrenergic receptors are coupled intracellularly with the second-messenger cAMP system, whose functional state can serve as a marker of beta-receptor activity. Sulser and Ventulani studied the effects of chronic *in vivo* antidepressant treatment on the NE-stimulated adenyl cyclase systems in the rat limbic forebrain (Sulser & Vetulani, 1977; Vetulani, Stawarz, & Sulser, 1976). They found that most, if not all, antidepressant treatments reduced the sensitivity of the NE-stimulated adenyl cyclase systems. Treatments found to be effective in inducing this subsensitivity included tricyclic antidepressants, "atypical" antidepressants, MAO inhibitors, and electroconvulsive therapy (ECT). Of particular interest is the finding that receptor subsensitivity was produced by the MAO inhibitor clorgyline, but not the MAO inhibitor deprenyl. Clorgyline has been shown to increase brain NE levels; thus it has CNS activity and is an effective antidepressant. Deprenyl, on the other hand, does not alter CNS NE activity and has dubious clinical efficacy (Finberg & Youdim, 1983). Such selective action supports the produced subsensitivity as a mode of antidepressant action in the CNS.

Elegant studies by Frazer (Frazer, 1980; Frazer & Lucki, 1982; Frazer *et al*., 1974) have replicated the findings that modification of the beta-adrenergic receptors by antidepressants results in a functional change in the second-messenger cAMP, and have demonstrated this effect in a biologically functional manner. In these studies, Frazer used the rat pineal gland as a model. The pineal gland has beta-receptors that are coupled to cAMP, which, when activated, stimulates the synthesis of the neurohormone melatonin. While acute treatment with a tricyclic antidepressant had no effect on this system, chronic treatment produced a subsensitivity in beta-receptors. This reduction in beta-receptor sensitivity was functionally reflected by (1) a decrease in cAMP production; (2) a decrease in the ability of a beta-receptor stimulant, isoproterenol, to elevate melatonin production; and (3) a decrease in the naturally occurring rise of melatonin that occurs as a component of the circadian rhythm during the nightime phase.

In the search for the biological substrates of depression, one ideally looks for mechanisms or effects common to all agents having antidepressant properties. This induced subsensitivity of the NE-stimulated beta-adrenergic adenyl cyclase system appears to have such commonality, suggesting that specific receptor abnormalities may be a key factor in the underlying biochemistry of depression. Adding support to this suggestion are studies that, by utilizing radioligand binding techniques, confirm the cAMP evidence of an induced beta-receptor subsensitivity. The results of radioligand binding indicate decreased beta-receptor binding in the rat brain after semichronic treatment with various types of antidepressant treatments (Sugrue, 1981).

In addition, the development of specific binding techniques for studying beta-receptors on circulating human leukocytes has allowed beta-receptors to be studied *in vivo* in humans. Using this leukocyte model, the effects of physiological changes on beta-receptor density can be evaluated in humans in an attempt to predict and define the factors responsible for *in vivo* alteration in receptor sensitivity and density in other less accessible tissues (e.g., CNS tissue). One such study (Wood, Feldman, & Nadeau, 1982) found that the beta-receptors in normal healthy subjects are in a chronic state of down-regulation and that the degree of down-regulation parallels the catecholamine concentrations. Alterations of catecholamines within the physiological range were found to be associated with modulation of beta-receptor density.

Charney, Menkes, and Heninger (1981) have also suggested that, in addition to beta-adrenergic receptor down-regulation, up-regulation of the postsynaptic alpha-1-adrenergic receptors (as well as the 5-HT receptors) may be a key regulatory mechanism by which antidepressants exert their effects. This hypothesis has support from both electrophysiological (Aghajanian, 1981; Menkes & Aghajanian, 1981) and behavioral (Maj, Mogilnicka, & Klimek, 1979) studies, which report enhanced activation of central alpha-1-receptors after semichronic antidepressant treatment. Recently, Sitaram *et al.* (1983), using the human iris as a model, concluded that up-regulation of alpha-1-adrenergic receptors is a significant regulatory mechanism of antidepressant action. Sugrue (1981), using radioligand binding techniques, has reported that alpha-1-receptor binding in the brain is unchanged after semichronic antidepressant treatment. This suggests that antidepressants can produce an enhanced functional responsiveness of central alpha-1-receptors, indicating a possible mode of antidepressant action, as well as raising the possibility that a subsensitivity of alpha-1-adrenergic receptors may be involved in depression. The finding that this enhanced functional responsiveness is not attributable to a change in receptor binding indicates that this enhanced state may be due to a modification of receptor-transmitter coupling rather than a change in receptor number.

The presynaptic alpha-2-adrenergic receptors are also gaining increasing attention with respect to the role adrenergic receptors may play in depression. Often referred to as "autoreceptors," they play an important part in the regulation of transmitter release from the presynaptic neurons. The mechanism by which alpha-2-receptors regulate the release of NE appears to be feedback inhibition. Specifically, released NE present in the synaptic cleft, as a result of neuronal excitation, activates the presynaptic alpha-2-receptors, which in turn inhibit further release of NE. This system of autoregulation may have important implications for our understanding of the etiology of depression, as well as of the mode of action of antidepressants. For example, Garcia-Sevilla, Zis, Hollingsworth, Greden, and Smith (1981), studying blood platelets of depressed patients, have shown that chronic administration of several antidepressants (including "atypicals") causes a subsensitivity of the alpha-2-receptors. With a reduction in alpha-2-receptor activation, there is less inhibition, resulting in increased NE release into the synaptic cleft. Studies using experimental animals and a variety of antidepressant treatments, such as clorgyline, amitriptyline, and iprindole, have reported findings consistent with those of Garcia-Sevilla *et al.* (Cohen, Campbell, Dauphin, Tallman, & Murphy, 1982; Crews & Smith, 1980; Smith, Garcia-Sevilla, & Hollingsworth, 1981). Stanford and Nutt (1982) showed a decrease in the number of alpha-2-receptors on neuronal membrane isolated from rat cerebral cortex, hippocampus, and hypothalamus, following repeated ECT. Recently, Smith, Hollingsworth, Garcia-Sevilla, and Zis (1983) found specific binding of platelet alpha-2-receptors to be significantly higher in depressed patients than in controls. These findings imply that a supersensitivity of central alpha-2-adrenergic receptors may exist in depressive disorders, and that effective forms of antidepressant treatment may act by decreasing the sensitivity of these receptors with semichronic or chronic administration.

As stated previously, 5-HT, as well as other neurotransmitters besides the catecholamines, may be involved in the biochemistry of the depressive disorders. Using radioligand binding techniques, two discrete serotonergic receptors have been characterized. 5-HT-1 receptors are labeled selectively by [^{3}H]5-HT, while 5-HT-2 receptors bind selectively with [^{3}H]spiroperidol (Peroutka & Synder, 1979; Synder & Peroutka, 1982). Furthermore, Synder and Peroutka (1982) propose that 5-HT-1 receptors may be associated with a cyclic nucleotide second-messenger system (cyclic guanine monophosphate, or cGMP), whereas 5-HT-2 receptors are not. If this selective association with a cGMP system exists, it could serve as a measurement technique used in conjunction with radioligand binding to differentiate the characteristics of these serotonergic receptors. Chronic administration of tricyclic antidepressants and MAO inhibitors causes a reduction in 5-HT-2 receptors (Fuxe *et al.*, 1983; Peroutka, Lebovitz, & Synder, 1981). This reduction in 5-HT-2 receptor concentration is comparable to (or greater than) that seen with beta-adrenergic receptors. Only a few antidepressants are found to reduce the numbers of 5-HT-1 receptors, and when down-regulation does occur, it is much less than that seen with 5-HT-2 receptors. Of particular interest is the finding that 5-HT-2 receptors appear to be associated with the behavioral effects of most serotonergic drugs (Peroutka & Synder, 1980). Such an association could indicate a reduction in central 5-HT-2 receptors as a critical action of antidepressant activity and 5-HT-2 receptor hypersensitivity as a possible underlying element of depression. However, the reported finding that repeated ECT produces an increase in central 5-HT-2 receptors ([^{3}H]spiroperidol binding sites) is in apparent conflict with such an indication (Kellar, Cascio, Butler, & Kurtzke, 1981; Vetulani, Lebrecht, & Pilc, 1981).

In summary, the biogenic amine hypothesis of depression postulates that the biological basis of endogenous depression is a lack of adequate levels of amine transmitters such as NE and 5-HT at the synaptic level. In recent years, receptor research has been important in implicating both presynaptic and postsynaptic receptors, not only as integral parts of synaptic function, but also as playing potentially key roles in the etiology and treatment of depression. The detailed extent to which this research has proceeded has depended upon newly developed techniques, such as radioligand binding and microiontophoresis. These techniques for measuring receptor function and characteristics have been used in conjunction with a variety of study models. Leukocytes for beta-receptor study (Wood *et al.*, 1982), and platelets for alpha-2-receptor study (Garcia-Sevilla *et al.*, 1981) are just two examples of effective models for the study of receptors and depression. While all these techniques and receptor models have their limitations, they have permitted researchers to examine and illuminate many of the potentially crucial receptor processes that may be involved in synaptic abnormalities underlying the behavioral profiles of depression.

With regard to the original biogenic amine hypothesis of depression, the research findings discussed can be summarized as follows: The supersensitivity of the beta-receptors in depression is a compensatory response to the NE deficiency that brings about a hyperfunctioning of the neuronal system. The depressive symptoms are ameliorated via the antidepressants because of the possible down-regulation of the postsynaptic neuronal response and the possible down-regulation of the alpha-2-receptors. Such a down-regulation would increase the NE released, thereby directly overcoming the deficiency that exists in depression.

Also to be considered is that the mechanism of action of most, if not all, antidepressant treatments is the reduction in number of both the beta-adrenergic and the 5-HT-2 serotonergic receptors following chronic or semichronic antidepressant administration. Such an evidenced commonality may point toward a common site of action, and, as such, toward an underlying pathophysiology of depression involving both the adrenergic and the serotonergic neurotransmitter systems.

While such theoretical interpretations may offer some consistency, this brief discussion on receptor research has also highlighted the fact that some findings do not appear to fit readily into such interpretations, underscoring our need for further research and understanding in this area. For example, there are the principally opposite changes that have been noted in the postsynaptic alpha-1-adrenergic and beta-adrenergic receptor sensitivity. What is the significance, if any, of this interrelationship? How does this fit in with the down-regulation of presynaptic alpha-2-receptors? And although there is general agreement on the role of presynaptic alpha-2-receptors in the inhibition of neurotransmitter (NE) release, Ariens and Simonis (1983) raise the question of whether this inhibition is predominantly caused by feedback of the neurotransmitter itself, or whether it may be due to catecholamines (namely, E) reaching the alpha-2-receptors from outside the synaptic junction. Also to be reconciled is the 5-HT-2 receptor up-regulation by ECT, which is in contrast to the "common mechanism" of 5-HT-2 receptor down-regulation produced by most other antidepressant treatments. These and other findings may reflect not only yet-to-be-understood characteristics of receptor function, but also other, potentially vital, aspects of neurophysiology. Two such aspects — cotransmission, involving the neuroactive peptides, and neurotransmitter interactions, involving potentially important balances between systems — are discussed in a later section. But before this discussion on receptor measurement and research pertinent to depression can be concluded, several points are left to be made.

First, it is important to keep in mind that much of this research has been carried out in animal models (e.g., healthy rats) or in models using peripheral human tissues (e.g., blood platelets). While these are valuable and accurate approaches to the preclinical studies of the mechanism of action of pharmacological agents, they do not directly study the pathological condition of interest. In reality, all human systems are finely tuned and have multiple regulatory and control mechanisms to maintain the normal homeostatic condition. Animal studies can therefore be expected to offer key pieces of information about the different neuronal mechanisms that may be aberrant in depression; this information in turn will direct the steps of further research and contribute to the final comprehensive explanation. In addition, these studies can be expected to offer the pharmacologist concepts to design more specific drugs with which to treat this disorder.

Another aspect that is becoming evident from receptor research is that in reality there may not be "atypical" antidepressant drugs. What in fact may be the case is that there are multiple molecular mechanisms whereby antidepressant drugs may produce their effects, all via some final common pathway. The list of all potential sites is currently unknown. Based on our current knowledge, we know that antidepressants can alter (1) reuptake; (2) metabolism; (3) number of receptor sites; (4) affinity of the receptor site for the neurotransmitter; (5) cAMP production; and (6) the yet-to-be-defined cascade of events that take place in the postsynaptic neuron, including enzymatic phosphorylation and specific ion channel modifications, necessary for the production of an action potential.

It would be highly surprising if the sites and mechanisms of action of antidepressant agents were, although complex, as simple as stated above. Preclinical research in animals and tissue models has uncovered a number of other receptor sites specific for each neurotransmitter through which antidepressants may function. For a more complete and in-depth discussion of neurotransmitter receptors, the reader is referred to two recent publications: a special issue of *Advances in Biochemical Psychopharmacology* (Segana, Yamamura, & Kusiyawa, 1983), and the earlier-cited paper by Charney *et al.* (1981).

ALTERNATIVE NEUROTRANSMITTER SYSTEMS

An important point to be made in this discussion of neurotransmitters and their measurement in depression is that a two-way relationship exists between hypothesis formation and technical development. Not only does the formation of a hypothesis, and the subsequent desire to test it, act as a guiding impetus for biotechnical development, but the reverse also holds true. This has been particularly evident in the study of depression. In the search for the biological basis of depression, consideration of the central monoamines has, by far, dominated this field of research. Such consideration has been based in part on the conviction that monoaminergic systems do play a dominant role in mood regulation and affect. But it has also been based on the fact that the technical means with which to measure the monoamine and monoamine metabolite concentrations with relative accuracy were available when accurate measurement techniques for other central neurotransmitter systems were not. In other words, the large volume of research that exists for the monoamines in the study of depression has been based on technical, as well as theoretical, considerations. This section discusses several of the alternative neurotransmitter systems that have recently come under investigation in the study of depression. In addition, where warranted, these neurotransmitter systems are discussed in the context of the emerging view that behavioral disorders may not be the exclusive domain of one system or the other, being instead due to interactions and/or balances existing between the neurotransmitter systems.

Dopamine

DA functions both as a precursor of NE and as a CNS neurotransmitter. The finding that NE and DA can function separately in the brain, influencing different neural processes, emerged from the findings that NE and DA can be located in seperate nuclei and neurons, and that the noradrenergic and dopaminergic systems have their own specific receptors. DA is found to be widely distributed in the brain and appears to be able to influence a wide variety of physiological functions. One well-known major dopaminergic tract is the nigrostriatal tract, which influences initiation and execution of movement. Loss of function of this tract produces the akinesia and rigidity of Parkinson disease. Another major dopaminergic tract is the mesolimbic tract, which appears to have influence over emotional function and thought organization. This tract, contained as part of the mesolimbic-mesocortical complex, has been implicated in DA theories of schizophrenia.

With respect to the affective disorders, early pharmacological evidence had dissuaded researchers from considering dopaminergic function as a potentially important factor in the biology of depression. Amphetamines, which are primarily DA releasers, proved to be ineffective in the treatment of depression. Benztropine has as one of its functions the selective inhibition of DA reuptake, but it too proved to be ineffectual as an antidepressant agent. There have been reports of low CSF HVA, the major metabolite of DA, in depression (Bowers, 1974; Goodwin *et al.*, 1973; Korf & van Praag, 1971; van Praag, Korf, & Puite, 1970), but the probenecid technique was used in many of these past studies; as such, the results must be interpreted with caution. Other studies have reported no such metabolite alteration (Berger *et al.*, 1980). More recent studies have been more promising, reporting behavioral (Serra, Argiolas, Klimek, Fadda, & Gessa, 1979) and neurophysiological (Chiodo & Antelman, 1980a, 1980b) changes following chronic antidepressant administration that appear to be associated with a decrease in sensitivity of the presynaptic DA receptors.

Like the NE presynaptic receptors, the activation of DA presynaptic receptors is believed to inhibit the further release of DA. A subsensitivity of these receptors would then have the effect of increasing the DA levels in the synaptic cleft. These findings have also gained support from ECT studies and specific drug studies. For example, Shopsin and Gershon (1978) reported moderate antidepressant effects with piribedil, a DA-mimetic drug. ECT has been found to alter both postsynaptic and presynaptic DA receptors, with the net result being enhanced dopaminergic function (Chiodo & Antelman, 1980a; Wielosz, 1981). The wide distribution of DA in the brain areas concerned with affect and thought organization, coupled with the recent findings of dopaminergic changes associated with chronic antidepressant treatments, has suggested that DA may play a role in the mechanism of action of antidepressants and possibly in the biological profile of depression.

Gamma-Aminobutyric Acid

In 1950, utilizing the then-new technique of paper chromatography, researchers identified the presence of high concentrations of gamma-aminobutyric acid (GABA) in the brain (Otusaka, 1973; Ryall, 1975). Its potency as a CNS inhibitory transmitter came to be appreciated when microiontophoretic studies, using such models as the crustacean stretch receptor, demonstrated GABA's ability to mimic the effects of the inhibitory nerve (Krnjevic & Schwartz, 1966). Subsequent studies identified GABA as the exclusive inhibitory amino acid in the inhibitory nerve and showed, via intracellular recordings, that the inhibitory nerve and GABA produced identical increases in chloride (Cl^-) conductance in muscle tissue (Hosli & Hosli, 1979). The determination of the specific locations of this neurotransmitter in the brain has been aided by immunocytochemical methods for identifying the synthesizing enzyme, glutamic acid decarboxylase. Most GABAergic neurons are intrinsic, being contained within specific regions such as the cortex, hippocampus, and cerebellum. In regions such as these, GABA can be found in concentrations as high as 1,000 times that found for the monoamines. Though the GABA distribution in the CNS appears to be ubiquitous, as well as intrinsic, [^{3}H]GABA autoradiographic techniques have shown GABA to be localized not only to areas such as the cerebellum, brain stem, spinal cord, and dorsal root ganglia, but also to the glial cells, implicating these cells in the GABA metabolic process (Hosli & Hosli, 1979).

It has been suggested that this potent, highly concentrated, and widely distributed inhibitory neurotransmitter may play a role in the pathophysiology of the affective disorders. GABA has been reliably measured in the CSF and appears to provide an available index of brain GABA function, with little contribution from the periphery (Bohlen, Huot, & Palfreyman, 1979; Grove *et al.*, 1980). Kasa *et al.* (1982), using the RRA method, demonstrated significantly lower CSF GABA levels in depressed patients than in healthy controls. This result confirmed the finding of lower CSF GABA levels by Gerner and Hare (1981), but not of Post *et al.* (1980).[1] Animal studies have shown that ECT and carbamazepine, which are used effectively to treat both mania and

1. Post *et al.* (1980) measured CSF GABA levels by modified cation-exchange chromatography; they reported that, with the exception of one case, the CSF GABA levels of depressed patients did not differ significantly from normal volunteers. It has been suggested by Berrettini *et al.* (1983) that this finding may be related more to a problem of methodology then to a patient population characteristic. They put forth that the nonsignificantly lower CSF GABA levels in depressed patients might have been related to the aliquot of CSF used for the analysis. Post *et al.* used 1 ml from a pool of the 15th-26th cc removed. Gerner and Hare (1981), using a similar pool of the 15th-26th cc removed, also found nonsignificant lower values in depressed subjects when compared to controls. When they then analyzed samples from a pool consisting of the 1st-12th cc removed, they found significantly lower values in the depressed patients.

depression, decrease GABAergic turnover (Bernasconi & Martin, 1979; Green *et al.*, 1978).[2] In a study of the "learned helplessness" model of depression the "learned helplessness" behavior was defined here as the significantly reduced ability to acquire a response for appetitive reinforcement following exposure to inescapable shock, desipramine and GABA acted in a similar fashion to reverse and prevent the behavior, implicting GABA in the therapeutics of the tricyclic antidepressants (Sherman & Petty, 1980). While there appears to be preliminary evidence supporting a GABAergic role in the affective disorders, it has been suggested that its role may be to influence the actions of other neurotransmitter systems, such as the noradrenergic system, that underlie the pathophysiology of depression. This "interactional" approach to GABAergic influence is discussed in a later section.

Acetylcholine

Acetylcholine (ACh) was the first chemical substance to be identified as a neurotransmitter, and has served as a basis of study through which researchers have come to understand many of the key principles of neurotransmission. In spite of this, we are just now coming to understand the complexity of this neurotransmitter. ACh has proven to be very difficult to measure and associate with behavioral effects, due to a variety of factors. For example, the establishment of ACh turnover rates has been very difficult because choline acts as both a precursor and a metabolite of ACh. Pharmacological tools by which to study relationships between ACh and behavior are improving, but are still inadequate. What is well known is that peripherally ACh acts as a neurotransmitter for motor neurons projecting to glands, muscles, and ganglia. Centrally, ACh tends to be localized in specific cell populations where its actions can be brief or prolonged, excitatory or inhibitory, and distant or local.

A number of studies using a variety of experimental approaches have suggested that ACh may play a role in the affective disorders. In 1974, Janowsky, El-Yousef, and Davis utilized physostigmine, which increases intracerebral ACh concentrations by inhibiting the enzyme involved in ACh catabolism (cholinesterase). The effects of physostigmine were compared with those of a placebo and of neostigmine. Neostigmine is also a cholinesterase inhibitor, but it acts peripherally and does not readily enter the brain. This work was an attempt to study the influence of increased ACh levels in the CNS (due to the action of physostigmine) on mood, drive level, and psy-

2. Post and colleagues have reported other studies in which there was no observed decrease in GABA turnover after carbamazepine administration (Post, Uhde, Rubinow, Ballenger, & Gold, 1983).

chomotor activity in depressed patients, manic patients, and schizoaffective patients. Physostigmine induced significant motor retardation in all patient populations studied, and induced mood shifts in a depressive direction in patients with an affective component to their illness. Such induced effects were not observed with the placebo or neostigmine. Furthermore, these induced effects diminished immediately after an anticholinergic was administered. In another study, physostigmine was shown to induce depressive symptoms in normals as well (Risch *et al.*, 1981).

Other responses to cholinergic agonists have been reported in a number of studies to be more profound in depressed patients than in controls. Exposure to organophosphate insecticides, which are irreversible cholinesterase inhibitors, has been reported to be associated with depressive symptoms (Gershon & Shaw, 1961). Decreased rapid eye movement (REM) latency and neuroendocrine responses (i.e., increased prolactin) have been reported in a number of studies to be significantly different in depressed patients when compared to controls (Jones *et al.*, 1986; Sitaram, Nurnberger, Gershon, & Gillin, 1980). Consistent with this proposed increase in CNS ACh levels in depression is the finding that choline, when orally administered as a treatment for tardive dyskinesia, produced profound depressive symptoms in approximately 50% of the treated patients (Tamminga, Smith, Ericksen, Chang & Davis, 1977). While the evidence cited is indirect, it implicates the cholinergic neurotransmitter in depression. The evidence itself is reminiscent of the early observations with reserpine and iproniazid that led to the biogenic amine hypothesis of depression.

This discussion of DA, GABA, and ACh as neurotransmitter systems other than NE and 5-HT that may be involved in depression has been brief. The peptides, the trace amines, histamine, and glycine are examples of other alternative neuroactive substances that are currently under investigation, but space restrictions preclude their discussion here. The purpose of this section has been to cite specific examples of alternative neuroactive substances, to highlight researchers' improved ability to measure and characterize such substances, and to introduce yet another avenue by which researchers are coming to appreciate the complexity of depression's underlying neurobiochemistry. In the sections to follow some of these substances are again discussed, but in the context of system interactions and balances.

THE NIMH COLLABORATIVE PROGRAM ON THE PSYCHOBIOLOGY OF DEPRESSION

Up until this point in this chapter, we have reviewed the origins of the catecholamine deficiency hypothesis and have highlighted how the field of basic neuroscience research has made large strides in terms of understanding new neuromechanisms and neurotransmitters. We have related this to possible ways in which the brain may normally function and to the mechanisms that may be affected by psychopathological processes. An obvious question to ask at this juncture is whether our present knowledge of neurotransmitters, neuromodulators, and their mechanisms is consistent with the hypothesis of a deficiency in biogenic amines in depression. Perhaps a more important question is whether the biogenic amine hypothesis is accurate and reliable enough to justify continued exploration.

Over the course of the years since its conception, there have been conflicting reports in the literature about the evidence for this hypothesis. This subject was a major consideration of the Williamsburg Conference on Depression, held in 1969 by the National Institute of Mental Health (NIMH). Following that conference, NIMH convened a study group to summarize the conclusions reached by the conference, and to report to NIMH the major obstacles to the advancement of depression research, and suggest ways to overcome these obstacles. Of major concern at the time was the small sample size in many studies of the biogenic amine hypothesis. In addition, the various laboratories that had performed these studies had used different diagnostic schemes, making comparison between different laboratories difficult if not impossible. Furthermore, no one study had measured multiple neurotransmitters in the same subjects. Therefore, this advisory committee to NIMH recommended that a collaborative study program be undertaken, involving a number of investigators throughout the country at clinical research centers, to examine the biological etiology of depression. The program should be designed to measure, in the same subjects, neurotransmitter, neuroendocrine, electrolyte, enzyme, and behavioral function in depression. This program should also study a large number of subjects and should include healthy controls for comparison. The explicit details of the program have been previously published, and the reader is referred to these publications for further information about the overall program (Katz, Secunda, Hirschfeld, & Koslow, 1979; Mass *et al.*, 1980; Secunda *et al.*, 1980).

We now discuss salient findings from the Biological Studies component of the NIMH Collaborative Program, presenting data only on drug-free depressed and healthy control subjects in order to test the hypothesis of the deficiency of biogenic amines in depression. A more detailed presentation can be found elsewhere (Koslow *et al.*, 1983). The biogenic amines and the metabolites measured are reported in Table 5-4.

Overall, the results of the Collaborative Program suggest a hyper-adrenergic state, not a deficiency in depression. Possible methodological and other reasons for this have been listed in Tables 5-1 and 5-2, and deserve further comment here. For example, the use of an appropriate control group is extremely important if one is to ask the question of whether there is an increase or a decrease in a function, in a particular state of psychopathology. In a number of previous reports, a neurological control group was utilized for comparison with depressed subjects. Figure 5-2 shows the values for one

TABLE 5-4 Neurotransmitter Measures Employed in the NIMH Collaborative Program on the Psychobiology of Depression, Biological Studies

Transmitter	Measure	Tissue
DA	HVA	CSF
NE	MHPG	
5-HT	5-HIAA	
NE/E	MPHG	Plasma
	MAO	
	Catechol-*O*-methyltransferase	
NE	VMA	
	MHPG	Urine (average of two) 24-hour collections)
	NE	
	NM	
	E	
	M	

neurotransmitter metabolite — 5-HIAA, the metobolite of 5-HT — that was measured in healthy control subjects, depressed subjects, and neurological controls. As can be seen, the overall results show that in neurological controls the 5-HIAA was elevated in comparison to the two other subject groups. This study provides one reason why in clinical studies where neurological controls were used, a finding of such a deficiency would be supported. Why there were

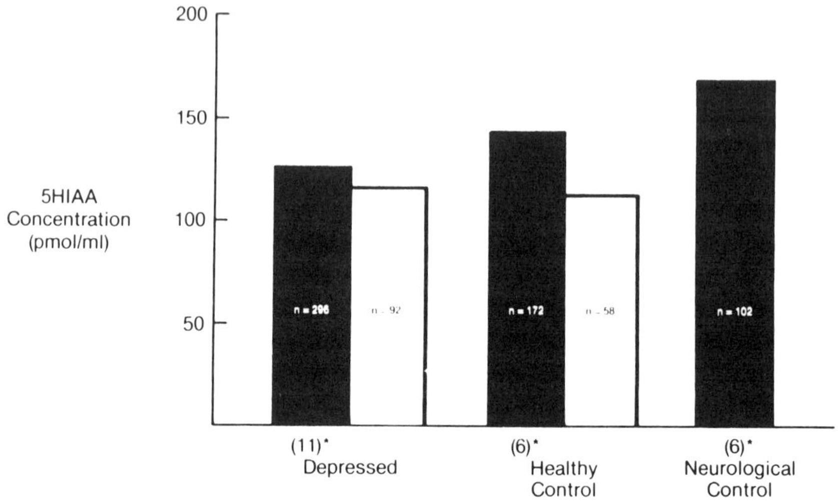

FIGURE 5-2 Overall CSF 5-HIAA weighted (■) and Collaborative Program study (□) (Koslow *et al.*, 1983) means for depressed subjects, healthy controls, and neurological controls. (Weighted means are from references cited in text.)

higher values in neurological controls is unclear. In some cases it was reported that the neurological controls were the healthy family members of subjects who would come in for a neurological exam; in other cases, it was reported that these were results from neurological controls who turned out to have no known neurological disease. Evidently, the argument is not valid in terms of their being normal, based on the values that were reported for 5-HIAA. Other measurements showed similar findings.

A second issue of major importance is the analytical method used for measuring the substance of interest. In some early studies, the analytical methods available were insufficient to measure the low concentrations of metabolites in CSF; therefore, probenecid was used — not only as a means of measuring dynamic states, but also as a means to elevate the levels of the monoamine metabolites of interest. As outlined earlier in this chapter, probenecid has a number of shortcomings and probably should not be used to study neurotransmitter dynamics. Furthermore, as the methodology has improved, so has the accuracy of the actual measurement of the neurotransmitter metabolites (see Figure 5-3).

Although there have not been many studies using GC-MS techniques, the level of agreement is clearly higher than that possible with fluorometric or GC techniques. The findings in Figure 5-3 cannot totally be ascribed to analytical method, but are more complex; in addition, there are probably contributions

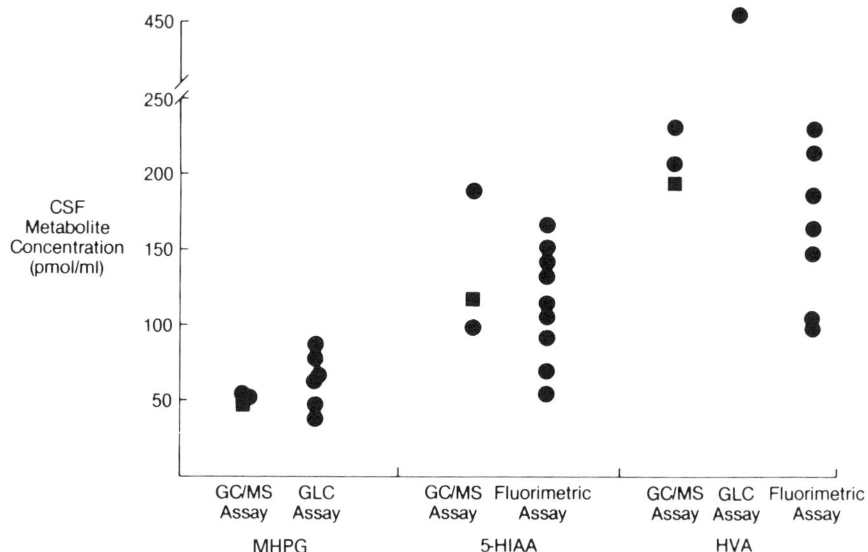

FIGURE 5-3 Reported mean CSF MHPG, 5-HIAA, and HVA concentrations in depressed patients by assay method. ■, Collaborative Program study (Koslow *et al.*, 1983) means; ●, other studies (referenced in text).

in the data that are due to differences in diagnosis, age, sex effects, and so on. The NIMH Collaborative Program on the Psychobiology of Depression attempted to overcome many of these earlier problems in its design. Although it is impossible to resolve all of the issues at hand, many of them were appropriately dealt with in the Collaborative Program. Table 5-5 shows some of the major assets of this multicenter study program.

An overall summary of the results for monoamine level concentrations in depressed subjects as compared to healthy control subjects is shown in Table 5-6; these findings support a state of hyperadrenergic function in depression for NE and 5-HT. As noted in this table, for the three CSF monoamine metabolites, both 5-HIAA and HVA showed strong gender effects and therefore were analyzed separately. The results found were that 5-HIAA was only elevated in females, while HVA was decreased only in males. The 5-HIAA data were examined for a bimodality in distribution, as previously reported by Asberg *et al.* (1976). The data failed to reproduce this effect. In Asberg's report no sex effects were found, and therefore males and females were analyzed together. Figure 5-4 shows a plot of the data from the Collaborative Program for 5-HIAA, where males and females were differentiated, and compares it to the data from Asberg *et al.*, where genders were not segregated. Certainly combining the sexes could produce a bimodal distribution if, in fact, male and female 5-HIAA values are not distributed in the same way.

While MHPG failed to show a sex effect, there were strong positive correlations of MHPG with age ($r = .41$, $p < .001$) This raised the issue of whether something was uniquely occurring with MHPG and maturation. One obvious point of differentiation in the aging process is menopause. Therefore the data were examined from the point of view of postmenopausal and premenopausal status in women. Since all the women in this study who were

TABLE 5-5 Experimental Design Advantages of the NIMH Collaborative Program on the Psychobiology of Depression, Biological Studies

- Patients excluded who were treated in last 2 months with depot medication
- Drug-free washout period of 10 days to 2 weeks
- Completeness of urinary collections assessed by sampling 4 successive days and measuring volume and creatinine
- Samples collected same time every day
- State-of-the-art quantitative measures used — GC-MS and GC
- Large sample of depressed subjects (n = 132); therefore age, sex effects, etc., could be accounted for
- Large sample of age-matched normal healthy control subjects (n = 80) for comparison (hospitalized and nonhospitalized)
- Rigorous, reliable psychiatric diagnostic procedure (SADS; RDC)
- Rigorous general health screen, with exclusion of subjects with any concomitant major medical illness
- Multiple measures of amine system; should adequately test hypothesis put forth

TABLE 5-6 Alterations in Monoamine Concentrations in Depressed Subjects as Compared to Healthy Controls

Monoamine concentration	Difference from controls
CSF	
MHPG	↑ females
5-HIAA	↑ females
HVA	↓ males
Urinary	
MHPG	↔
VMA	↑
NM	↑
M	↑
E	↑ [a]
NE	↑ [b]

Note. ↑, ↓, and ↔ indicate increased, descreased, and no change, respectively. Data from Koslow *et al.* (1983).

[a] Levels for unipolar depressives were greater than those for bipolars.

[b] Increased for unipolars only; bipolars were not significantly different from controls.

postmenopausal were also over the age of 50, the men in this study were classified as younger or older than 50 years of age. The results of these analyses are reported in Figure 5-5.

Two sets of statistical analyses were performed on these four age-sex groups (premenopausal women; postmenopausal women; men less than or equal to 50 years of age; men greater than 50 years of age). First, analysis of variance (ANOVA) was used to compare the four groups within each subject category (controls and depressed). Second, *t* tests were used to compare the depressed and control subjects within the categories of premenopausal-postmenopausal women, or men less than or greater than 50 years of age. The ANOVA in controls showed no significant findings, while in the depressed subjects the ANOVA showed a significant difference ($p < .001$), which was due to the postmenopausal women and men 50 years or older. When the *t* tests within subgroups were analyzed, the only significant finding was for postmenopausal depressed women, who were significantly higher in CSF MHPG than control postmenopausal women (two-tailed *t*; $p < .002$). Postmenopausal women from both the control and the depressed groups were removed from the analysis to see whether CSF MHPG would still be elevated. When this analysis was performed, no significant difference was found for CSF MHPG ($p > .20$).

Similar analyses were conducted for 5-HIAA and HVA, even though the analyses had already been done individually by sex (see Figures 5-6 and 5-7). For 5-HIAA, the ANOVA within the depressed group showed that the

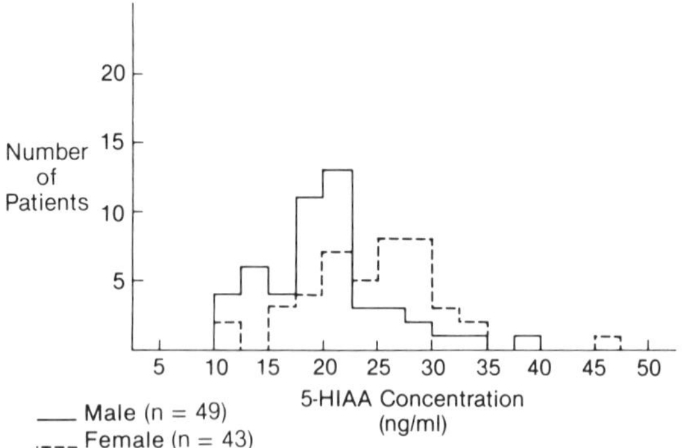

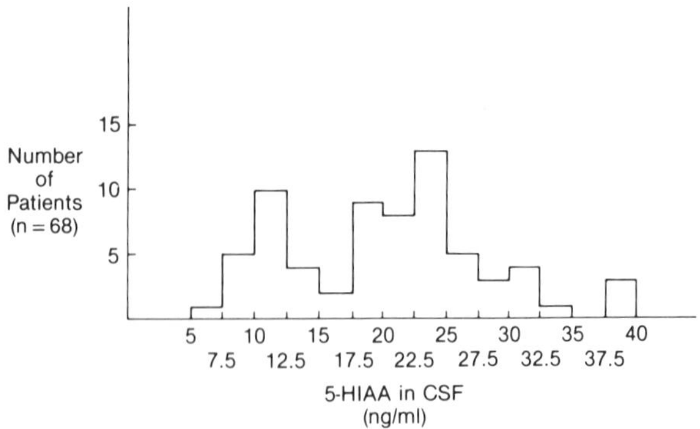

FIGURE 5-4 Comparison of 5-HIAA values obtained from NIMH Collaborative Program on the Psychobiology of Depression (Koslow *et al.*, 1983) (upper graph) with those reported by Asberg *et al.* (1976) (lower graph).

concentrations for postmenopausal women were significantly greater than for all other groupings. Within controls, the ANOVA just missed signficance (p = .054), which was again probably due to the influence of postmenopausal women on the data. Unlike the finding with MHPG, t tests between control and depressed groups within the four groupings failed to show any significant differences for 5-HIAA. However, the comparison between control and depressed premenopausal women just missed significance (p = .056). These data show that the overall effect in 5-HIAA was not solely restricted to one age group within women, be they premenopausal or postmenopausal.

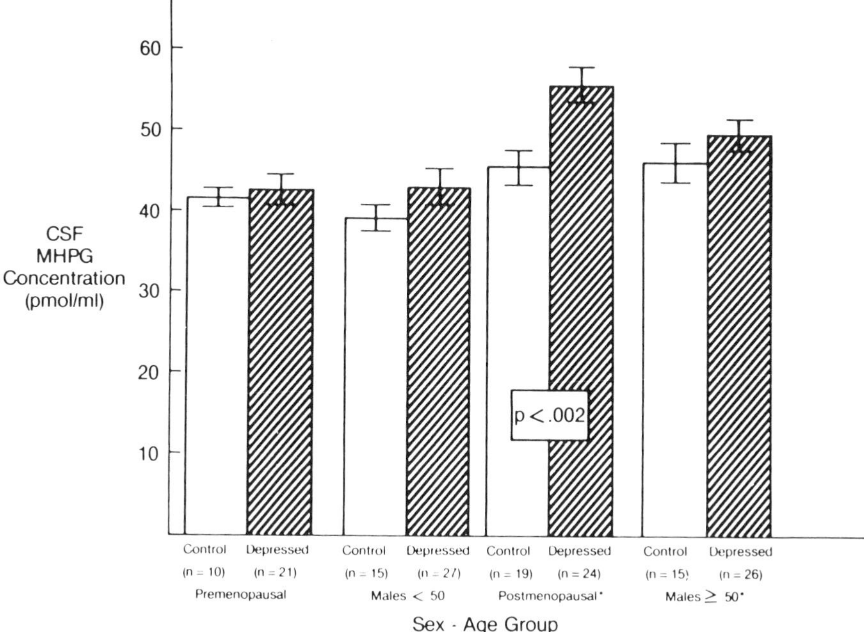

FIGURE 5-5 Depressed-control comparisons of CSF MHPG across four sex-age groups (ANOVA). Data from Koslow *et al.* (1983).

For HVA, an ANOVA within the control and depressed groups failed to find significant differences, although there were trends toward significance. In comparing control and depressed subjects within each category, the older depressed men had significantly lower values for HVA than did controls ($p < .009$), while the younger men were not significantly different ($p = .21$). For the female subjects, the postmenopausal women just missed significance ($p = .06$), with the depressed women being lower than the healthy control women, while the values for premenopausal women were not significant ($p = .99$). Overall, the data for HVA would suggest that there is a trend for HVA to be elevated in both older control and depressed groups. Within this older population of men and women, the depressed patients have lower concentrations of HVA compared to normal controls. However, it is important to note that the only significant finding was for the male population, and it was predominantly due to the men greater than 50 years of age.

Taken together, these data are provocative and at the moment are difficult to totally interpret and comprehend. They do, however, highlight the need for careful control of age and sex effects when analyzing data in depression. What are striking are the variations that occur in postmenopausal women. They suggest that there are strong neuroendocrine interactions with these neuro-

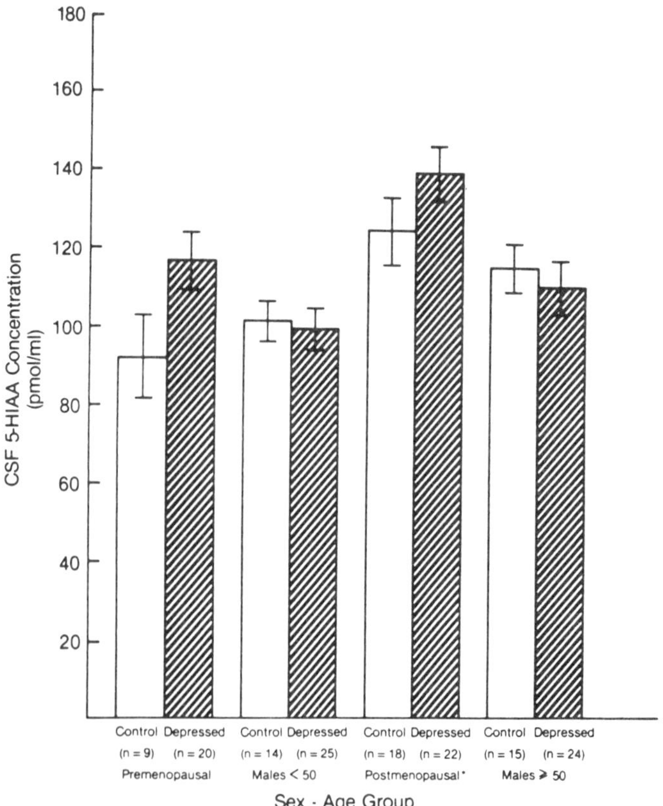

FIGURE 5-6 Depressed-control comparisons of CSF 5-HIAA across four sex-age groups (ANOVA). Data from Koslow *et al.* (1983).

transmitter systems. The higher prevalence of depression in women may be associated with the interactions occurring between neuroendocrine and neurotransmitter systems. This issue will, however, require much further examination in terms of both basic and clinical research.

As can be seen in Table 5-6, the analysis of urinary monoamines and metabolites provides the strongest data for the existence of an overall hyperadrenergic state in the depressed subjects. In comparison to control subjects, the depressed subjects as a group showed a 57% increase for NE, a 32% increase for E, a 42% increase for NM, a 39% increase for M, and a 23% increase for VMA; MHPG showed essentially no change (3%). One surprising finding was that there was no alteration in the 24-hour urinary levels of MHPG, though higher concentrations were found for the biogenic amines and the other metabolites excreted over the same time period. While much of the

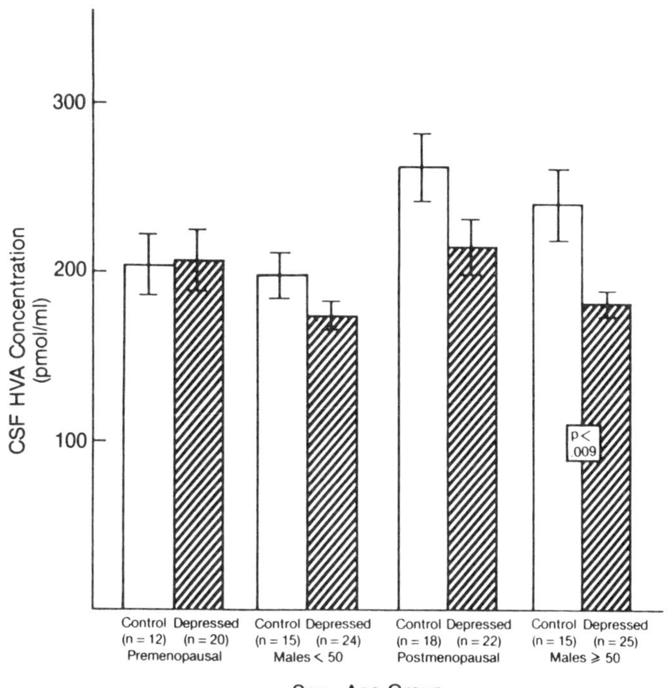

FIGURE 5-7 Depressed-control comparisons of CSF HVA across four age-sex groups (ANOVA). Data from Koslow *et al.* (1983).

literature has pointed to the alterations in MHPG, numerous inconsistencies have been reported. Very few studies have compared excretion of urinary MHPG by depressed subjects with that by normal controls. There may, in fact, be subgroups of depressed subjects who do have low levels of MHPG, but this aspect of the data has not yet been analyzed.

It was not possible to discriminate, from a neurotransmitter/metabolite perspective, any differences between unipolar and bipolar depression, with the exception of the measures for E and NE. NE and E had significantly different levels of excretion in urine not only in unipolars and bipolars, but also in manic subjects (Table 5-7). NE levels were significantly higher in unipolar subjects than in bipolar subjects or healthy controls ($p < .0001$). For E, the unipolar subjects were significantly higher than controls ($p < .0001$) and bipolar subjects ($p < .03$). Bipolar subjects, on the other hand, showed significantly greater concentrations only for E secretion when compared to healthy control subjects ($p < .0001$). Although not a major subject of this discussion, it is of interest to mention at this point that the manic subjects only showed significantly elevated levels for NE when compared to bipolar and control subjects ($p < .0001$).

TABLE 5-7 Summary of Urinary NE and E Values for Depressed Subjects as Compared to Healthy Controls

Depressive subgroup	Difference in NE from controls	Difference in E from controls
Unipolar depressed	↑	↑
Bipolar depressed		↑
Manic	↑	

Note. ↑ indicates significantly increased values as compared to healthy controls. Data from Koslow *et al.* (1983).

Although there is great variance in the data, as can be seen in the individual data points, and as reflected in the standard deviation, these data suggest that NE and E levels may be state-dependent in affective disorders. That is, in bipolar illness, E is elevated in the depressed state, while NE is elevated in the manic state. It would be most interesting to see whether this holds up in the same subject when he or she goes from one state to the other. In unipolar subjects, however, both NE and E are elevated, with the NE elevation possibly being a trait reflection rather than a state reflection.

To summarize the findings to date, the analyses of these data do support the view that there is an alteration in biogenic amines. However, the overwhelming direction of the change does not favor the deficiency hypothesis, but rather favors a hypothesis of hyperadrenergic function. In CSF, the metabolites of NE and 5-HT, while elevated, were elevated only in females. This finding favors hyperbiogenic amine function in the CNS, but does not provide direct support for its association with depression, since it is gender-specific. It is possible that this gender specificity may, in fact, be related to depression, since there is a higher rate of depression in females than in males, and it may relate to neuroendocrine interactions with neurotransmitter systems.

The analysis of the urinary data strongly supports a hyperadrenergic function. Both the neurotransmitter released from sympathetic nerves (NE) and that released from the adrenal glands (E) were found to be greatly elevated in depression, as were most of their metabolites. The one exception was MHPG, which was not elevated in depressed subjects as compared to controls. While this finding about MHPG is not understood at this point, it does argue for the measurement of as many measures of neurotransmitter functions as possible. If this assessment of the urinary data is applied to the CSF measures, then perhaps these measures are not the best reflection of the neurotransmitter systems function in the brain. Since, in urinary measures, no change in MHPG was detected while large changes in NE, E, and their metabolites (other than MHPG) were seen, what appears to be needed is a more direct assessment of these two catecholamines and metabolites than that provided by MHPG. The higher excretion rates of catecholmines and metabolites in depression may be a reflection of increased release, increased synthesis, differential disposition, or a combination of these phenomena.

The peripheral measures do suggest that there may be a hyperfunctional central state, since both the sympathetic nerves, which release NE, and the adrenal glands, which release E, are under central control. There may be a hyperadrenergic state, both centrally and peripherally, in depression. While this discussion has analyzed depressed subjects in comparison to controls from an overall population viewpoint, it is strongly believed that depression is a heterogeneous group of disorders. These data would support this notion in that there is a larger variation in biogenic amine concentration in both the CSF and urinary amines and metabolites measured in depressed subjects when compared to those measured in normal healthy controls. The distributions of the values in depression had a much wider range than that seen in healthy controls. Future analyses, taking into consideration the relationship of biogenic amines and their metabolites to depressive subtypes, clinical state symptoms, and behaviors in other chemical characteristics, may in fact yield subtypes of depression that are strictly hyperadrenergic, as well as subtypes of depression characterized by normal adrenergic function or hypoadrenergic function.

THE NEW BIOLOGY

The next decade promises to be one of great progress because of the newer technologies that offer the promise of expanding both our anatomical and our molecular understanding of nerve function. The vastly improved brain-imaging techniques have sufficient resolution not only to permit the study of the functioning human at a resolution of slightly greater than 1 cm, but also to allow the study of very specific brain regions. The use of short-lived isotopes, which emit positrons when chemically incorporated into the structure of pharmacological agents or chemical precursors, can be visualized in specific brain regions using the technique of positron emission transaxial tomography. The compound deoxyglucose has been used in this manner to measure "neuronal activity."[3] Dopa, the precursor for the neurotransmitters DA, NE,

3. The energy requirements of cerebral tissue are derived almost entirely from glucose catabolism under normal circumstances. Alterations in functional neuronal activity, in any particular region of the CNS, appears to be associated with changes in energy consumption in that area (Sokoloff, 1977). In this way, measuring the rate of cerebral glucose consumption can provide insight into the functional activity of the CNS.

and E, has been shown to be an effective measurement tool, as has the DA receptor binding agent spiperone. Through the use of these compounds in human subjects, new insights into the brain areas, neurotransmitters, and receptor systems involved in depression will be gained and used to focus on the etiology of this disorder. In a similar way, it is expected that the imaging technique of nuclear magnetic resonance will soon be used to measure functional brain activity in specific brain regions, eliminating the need to use radioisotopes to study human brain function.

The techniques of cellular and molecular biology are rapidly being mainstreamed into the neuroscience research approaches to brain function. This affords scientists the opportunity to begin to understand the genomic control of the various elements within the nervous system. The use of these techniques allows for the circumvention of the often laborious and almost impossible task of the isolation of pure proteins — for example, of receptors, biosynthetic enzymes, or ion channels. It is now possible through the molecular biology approach to isolate the genes or messenger ribonucleic acids coding for specific proteins, and then to produce the purified molecular protein of interest.

Many of these new developments are just now being applied extensively in biopsychiatric research, and their full value for the study of depression has yet to be realized. Several areas of research are already yielding valuable new insights concerning the processes and principles of neurotransmission, and, as such, are yielding potentially valuable insights into the neuronal processes underlying depression.

Neuropeptides

One of the greatest explosions of new knowledge that has occurred is the discovery of multiple peptides that are found in the CNS in specific neuronal systems and apparently function as neurotransmitters or neuromodulators. The discovery of these neuropeptides is of importance to the study of depression, because it represents a new approach to the biochemistry of human brain and behavior research — one that may provide additional information about the neurobiochemical functions that are impaired in depression.

Neuropeptides are small proteins consisting of 2-40 amino acids; they are produced in the CNS and exert direct effects on the CNS. Many of these peptides were originally identified in peripheral organs decades ago, and have only recently been identified in the CNS. Many of these neuropeptides show peripheral endocrine activity, but their effect on the CNS is independent of this. During the last 10 years, literally hundreds of peptides have been identified in the CNS, with 30-40 of them being considered as peptide neurotransmitters (Snyder, 1980). RIA techniques have shown the neuropeptides to be widely distributed throughout the brain, with many of them, like the biogenic amines, being localized in brain areas involved in the regulation of emotion and affect (i.e., the limbic areas). Krieger (1983) emphasizes the potential importance of peptides in CNS function, and discusses 15 selected brain peptides in selected CNS areas. Table 5-8 lists these peptides and their brain regions of highest concentration, as well as the regions where intracellular peptides have been demonstrated. It is of interest to note the obvious clustering of peptides in some regions and almost an absence of peptides in others.

Though the field of neuropeptide research is still in its infancy, a vast amount of information has already accumulated about CNS function and the

TABLE 5-8 Relative Concentrations of Selected Neuropeptides in Selected CNS Areas

	Relative concentrations			
	Very high-high		Moderate-low	
Area	Cell bodies	Other neural elements	Cell bodies	Other neural elements
Hypothalamus	TRH, SRIF, ACTH, α-MSH, β-LPH, β-EP, sub P, NT, ENK	Insulin	LHRH, CCK-8, VIP, ANG	
Limbic areas (including amygdala, hippocampus)	sub P, VIP	CCK-8	LHRH, SRIF, ENK, NT	TRH, ACTH, α-MSH, β-EP, β-LPH, VP
Median eminence		LHRH, TRH SRIF, ACTH, α-MSH, β-LPH, NT, VP		β-EP, ENK, ANG, sub P, CCK-8
Medulla and pons	ENK, sub P		TRH, SRIF	ACTH, α-MSH, ANG, β-LPH, β-EP, VIP, NT, CCK-8, VP
Mesencephalon	sub P		ENK, VIP	LHRH, TRH, NT CCK-8, SRIF, α-MSH, ANG, VP, β-LPH, β-EP
Neocortex	CCK-8, VIP		SRIF, insulin	TRH, ACTH, VP, α-MSH, β-LPH
Thalamus			sub P	SRIF, ACTH, VP, α-MSH, β-EP, NT, insulin, CCK-8, VIP, ENK

Note. Abbreviations: ACTH, adrenocorticotropic hormone; ANG, angiotensin; α-MSH, alpha-melanocyte-stimulating hormone; β-EP, beta-endorphin; β-LPH, beta-lipotropin; CCK-8, cholecystokinin-8; ENK, enkaphalin; LHRH, luteinizing-hormone-releasing hormone; NT, neurotensin; SRIF, somatostatin; sub P, substance P; TRH, thyrotropin-releasing hormone; VIP, vasoactive intestinal polypeptide; VP, vasopressin. Adapted from Krieger (1983).

neuropeptides. It is not possible to discuss this material in depth here, but several key points should be made. First, while much of the neuropeptide research is not directly applicable to the study of depression, there are preliminary but inconclusive reports of neuropeptide involvement in the neurobiochemical etiology of depression. For example, thyrotropin-releasing hormone (TRH) is a peptide found in the hypothalamus that controls the release of thyroid-stimulating hormone. Examination of the effects of TRH on CNS function and behavior was prompted by the discovery that as much as 80% of the TRH in the brain is located outside the hypothalamus. It has been reported that there is an increased metabolism of DA and NE (Rastogi, 1979), as well as increased release of radioactively labeled DA and NE from rat synaptosomes (Horst & Spirt, 1974), following TRH treatment. The ability of TRH to increase DA turnover is consistent with the biogenic amine hypothesis of depression. In fact, in 1972, Prange, Lara, Wilson, Alltop, and Breese presented data implicating a possible role of TRH in depression. These researchers treated 10 women with unipolar depression with a single dose of TRH and observed a significant reduction (approximately 50%) in depressive symptomatology after a few hours. Three other examples of preliminary research indicating a possible role of specific peptides in depression are as follows:

1. Kline and his associates (1977) reported improvement in the symptoms of depression after acute administration of the endogenous opiate peptide beta-endorphin.
2. Gold *et al.* (1980) reported that nonpsychotically depressed bipolar patients had significantly lower levels of CSF vasopressin when compared to manic patients.
3. Post *et al.* (1982) reported that bipolar patients, especially when in the depressed state, had significantly lower levels of CSF oxytocin when compared to healthy controls.

These studies represent an expansion of the approach to the neurobiochemical study of depression and a departure from the almost exclusive emphasis on the monoamine neurotransmitters in depression research. Neuropeptide research is causing a reformulation of some of the most basic concepts of neurotransmission. It was originally believed that all neurons and nerve systems contained only one neurotransmitter. Now, however, it has been demonstrated that neuropeptides can exist in neurons along with classical neurotransmitters or with other peptides (Chan-Palay, Jonsson, & Palay, 1978; Hokfelt *et al.*, 1978; Hokfelt, Johansson, Ljungdahl, Lundberg, & Schultzberg, 1980; Hokfelt *et al.*, 1982; Krieger, 1983). This neuronal coexistence of a biogenic amine transmitter with a biologically active peptide in the CNS was first identified in descending serotonergic pathways in the spinal cord of the rat. Specifically, 5-HT-containing cell bodies in the medullary raphe nuclei and other adjacent cell groups were shown to possess substance-P-like immunoreactivity (Chan-Palay, 1979; Chan-Palay *et al.*, 1978; Hokfelt *et al.*, 1978). Subsequent evidence has shown that coexistence occurs in both central and peripheral neurons, and that ACh and GABA can be involved as well as the catecholamines and 5-HT (Glazer, Steinbusch, Verhofstad, & Basbaum, 1981; Hokfelt *et al.*, 1977; Johansson *et al.*, 1981). In fact, coexistence is becoming so well documented that some researchers even speculate that neurons containing only one classical neurotransmitter may prove to be the exception rather than the rule (Costa, 1982, Hokfelt *et al.*, 1982).

Though much of the functional significance of coexistence of peptides and neurotransmitters is yet to be understood, findings suggest that peptides may both enhance the action of the classical transmitters and act as transmitters themselves. The coexistence of peptides and classical transmitters in nerve endings makes it possible for both to interact in chemical transmission. This has added credence to an area of research that may yield neurobiochemical information having far-reaching implications not only for depression research, but also for the entire field of brain and behavior research. Increasingly, there are reports of interactional effects of one central neurotransmitter or neuropeptide with another.

Understanding the etiology of depression requires an appreciation of the complexity of both normal and impaired brain function. The study of interactional effects between central neuroactive substances may be an avenue to that understanding. At the very least, it represents a research frontier of modern neurobiology that breaks with the generally static, linear, one-system approach to brain function of the past, and provides researchers with a more dynamic and perhaps more realistic approach to brain function and the study of depression. While many of the findings in this area are preliminary and result from studies designed to investigate many different aspects of brain function, they may nevertheless represent the doorway to a new understanding of the neurobiochemical events underlying depression. The rest of this chapter is devoted to highlighting this area of research, relating it, where possible, to the affective disorder of depression.

Neuroactive Interactional Systems and Effects

The extrapyramidal system of the CNS plays an important role in motor control. Interaction and balance of the neuroactive substances in the CNS are becoming increasingly central focal concepts in the understanding of pyramidal function. It has become evident that the interaction of striatal DA, ACh, and GABA neurons (which are part of the pyramidal system) plays a key role in determining striatal function under normal physiological conditions, as well as in neurological disorders such as Huntington chorea and Parkinson disease. In the nigrostriatal system, dopaminergic agonists (e.g., apomorphine) and antipsychotics (e.g., haloperidol) can elicit functional alterations in GABAergic (van der Heyden, Venema, & Korf, 1980), cholinergic (Costa & Cheney, 1978; Racagni, Cheney, Trabucchi, & Costa, 1976), and peptidergic systems (Hong, Yang, Fratta, & Costa, 1978; Marco, Mao, Revuelta, Peralta, & Costa, 1978), which are initiated by their primary action on dopaminergic receptors.

The enkephalins and endorphins are endogenous opioid peptides that are present in the CNS and possess morphine-like pharmacological activity. A number of studies have suggested functional interactions between these opioid peptides and classical neurotransmitters in the CNS (Harsing & Yang, 1984; Hong, Yang, Gillin, DiGiulo, Fratta, & Costa, 1979; Hong, Yang, Gillin, Fratta, & Costa, 1979). For example, Jakubovic (1982) concluded that CNS DA, NE, 5-HT, and other related compounds may modulate the levels and physiological functions of endogenous peptide opioids in the CNS by their direct interaction with the enzymatic degradation of these peptides.

Cholecystokinin (CCK), one of the identified central neuropeptides, has been shown to increase the activity in dopaminergic neurons (Skirboll *et al.*, 1981) and to interact with DA at the DA receptor level (Fuxe *at al.*, 1981). Specific CNS neurons containing both DA and CCK-like substance have significant projections to the limbic areas of the forebrain. This localization of nerve endings having DA-CCK coexistence is noteworthy in light of their postulated interactional effects, the implicated involvement of dopaminergic involvement in depression, as well as, the reported overactivity of dopaminergic systems in schizophrenia (Matthysse & Kety, 1975).

In the earlier discussion of receptor research relevant to the study of depression, the effects of chronic antidepressant treatment have been emphasized. It was stated that different receptor components may be involved in the adaptive changes occurring in NE neurons following chronic exposure to antidepressant treatments. Racagni *et al.* (1983) have attempted to study some of the presynaptic and postsynaptic biochemical events that may be involved in the development of the subsensitivity of the NE system following chronic antidepressant treatment. One conclusion drawn from this study is that resultant subsensitivity of NE neurons could be indicative of a local regulation of NE release by other neurotransmitters, specifically 5-HT. Sulser (1983) cites evidence supporting both the importance of NE signal input and the corequirement of intact 5-HT neurons for beta-adrenergic down-regulation. He states that this, as well as a wealth of other evidence demonstrating a functional link between serotonergic and noradrenergic neuronal systems involving the regulation of NE receptors, provides a scientific basis for a "serotonin-norepinephrine-link-hypothesis of affective disorders" (1983, p. 303) Consistent with this position are studies indicating that serotonergic neurons may regulate NE release (Crespi, Buda, McRae-Degueurceing, & Pujol, 1980; Renaud, Buda, Lewis, & Pujol, 1975) and biochemical and electrophysiological evidence supporting the existence of presynaptic serotonergic receptors on NE nerve terminals (Samanin, Quattrone, Consolo, Ladinsky, & Algeri, 1978; Wang, DeMontigny, Gold, Roth, & Aghajanian, 1979).

In 1972, Janowsky and colleagues proposed that a balance between central cholinergic and adrenergic neurotransmitter activity may play a role in the etiology of the affective disorders, with depression being a disease of cholinergic dominance. This proposition was based, in large part, on research findings resulting from the use of physostigmine. This compound is a reversible cholinesterase inhibitor that increases central ACh levels and thus disturbs the proposed cholinergic-adrenergic balance. This drug has been shown to act as an antimanic agent, to induce depression, and to produce effects that are opposite to those seen with adrenergic stimulation (Janowsky, El-Yousef, Davis, & Sekerke, 1972a, 1972b, 1973). As an extension of this original work, Shopsin, Janowsky, Davis, and Gershon (1975) proposed that an imbalance among adrenergic, dopaminergic, and cholinergic central neurotransmitters may be responsible for psychotic symptoms, including mania, depression, and schizoaffective psychosis. Depression was again cited as specifically resulting from a preponderance of adrenergic activity. In 1983, Janowsky, Risch, and Gillin, reaffirming their earlier postulations, reported evidence that cholinergic compounds, alone and in combination with antiadrenergic drugs, may be effective in the rapid treatment of mania. Furthermore, they offered evidence that anticholinergic agents may have potential antidepressant effects.

What is seen here, through these examples of relatively recent experimental investigations, is an ever-evolving understanding of the complexity of the CNS as a whole and of the neurobiochemical profile of depression in particular. The study of neurotransmitter-neuropeptide interactions and their importance in depression is, at present, speculative and pioneering in nature. But it is an endeavor that, encouraged by preliminary evidence, calls for further investigation. It will be the task of future research to determine to what extent the balance between multiple synaptic messengers is disturbed in the various mental disorders and how drugs of various types may affect the complex interplay between the compounds released at synapses.

References

Aghajanian, G. K. (1981). Tricyclic antidepressants and single-cell responses to serotonin and norepinephrine: A review of chronic studies. In E. Usdin, W. E. Bunney, & J. M. Davis (Eds.), *Neuroreceptors — basic and clinical aspects* (pp. 27-35). New York: Wiley.

Ariens, E. J., & Simonis, A. M. (1983). Physiological and pharmacological aspects of adrenergic receptor classification. *Biochemical Pharmacology, 32* (10), 1539-1545.

Asberg, M., Thoren, P., Traskman, K., Bertilsson, L. & Ringberger, V. (1976). "Serotonin depression" — a biochemical subgroup within the affective disorders? *Science, 191*, 478-480.

Ashcroft, G. W., Crawford, T. B. B., Eccleston, D., Sherman, D. F., McDougall, E. Y., Stanton, T. B., & Binns, T. R. (1966). 5-Hydroxyindole compounds in the cerebrospinal fluid of patients with psychiatric or neurological diseases. *Lancet, 2*, 1049-1052.

Ayd, F. J. (1958). Drug-induced depression: Fact or fallacy? *NY State Journal of Medicine, 58*, 354-356.

Baldessarini, R. J. (1975). Biogenic amine hypothesis in affective disorders. In F. F. Flach & S. Draghi (Eds.), *The nature and treatment of depression* (pp. 347-385). New York: Plenum Press.

Beckmann, H., & Goodwin, F. K. (1980). Urinary MHPG in subgroups of depressed patients and normal controls. *Neuropsychobiology, 6*, 91-100.

Berger, P. A., & Barchas, T. D. (1977). Monoamine oxidase inhibitors. In E. Usdin & I. S. Forrest (Eds.), *Psychotherapeutic drugs* (pp. 1173-1216). New York: Marcel Dekker.

Berger, P. A., Faull, K. F., Kilkowski, J., Anderson, P. J., Kraemer, H., Davis, K., & Barchas, J. D. (1980). CSF monoamine metabolites in depression and schizophrenia. *American Journal of Psychiatry, 137*, 174-180.

Bernasconi, R., & Martin, P. (1979). Effects of antiepileptic drugs on the GABA turnover rate. *Archives of Pharmacology, 307*, 251.

Berrettini, W. H., Nurnberger, J. I., Jr., Hare, T. A., Simmons-Alling, S., Gershon, E. S. & Post, R. M. (1983). Reduced plasma and CSF gamma-aminobutyric acid in affective illness: Effects of lithium carbonate. *Biological Psychiatry, 18* (2), 185-194.

Bohlen, P., Huot, S., & Palfreyman, M. (1979). The relationship between GABA concentrations in brain and cerebrospinal fluid. *Brain Research, 167* 297-305.

Bowers, M. B., Jr. (1974). Lumbar CSF 5-hydroxyindoleacetic acid and homovanillic acid in affective syndromes. *Journal of Nervous and Mental Disease, 158*, 325-330.

Bunney, W. E., Jr., & Davis, J. M. (1965). Norepinephrine in depressive reaction: A review. *Archives of General Psychiatry, 13*, 483-494.

Chan-Palay, V. (1979). Combined immunocytochemistry and autoradiography after in vivo injection of monoclonal antibody to substance P and ^{3}H-serotonin: Coexistence of two putative transmitters in single raphe cells and fibre plexus. *Anatomy and Embryology, 156*, 241-254.

Chan-Palay, V., Jonsson, G., & Palay, S. L. (1978). Serotonin and substance-P coexist in neurons of rat's central nervous system. *Proceedings of the National Academy of Sciences USA, 75*, 1582-1586.

Charney, D. S., Menkes, D. B., & Heninger, G. R. (1981). Receptor sensitivity and the mechanism of action of antidepressant treatment: Implications for the etiology and therapy of depression *Archives of General Psychiatry, 38*, 1160-1180.

Chiodo, L., & Antelman, S. M. (1980a). Electroconvulsive shock: Progressive dopamine autoreceptor subsensitivity independent of repeated treatment. *Science, 210*, 799-801.

Chiodo, L., & Antelman, S. M. (1980b). Repeated tricyclics induce a progressive dopamine autoreceptor subsensitivity independent of daily drug treatment. *Nature, 287*, 451-454.

Cohen, R. M., Campbell, I. C., Dauphin, M., Tallman, J. F., & Murphy, D. L. (1982). Changes in alpha and beta receptor densities in rat brain as a result of treatment with monoamine oxidase inhibiting antidepressants. *Neuropharmacology, 21*, 293-298.

Coppen, A., Prange, A. J., Whybrow, P. C., & Noguera, R. (1972). Abmormalities of indoleamines in affective disorders. *Archives of General Psychiatry, 26*, 474-478.

Coppen, A., Shaw, D. M., Herzberg, B., & Maggs, R. (1967). Tryptophan in treatment of depression. *Lancet, 2*, 1178-1180.

Costa, E. (1982). Coexistence of putative neuromodulators in the same axon: Pharmacological consequences at receptors. In A. Cuello (Ed.), *Cotransmission* (pp. 25-50). London: Macmillan.

Costa, E., & Cheney, D. L. (1978). Regulation of cholinergic neurons by dopaminergic terminals: Influence of cataleptogenic and noncataleptogenic antipsychotics. S. Garattini, I. F. Pujol, & R. Samanin (Eds.), *Interactions between putative neurotransmitters in the brain* (pp. 23-38). New York: Raven Press.

Crespi, F., Buda, M., McRae-Degueurce, A., & Pujol, J. F. (1980). Alteration of tyrosine hydroxylase activity in the locus coeruleus after administration of p-chlorophenylalanine. *Brain Research, 191*, 501-509.

Crews, F. T., & Smith, C. B. (1980). Potentiation of responses to field stimulation of isolated rat left atria during chronic tricyclic antidepressant administration. *Journal of Pharmacology and Experimental Therapeutics, 25*, 143-149.

Dencker, S. J., Malm, V., Roos, B. E., & Werdinius, B. (1966). Acid monoamine metabolites of cerebrospinal fluid in mental depression and mania. *Journal of Neurochemistry, 13*, 1545-1548.

Edwards, D. J., Spiker, D. G., Neil, J. F., Kupfer, D. J., & Rizk, M. (1980). MHPG excretion in depression. *Psychiatry Research, 2*, 295-305.

Finberg, J. P. M., & Youdim, M. B. H. (1983). Selective MAO A and B inhibitors: Their mechanism of action and pharmacology. *Neuropharmacology, 22* (3B), 441-446.

Frazer, A. (1980). Antidepressant drugs: effect on adrenergic responsiveness and monoamine receptors. *Psychopharmacology Bulletin, 16*, 77-78.

Frazer, A., & Lucki, I. (1982). Effects on beta-adrenergic and serotonineregic receptors. *Advances in Biochemical Psychopharmacology, 31*, 69-90.

Frazer, A., Pandley, G., Mendels, J., Neeley, S., Kane, M., & Hess, M. E. (1974). The effect of triiodothyronine in combination with imipramine on [^{3}H]-cyclic AMP production in slices of rat cerebral cortex. *Neuropharmacology, 13*, 1131-1140.

Fuxe, K., Agnati, L. F., Kohler, C., Kuonen, D., Ogren, S.-O., Andersson, K., & Hokfelt, T. (1981). Characterization of normal and supersensitive dopamine receptors: Effects of ergot drugs and neuropeptides. *Journal of Neural Transmission, 51*, 3-37.

Fuxe, K., Ogren, S.-O., Agnati, L. F., Benfenati, F., Fredholm, B., Andersson, K., Zini, I., & Eneroth, P. (1983). Chronic antidepressant treatment and central 5-HT synapses. *Neuropharmacology, 22* (3B), 389-400.

Garcia-Sevilla, J. A., Zis, A. P., Hollingsworth, P. J., Greden, J. F., & Smith, C. B. (1981). Platelet alpha$_2$-adrenergic receptors in major depressive disorders. *Archives of General Psychiatry 38*, 1327-1332.

Gerner, R. H., & Hare, T. A. (1981). CSF GABA in normal subjects and patients with depression, schizophrenia, mania and anorexia nervosa. *American Journal of Psychiatry, 138*, 1098-1101.

Gershon, S., & Shaw, F. H. (1961). Psychiatric sequelae of chronic exposure to organophosphorous insecticides. *Lancet, 1* 1371-1374.

Glazer, E. J., Steinbusch, H., Verhofstad, A., & Basbaum, A. I. (1981). Serotonin neurons in nucleus raphe dorsalis and paragigantocellularis of the cat contain enkephalin. *Journal of Physiology* (Paris), *77*, 241-245.

Gold, P. W., Goodwin, F. K., Ballenger, J. C., Weingartner, H., Robertson, G. L., & Post, R. M. (1980). Central vasopressin function in affective illness. In D. de Wied & P. Van Keep (Eds.), *Hormones and the brain* (pp. 241-252). Lancaster, England: MTP Press.

Goodwin, F. K., Post, R. M., Dunner, D. L., & Gordon, E. K. (1973). Cerebrospinal fluid amine metabolites in affective illness: The probenecid technique. *American Journal of Psychiatry, 130*, 73-79.

Gordon, E. K., & Oliver, J. (1971). 3-Methoxy-4-hydroxphenylethylene glycol in human CSF. *Clinica Chimica Acta, 35*, 145-150.

Green, A. R., Peralta, E., Hong, J. S., Mao, C. C., Alterwill, C. K., & Costa, E. (1978). Alterations in GABA metabolism and met-enkephalin content in rat brain following repeated electroconvulsive shocks. *Journal of Neurochemistry, 31*, 607-618.

Greengard, P. (1978). *Cyclic nucleotides, phosphorylated proteins, and neuronal function*. New York: Raven Press.

Grove, J., Tell, G., Schechter, P. J., Koch-Weser, J., Warter, J. M., Marescaux, C., & Rumbach, L. (1980). Increased CSF gamma-aminobutyric acid after treatment with gamma-vinyl GABA. *Lancet, 2*, 647.

Harsing, L. G., & Yang, H-Y. T. (1984). Serotonergic regulation of hypothalamic met$_5$-enkephalin content. In I. Hanin (Ed.), *Dynamics of neurotransmitter function* (pp. 169-176). New York: Raven Press.

Hokfelt, T., Elfvin, L. G., Elde, R., Shultzberg, M., Goldstein, M., & Luft, R. (1977). Occurrence of somatostatin-like immunoreactivity in some peripheral sympathetic noradrenergic neurons. *Proceedings of the National Academy of Sciences USA, 74*, 3587-3591.

Hokfelt, T., Johansson, O., Ljungdahl, A., Lundberg, J. M., & Schultzberg, M. (1980). Peptidergic neurones. *Nature, 284*, 515-521.

Hokfelt, T., Ljungdahl, A., Steinbush, H., Verhofstad, A., Nilsson, G., Brodin, E., Pernow, B., & Goldstein, M. (1978). Immunohistochemical evidence of substance P-like immunoreactivity on some 5-hydroxytryptamine-containing neurons in the rat central nervous system. *Neuroscience, 3*, 517-538.

Hokfelt, T., Lundberg, J. M., Skirboll, L., Johansson, O., Schultzberg, M., & Vincent, S. R. (1982). Coexistence of classical transmitters and peptides in neurones. In A. Cuello (Ed.), *Cotransmission* (pp. 77-125). London: Macmillan.

Hollister, L. E. (1981). Excretion of 3-methoxy-4-hydroxyphenylglycol in depressed and geriatric patients and normal persons. *International Pharmacopsychiatry, 16*, 138-143.

Hollister, L. E., Davis, K. L., & Berger, P. A. (1980). Subtypes of depression based on excretion of MHPG and response to nortriptyline. *Archives of General Psychiatry, 37*, 1107-1110.

Hong, J. S., Yang, H.-Y. T., Fratta, W., & Costa, E. (1978). Rat striatal methionine-enkephalin content after chronic teatment with cataleptogenic and noncataleptogenic antischizophrenic drugs. *Journal of Pharmacology and Experimental Therapeutics, 205*, 141-147.

Hong, J. S., Yang, H.-Y. T., Gillin, J. C., DiGiulio, A. M., Fratta, W., & Costa, E. (1979). Chronic treatment with halaperidol accelerates the biosynthesis of enkephalins in rat striatum. *Brain Research, 160*, 192-195.

Hong, J. S., Yang, H.-Y. T., Gillin, J. C., Fratta, W., & Costa, E. (1979). Participation of met_5-enkephalin in the action of antipsychotic drugs. In E. Usdin & W. E. Bunney, Jr. (Eds.), *Endorphins in mental health research*, (pp. 105-114). London: Macmillan.

Horst, W. D., & Spirt, N. (1974). A possible mechanism for the antidepressant activity of thyrotropin-releasing hormone. *Life Sciences, 15*, 1073-1082.

Hosli, L., & Hosli, E. (1979). Autoradiographic studies on the cellular localization of GABA and beta-alanine uptake by neurons and glial tissue in culture. *Advances in Experimental Medicine and Biology, 123*, 205-218.

Jakubovic, A. (1982). The effects of biogenic amines on cleavage of met-enkephalin by brain tissue extracts. *Progress in Neuro-Psychopharmacology and Biological Psychiatry, 6*, 399-402.

Janowsky, D. S., El-Yousef, M. K., & Davis, J. M. (1974). Acetylcholine and depression. *Psychosomatic Medicine, 36*, 248-257.

Janowsky, D. S., El-Yousef, M. K., Davis, J. M., & Sekerke, H. J. (1972a). A cholinergic-adrenergic hypothesis of mania and depression. *Lancet, 2*, 632-635.

Janowsky, D. S., El-Yousef, M. K., Davis, J. M., & Sekerke, H. J. (1972b). Cholinergic antagonism of methylphenidate-induced stereotyped behavior. *Psychopharmacology, 27*, 295-303.

Janowsky, D. S., El-Yousef, M. H., Davis, J. M., & Sekerke, H. J. (1973). Provocation of schizophrenia symptoms by intravenous administration of methylphenidate. *Archives of General Psychiatry, 28*, 185-191.

Janowsky, D. S., Risch, S. C., & Gillin, J. C. (1983). Adrenergic-cholinergic balance and the treatment of affective disorders. *Progress in Neuro-Psychopharmacology and Biological Psychiaty, 7*, 297-307.

Jensen, K. (1959). Depression in patients treated with reserpine for arterial hypertension. *Acta Psychiatrica et Neurologica Scandanavica, 34*, 195-204.

Johansson, O., Hokfelt, T., Pernow, B., Jeffcoate, S. L., White, N., Steinbusch, H. W. M., Verhofstad, A. A. J., Emson, P. C., & Spindel, E. (1981). Immunohistochemical support for the three putative transmitters in one neuron: Coexistence of 5-hydroxytryptamine, substance P and thyrotropin releasing hormone-like immunoreactivity in medullary neurons projecting to the spinal cord. *Neuroscience, 6*, 1857-1881.

Jones, D., Kelwala, S., Pohl, R., Dube, S., Jackson, E., & Sitaram, N. (1986). Cholinergic REM sleep induction response as a marker of endogenous depression. In I. Hanin (Ed.), *Dynamics of cholinergic function* (pp. 375-383). New York: Plenum Press.

Kasa, K., Otsuki, S., Yamamoto, M., Sato, M., Kuroda, H., & Ogawa, N. (1982). Cerebrospinal fluid gamma-aminobutyric acid and homovanillic acid in depressive disorders. *Biological Psychiatry, 17* (8), 877-883.

Katz, M. M., Secunda, S., Hirschfeld, R. M. A., & Koslow, S. H. (1979). The NIMH Clinical Research Branch Collaborative Program on the Psychobiology of Depression. *Archives of General Psychiatry, 36*, 765-771.

Kellar, K. J., Cascio, C. S., Butler, J. A., & Kurtzke, R. N. (1981). Differential effects of electroconvulsive shock and antidepressant drugs on serotonin-2 receptors in rat brain. *European Journal of Pharmacology, 69*, 515-518.

Kline, N. S., Li, C. H., Lehmann, H. E., Lajtha, A., Laski, E., & Cooper, T. (1977). Beta-endorphin-induced changes in schizophrenia and depressed patients. *Archives of General Psychiatry, 34*, 1111-1112.

Korf, J., & van Praag, H. M. (1971). Amine metabolism in human brain: Further evaluation of the probenecid test. *Brain Research, 35*, 221-230.

Koslow, S. H., Mass, J. W., Bowden, C. L., Davis, J. M., Hanin, I., & Javaid, J. (1983). Cerebrospinal fluid and urinary biogenic amines and metabolites in depression and mania: A controlled, univariate analysis. *Archives of General Psychiatry, 40*, 999-1010.

Krieger, D. T. (1983). Brain peptides: What, where, and why? *Science, 222*, 975-985.

Krnjevic, R. J., & Schwartz, S. (1966). Is gamma-aminobutyric acid an inhibitory transmitter? *Nature, 211*, 1372-1374.

Maas, J. W., Fawcett, J., & De Kirmenjian, H. (1968). 3-Methoxy-4-hydroxy phenylglycol (MHPG) excretion in depressive states. *Archives of General Psychiatry, 19*, 129-134.

Maas, J. W., Koslow, S. H., Davis, J. M., Katz, M. M., Mendels, J., Robins, E., Stokes, P. E., & Bowden, C. L. (1980). Biological component of the NIMH Clinical Research Branch Collaborative Program on the Psychobiology of Depression: I. Background and theoretical considerations. *Psychological Medicine, 10*, 759-776.

Maj, J., Mogilnicka, E., & Klimeki, V. (1979). The effect of repeated administration of antidepressant drugs on the responsiveness of rats to catecholamine agonists. *Journal of Neural Transmission, 44*, 221-235.

Mandell, A. J., Segal, D. S. & Kuczenski, R. (1974). Metabolic adaptation to antidepressant drugs — a neurochemical paradox. *Psychopharmacology Bulletin*, 10, 53-54.

Marco, E., Mao, C. C., Revuelta, A., Peralta, E., & Costa, E. (1978). Turnover rates of gamma-aminobutyric acid in substantia nigra, n. caudatus, globus pallidus and n. accumbens of rats injected with cataleptogenic and non-cataleptogenic antipsychotics. *Neuropharmacology, 17*, 589-596.

Matthysse, S. W., & Kety, S. S. (Eds.). (1975). *Catecholamines and schizophrenia.* Oxford: Pergamon Press.

Mendels, J., Frazer, A., Fitzgerald, R. G., Ramsey, T. A., & Stokes, J. W. (1972). Biogenic amine metabolites in cerebrospinal fluid of depressed and manic patients. *Science, 175*, 1380-1382.

Menkes, D. B., & Aghajanian, G. K. (1981). Alpha-1 adrenoceptor-mediated responses in the lateral geniculate nucleus are enhanced by chronic antidepressant treatment. *European Journal of Pharmacology, 74*, 27-35.

Oreland, L., Wilberg, A., Asberg, M., Traskman, L., Sjostrand, L., Thoren, P., Bertilsson, L., & Tybring, G. (1981). Platelet MAO activity and monoamine metabolites in cerebrospinal fluid in depressed and suicidal patients and in healthy controls. *Psychiatric Research, 4*, 21-29.

Otsuka, M. (1973). Gamma-aminobutyric acid and some other transmitter candidates in the nervous system. In G. H. Acheson (Ed.), *Pharmacology and the future of man: Proceedings of the Fifth International Congress on Pharmacology* (Vol. 4, pp. 186-201). Basel: Karger.

Papeschi, R, & McClure, D. J. (1971). Homovanillic and 5-hydroxyindoleacetic acid in cerebrospinal fluid of depressed patients. *Archives of General Psychiatry, 25*, 354-358.

Peroutka, S. J., Lebovitz, R. M., & Snyder, S. H. (1981). Two distinct central serotonin receptors with different physiological functions. *Science, 212*, 827-829.

Peroutka, S. J., & Snyder, S. H. (1979). Multiple serotonin receptors: Differential binding of (^{3}H)-5-hydroxytryptamine, (^{3}H)-lysergic acid diethylamide, and (^{3}H)-spirperidol. *Molecular Pharmacology, 16*, 687-699.

Peroutka, S. J., & Synder, S. H. (1980). Chronic antidepressant treatment decreases spiroperidol-labeled serotonin receptor binding. *Science, 210*, 88-90.

Pickar, D., Sweeney, D. R., Maas, J. W., & Heninger, G. R. (1978). Primary affective disorder, clinical state change, and MHPG excretion. *Archives of General Psychiatry, 35*, 1378-1383.

Post, R. M., Ballenger, J. C., Hare, T. A., Goodwin, F. K., Lake, C. R., Jimerson, D. C., Bunney,

W. E. (1980). Cerebrospinal fluid GABA in normals and patients with affective disorders. *Brain Research Bulletin, 5*, 755-759.

Post, R. M., Gold, P., Rubinow, D. R., Ballenger, J. C., Bunney, W. E., Jr., & Goodwin, F. K. (1982). Peptides in the cerebrospinal fluid of neuropsychiatric patients: An approach to central nervous system peptide function. *Life Sciences, 31*, 1-15.

Post, R. M., Gordon, E. K., Goodwin, F. K., & Bunney, W. E., Jr. (1973). Central norepinephrine metabolism in affective illness: MHPG in the CSF. *Science, 179*, 1002-1003.

Post, R. M., Uhde, T. W., Rubinow, D. R., Ballenger, J. C., & Gold, P. W. (1983). Biochemical effects of carbamazepine: Relationship to its mechanisms of action in affective illness. *Progress in Neuro-Psychopharmsiology and Biological Psychiatry, 7*, 263-271.

Prange, A. J., Jr., Lara, P. P., Wilson, I. C., Alltop, L. B., & Breese, G. R. (1972). Effects of thyrotropin-releasing hormone in depression. *Lancet, 1*, 999-1002.

Racagni, G., Cheney, D. L., Trabucchi, M., & Costa, E. (1976). In vivo actions of clozapine and haloperidol on the turnover rate of acetylcholine in rat striatum. *Journal of Pharmacology and Experimental Therapeutics, 196*, 323-332.

Racagni, G., Mocchetti, I., Calderini, G., Battistella, A., & Bruenello, N. (1983). Temporal sequence of changes in central noradrenergic system of rat after prolonged antidepressant treatment: Receptor desensitization and neurotransmitter interactions. *Neuropharmacology, 22* (3B), 415-424.

Rastogi, R. B. (1979). Thyrotropin-releasing hormone influences on behavior: Possible involvement of brain monoaminergic systems. In R. Collu, J. A. Barbeau, J. G. Rochefort, & J. R. Ducharme (Eds.), *Central nervous system effects of hypothalamic hormones and other peptides* (pp. 123-140). New York: Raven Press.

Renaud, B., Buda, M., Lewis, B. D., & Pujol, J. F. (1975). Effects of 5, 7-dihydroxytryptamine on tyrosine-hydroxylase activity in central catecholaminergic neurons of the rat. *Biochemical Pharmacology, 24*, 1739-1742.

Risch, S. C., Cohen, P. M., Janowsky, D. S., Kalin, N. H., Insel, T. R., & Murphy, D. L. (1981). Physostigmine induction of depressive symptomatology in normal volunteer subjects. *Journal of Psychiatric Research, 4*, 89-94.

Roos, B. E., & Sjostrom, R. (1969). 5-Hydroxyindoleacetic acid (and homovanillic acid) levels in the cerebrospinal fluid after probenecid application in patients with manic depressive psychosis. *Pharmacology Clinics, 1*, 153-155.

Ryall, R. W. (1975). Amino acid reuptake in CNS: I. GABA and glycine in the spinal cord. In L. L. Iversen, S. N. Snyder, & S. D. Iversen (Eds.), *Handbook of psychopharmacology* (Vol. 4, Sec. 1, pp. 83-128). New York: Plenum Press.

Samanin, R., Quattrone, A., Consolo, S., Ladinsky, H., & Algeri, S. (1978). Biochemical and pharmacological evidence of the interaction of serotonin with other aminergic systems in the brain. In S. Garattini, J. F. Pujol, & R. Samanin (Eds.), *Interactions between putative neurotransmitters in the brain* (pp. 383-399). New York: Raven Press.

Schildkraut, J. J. (1965). The catecholamine hypothesis of affective disorders: A review of supporting evidence. *American Journal Psychiatry, 122*, 509-522.

Schildkraut, J. J. (1973). Norepinephrine metabolites as biochemical criteria for classifying depressive disorders and predicting responses to treatment: Preliminary findings. *American Journal of Psychiatry, 130*, 695-698.

Schildkraut, J. J., Orsulak, P. J., LaBrie, R. A, Schatzberg, A. F., Gudeman, J. E., Cole, J. O., & Rohde, W. A. (1978). Toward a biochemical classification of depressive disorders: II. Application of multivariate discriminant function analysis to data on urinary catecholamines and metabolites. *Archives of General Psychiatry, 35*, 1436-1439.

Schildkraut, J. J., Orsulak, P. J., Schatzberg, A. F., Gudeman, J. E., Cole, J. O., Rohde, W. A., & LaBrie, R. A. (1978). Toward a biochemical classification of depressive disorders: I. Differences in urinary excretion of MHPG and other catecholamine metabolites in clinically defined subtypes of depression. *Archives of General Psychiatry, 35*, 1427-1433.

Secunda, S. K., Koslow, S. H., Redmond, D. E., Garver, D., Ramsey, T. A., Croughan, J., Kocsis,

J., Hanin, I., Lieberman, K., & Casper, R. (1980). Biological component of the NIMH Collaborative Clinical Research Branch Collaborative Program on the Psychobiology of Depression: II. Methodology and data analysis. *Psychological Medicine, 10*, 777-793.

Segana, T., Yamamura, H. I., & Kusiyawa, K. (Eds.). (1983). Molecular pharmacology of neurotransmitter receptors [Special issue]. *Advances in Biochemical Psychopharmacology, 36*.

Serra, G., Argiolas, A., Klimek, V., Fadda, F., & Gessa, G. L. (1979). Chronic treatment with antidepressants prevents the inhibitory effect of small doses of apomorphine synthesis and motor activity. *Life Sciences, 25*, 415-424.

Shaw, D. M., O'Keefe, R., MacSweeney, D. A., Brooksbank, B. W. L., Norguera, R., & Coppen, A. (1973). 3-Methoxy-4-hydroxyphenylglycol in depression. *Psychological Medicine, 3*, 333-336.

Sherman, A. D., & Petty, I. (1980). Neurochemical basis of the action of antidepressants on learned helpessness. *Behavioral and Neural Biology, 30*, 119-134.

Shopsin, B. & Gershon, S. (1978). Dopamine receptor stimulation in the treatment of depression: Piribedil. *Neuropsychobiology, 4*, 1-14.

Shopsin, B., Janowsky, D., Davis, J., & Gershon, S. (1975). Rebound phenomena in manic patients following physostigmine: Towards an understanding of the aminergic mechanisms underlying affective disorders. In E. Domino & J. Davis (Eds.), *Neurotransmitter balances regulating behavior* (pp. 149-155). New York: Raven Press.

Shopsin, B., Wilk, S., Sathananthan, G., Gershon, S., & Davis, K. (1974). Catecholamines and affective disorders revised: A critical assessment. *Journal of Nervous and Mental Disease, 158*, 369-383.

Sitaram, N., Jones, D., Kelwala, S., Bell, J., Stevenson, J., & Gershon, S. (1983). *Progress in Neuro-Psychopharmacology and Biological Psychiatry, 7*, 273-286.

Sitaram, N., Nurnberger, J. I., Gershon, E. S., & Gillin, J. C. (1980). Faster cholinergic REM sleep induction in euthymic patients with primary affective illness. *Science, 208*, 200-202.

Sjostrom, R. & Roos, B. E. (1972). 5-Hydroxyindoleacetic acid and homovanillic acid in cerebrospinal fluid in manic-depressive psychosis. *European Journal of Clinical Pharmacology, 4*, 170-176.

Skirboll, L. Grace, A. A., Hommer, D. W., Rehfeld, J., Goldstein, M., Hokfelt, T., & Bunney, B. S. (1981). Petide-monoamine coexistence: Studies of the actions of cholecystokinin-like peptide on the electrical activity of midbrain dopamine neurons. *Neuroscience, 6*, 2111-2124.

Smith, C. B., Garcia-Sevilla, J. A., & Hollingsworth, P. J. (1981). Alpha-2 adrenoreceptors in rat brain are decreased after long-term tricyclic antidepressant drug treatment. *Brain Research, 210*, 413-418.

Smith, C. B., Hollingsworth, P. J., Garcia-Sevilla, J. A., & Zis, A. P. (1983). Platelet alpha-2 adrenoreceptors are decreased in number after antidepressant therapy. *Progress in Neuro-Psychopharmacology and Biological Psychiatry, 7*, 241-247.

Snyder, S. H. (1980). Brain peptides as neurotransmitters. *Science, 209*, 976-983.

Snyder, S. H., & Peroutka, S. J. (1982). A possible role of serotonin receptors in antidepressant drug action. *Pharmacopsychiatry, 15*, 131-134.

Sokoloff, L. (1977). Relation between physiological function and energy metabolism in the central nervous system. *Journal of Neurochemistry, 29*, 13-26.

Spiker, D. G., Edwards, D., Hanin, I., Neil, J. F., & Kupfer, D. J. (1980). Urinary MHPG and clinical response to amitriptyline in depressed patients. *American Journal of Psychiatry, 137*, 1183-1187.

Stanford, S. C., & Nutt, D. J. (1982). Comparison of the effects of repeated electroconvulsive shock on alpha$_2$- and beta-adrenoreceptors in different regions of rat brain. *Neuroscience, 7*, 1753-1757.

Subrahmanyam, S. (1975). Role of biogenic amines in certain pathological conditions. *Brain Research, 87*, 355-362.

Sugrue, M. F. (1981). Current concepts on the mechanisms of action of antidepressant drugs. *Pharmacology and Therapeutics, 13*, 219-247.

Sulser, F. (1983). Deamplification of noradrenergic signal transfer by antidepressants: A unified catecholamine-serotonin hypothesis of affective disorders. *Psychopharmacology Bulletin, 19* (3), 300-304.

Sulser, F., & Vetulani, J. (1977). The noradrenergic cyclic AMP generating system in the limbic forebrain: A functional postsynaptic norepinephrine receptor system and its modification by drugs which either precipitate or alleviate depression. In I. Hanin & E. Usdin (Eds.), *Animal models in psychiatry and neurology* (pp. 189-199). Oxford: Pergamon Press.

Tamminga, C. A., Smith, R. C., Ericksen, S. E., Chang, S., & Davis, J. M. (1977). Cholinergic influences in tardive dyskinesia. *American Journal of Psychiatry, 7*, 769-774.

van der Heyden, J. A. M., Venema, K., & Korf, J. (1980). Biphasic and opposite effects of dopamine and apomorphine on endogenous GABA release in the rat substantia nigra. *Journal of Neurochemistry, 34*, 119-125.

van Praag, H. M., & Korf, J. (1971). Retarded depression and the dopamine metabolism. *Psychopharmacology, 19*, 199-203.

van Praag, H. M., Korf, J., & Puite, J. (1970). 5-Hydroxyindoleacetic acid levels in the cerebrospinal fluid of depressive patients treated with probenecid. *Nature, 225*, 1259-1260.

van Praag, H. M., Korf, J., & Schut, d. (1973). Cerebral monoamines and depression: An investigation with the probenecid technique. *Archives of General Psychiatry, 28*, 827-831.

Vestergaard, P., Sorensen, T. Hoppe, E., Rafaelsen, O. J., Yates, C. M., & Nicolaou N. (1978). Biogenic amine metabolites in cerebrospinal fluid of patients with affective disorders. *Acta Psychiatrica Scandinavica, 58*, 88-96.

Vetulani, J., Lebrecht, V., & Pilc, A. (1981). Enhancement of responsiveness of the central serotonergic system and electroconvulsive treatment. *Europearn Journal of Pharmacology, 75*, 81-85.

Vetulani, J., Stawarz, R. J., & Sulser, F. (1976). Adaptive mechanisms of the noradrenenergic cyclic AMP generating system in the limbic forebrain of the rat: Adaptation to persistent changes in the availability of norephephrine (NE). *Journal of Neurochemistry, 27*, 661-666.

Wang, R. Y., DeMontigny, C., Gold, B. I., Roth, R. H., & Aghajanian, G. K. (1979). Denervation supersensitivity to serotonin in rat forebrain single cell studies. *Brain Research, 178*, 479-497.

Wielosz, M. (1981). Increased sensitivity to dopaminergic agonists after repeated electroconvulsive shock (ECS) in rats. *Neuropharmacology, 20*, 941-945.

Wilk, S., Shopsin, B., Gershon, S., & Suhl, M. (1972). Cerebrospinal fluid levels of MHPG in affective disorders. *Nature, 235*, 440-441.

Wood, A. J. J., Feldman, R., & Nadeau, J. (1982). Physiological regulation of beta-receptors in man. In I. H. Slater (Ed.), *Clinical and experimental hypertension* (Vol. A4 [4 + 5], pp. 807-817). New York: Marcel Dekker.

CHAPTER 6

The Neuroendocrine Measurement of Depression

PETER E. STOKES
Payne Whitney Psychiatric Clinic
New York Hospital-Cornell University Medical Center

INTRODUCTION

Measurements of neuroendocrine function in affective disorder have gained increasing popularity over the past 20 years. To a large extent, this is a reflection of the increasing availability of sensitive, reproducible assays for various hormones, and our increased knowledge of central nervous system (CNS) control mechanisms for hormone secretion from the pituitary gland. Parallel to this, and to some degree preceding it, has been our understanding and still progressing knowledge of biogenic amines and neurotransmitter systems within the CNS. With the knowledge that hypothalamic hormones are under the influence of various CNS amine systems, many investigators have pursued the concept that the measurement of hormones in various biofluids, or the response of hormones to pharmacological manipulations, might provide information about the CNS neurotransmitters or systems that are involved in or characteristic of particular behavioral states, syndromes, or diagnostic categories. In fact, pharmacological manipulations have further increased our understanding of neuroendocrine control mechanisms in the intact animal. Studies in humans are obviously much more difficult and hampered, because only indirect and peripheral measures can be obtained about CNS neurotransmitters and hormones. Nevertheless, as our pharmacological tools become more specific to the neurotransmitter systems affected, we will be able to refine our neuroendocrine response measures further.

This review focuses on related aspects of the past two decades' interest in neuroendocrinology and psychiatry, and attempts to address the following questions:

1. Do neuroendocrine measures provide a greater understanding of clinical psychiatric illness?

2. Will neuroendocrine tests provide to the study of psychiatric disease what the laboratory tools in other branches of medicine have provided to

those clinical specialties? In particular, are certain neuroendocrine findings associated with particular behavioral states, syndromes, or diagnostic categories?

3. Do these measures increase our abilities to define and characterize disease types?

4. Can neuroendocrine assays increase our predictive or prognostic ability? In particular patients, will neuroendocrine measures provide information about treatment outcome, detection of early response, failure or relapse, choice of treatment modality or drug therapy, risk of suicide, and so on?

5. Will neuroendocrine tests allow us to identify persons at risk for developing illness, especially currently well relatives of sick probands?

6. Will these neuroendocrine functions define new classes or types of psychiatric illness by identifying similar neuroendocrine dysfunction in patient groups that cut across currently accepted diagnostic entities?

7. Is it possible that multiple neuroendocrine measures may elucidate patterns of response that can provide us with guidelines to the questions raised above more clearly than can results from the study of a single neuroendocrine axis?

The answers to these questions are some of the hopes that all of us share, but while these are obviously important, we should not lose sight of the fact that our work is evolving and is still young compared to laboratory medicine in other fields. Furthermore, our endeavors to answer the questions posed above will gradually increase our ability to define the limits of our techniques and simultaneously to change and improve them, so that we may learn more about the control mechanisms of neuroendocrine function *and* how the measurement of these functions can assist us in understanding and treating psychiatric illness.

This review discusses selected neuroendocrine functions, concentrating mainly on data in humans, both normal and psychiatric.

GROWTH HORMONE

The control of growth hormone (GH) secretion is complicated and involves several monoaminergic systems in the CNS — norepinephrine, dopamine, and serotonin. It is also probable that at least under certain conditions cholinergic systems influence GH secretion (Mendelson, Jacobs, Sitaram, Wyatt, & Gillin, 1978).

A variety of stimuli have been shown to be associated with GH release in depressed patients and in normals. These include insulin hypoglycemia (Mueller, Heninger, & McDonald, 1972), administration of L-dopa (Sachar, Mushrush, Perlow, Weitzman, & Sassin, 1972), 5-hydroxytryptophan (5-HTP; Takahashi, Kondo, & Yoshimura, 1974a), apomorphine (Mendels, Frazer, & Carroll, 1974), and D-amphetamine (Langer, Heinze, Reim, & Matussek, 1976). However, much of the earlier work was subsequently shown to be inadequate because of a lack of control for factors that affect GH response, such as gender, age, and menstrual status. At present only the results with insulin hypoglycemia, D-amphetamine administration, and possibly L-dopa are worth considering, and these are controversial. Most reports up until recent times have suggested that depressed patients, or various subgroups of them, show diminished response to these stimuli.

Raiti, Davis, and Blizzard (1967) reported that intravenous (i.v.) arginine vasopressin and the insulin tolerance test (ITT) both cause GH release in children and are useful tests in the endocrine diagnosis of GH insufficiency. Of 31 pairs of arginine vasopressin and ITTs in 15 children aged 9 to 19 years, 22 showed GH increases greater than 5 ng/ml. However, the tests were not always concordant; 5 showed no GH response to arginine vasopressin, and 4 showed no increase to ITT. Thus different stimuli to the same neuroendocrine axis do not necessarily produce the same response in the same individual. This may result from different mechanisms of action of the different stimuli. Raiti *et al.* concluded that clinical GH deficiency cannot be diagnosed unless both tests show failure to respond. Furthermore, there are few data on test-retest reliability of GH response to any of these stimuli; Greenwood, Landon, and Stamp (1966) showed that repeat ITTs revealed marked GH response variability (from 22 to 64 ng/ml on repeat tests) in 5 control subjects (sex and menstrual status unspecified).

Sachar, Finkelstein, and Hellman (1971) studied the plasma GH response to insulin hypoglycemia, the endocrine test used to ascertain adequacy of GH secretion (Roth, Glick, Yallow, & Berson, 1963). The hypothesis that Sachar *et al.* proposed was tha since children with maternal deprivation syndrome (growth failure and lack of GH secretion during ITT) showed clinical features that they considered similar to the anaclitic depression of Spitz and Wolf (1946), perhaps adult depressed patients would also show inhibition of GH secretion. In this study of 13 depressed patients, 5 failed to secrete GH "adequately," while all 23 age-matched nondepressed subjects did.

However, Koslow, Stokes, Mendels, Ramsey, and Casper (1982), in a large sample of depressed patients, found no significant differences between insulin-induced GH response in postmenopausal depressed women vs age-matched healthy normals when blood sugar fall and other important variables were controlled. However, they did note again the interesting finding first reported by Mueller, Heninger, and McDonald (1969) that depressed unipolar subjects showed insulin resistance to the ITT. Garver, Pandey, Dekirmenjian, and DeLeon-Jones (1975) reported that peak GH response to insulin hypoglycemia correlated with preinsulin 24-hour urinary 3-methoxy-4-hydroxyphenylglycol (MHPG) excretion as a measure of CNS norepinephrine. However, these data are difficult to interpret because of the mixed population of premenopausal and postmenopausal patients and the inclusion of data from two patients with increased fasting GH levels. Other studies have reported inadequate GH response to insulin hypoglycemia in depressed patients, but all have been confounded by not excluding subjects on the basis of one or more factors now known to influence GH responsiveness. For example, some reports did not take into account menstrual status (Mueller *et al.*, 1969), weight and menstrual status (Casper, Davis, Pandey, Garver, & Dekirmenjian, 1977; Gregoire, Brauman, de Buck, & Corvilain, 1977), or adequate fall in plasma glucose after insulin (Gregoire *et al.*, 1977; Mueller *et al.*, 1969; Sachar *et al.*, 1971). Merimee and Fineberg (1971) have shown that GH response is related to the stage of the menstrual cycle and is increased during the preovulatory period, thus re-emphasizing the GH-release-enhancing effect of estrogens. Additionally, all the preceding studies except one (Koslow *et al.*, 1982) studied small numbers of patients, and the data available on test-retest reliability of the ITT are not good (Greenwood *et al.*, 1966).

Gruen, Sachar, Altman, and Sassin (1975) also reported decreased GH response to insulin hypoglycemia in 4 of 10 postmenopausal depressed women, compared to 10 healthy normal postmenopausal females. It was suggested that the differences in GH response to L-dopa versus insulin hypoglycemia might be based on different mechanisms of stimulation of catecholamine systems involved in GH release. Thus, since both dopaminergic and noradrenergic stimulation can release GH, the release of GH after L-dopa may primarily involve dopamine, while the GH response to hypoglycemia may involve norepinephrine. A second possibility suggested was that hypoglycemia involves release of endogenous dopamine and presumably requires adequate levels of the preformed amine for release into the synaptic cleft in order to have a normal GH response. In contrast, patients with blunted GH response after L-dopa were postulated to have inadequate synthesis of dopamine from this precursor.

Psychoendocrine studies with L-dopa derive from the observation by Boyd, Lebovitz, and Pfieffer (1970) that GH can be released *in vivo* in humans by administration of L-dopa. This produced suggestive evidence that dopamine and probably norepinephrine are important CNS neurotransmitters for the control of GH release in humans. A few years later, Sachar, Frantz, Altman, and Sassin (1973) suggested that the magnitude of GH response to L-dopa might be decreased in patients with unipolar depression, compared to normals or depressed patients with bipolar disease. However, Sachar and colleagues subsequently showed that there were no significant differences in GH response to L-dopa in these depressed patients when age and gender effects (menstrual status) were adequately controlled (Sachar *et al.*, 1975). The low GH response originally reported in postmenopausal depressed females was later shown to be secondary to their low estrogen level and the known effects of the high premenopausal estrogen levels in potentiating GH response. No difference in plasma L-dopa concentrations were found between the groups studied.

Apomorphine, a dopaminergic agonist, has been shown to increase GH release in a dose-dependent manner in normals (Lal, de la Vega, Sourkes, & Friessen, 1972). Responses in depressed patients have been reported as subnormal, but the effect of stress was not clearly eliminated in this test procedure, since even a low dose (0.75 mg) may produce nausea. In fact, current data would suggest that the GH response to the dopamine agonist apomorphine is not impaired in depression (Casper *et al.*, 1977; Christie, Whalley, Brown, & Dick, 1982; Frazer, 1975).

A subsequent study in humans reported no enhancement of GH response to the dopaminergic agonist apomorphine after 4 to 7 administrations of electroconvulsive therapy (ECT) (Christie *et al.*, 1982). However, it should be noted that a slight trend in the direction of post-ECT enhancement of GH response was present in this study. Furthermore, some of the apparent lack of enhancement of post-ECT GH response may have been secondary to the considerably elevated resting preapomorphine GH levels that occurred in at least a few of the 12 subjects studied. Elevated resting GH levels may exert a negative feedback effect on subsequent GH secretion (G. M. Brown, Seggie, Charmbers, & Ettigi, 1978). Examination of healthy normal volunteers and depressed patients in remission could provide further information regarding this question.

By now, the complexity and conflict surrounding GH secretion should be apparent. Evidence has accumulated that some stimuli for GH secretion can produce this effect by acting on tissues outside the blood-brain barrier. The median eminence of the basal hypothalamus, and the pituitary itself, lie outside the usual blood-brain barrier (G. M. Brown, Seemen, & Lee, 1976; Wislocki & King, 1936). Domperidone, a peripheral dopaminergic receptor blocker that only poorly crosses the blood-brain barrier (Laduron & Leysen, 1979), can induce prolactin (PRL) secretion because of its blockade of dopaminergic receptors located on the pituitary gland (Caron *et al.*, 1978; Gruen *et al.*, 1978). Lal *et al.* (1982) showed that domperidone simultaneously attenuated, but did not completely block, the GH release expected from administration of apomorphine. Thus, some of the apomorpohine-stimulated GH secretion is modulated by dopaminergic receptors located outside the blood-brain barrier. This is consonant with reports that have demonstrated increased GH secretion in association with infusion of dopamine, which by itself does not cross the blood-brain barrier (Burrow, May, Spaulding, & Donabedian, 1977; Kaptein, Kletzky, Spencer, & Nicoloff, 1980; Leebaw, Lee, & Woolf, 1978).

However, when L-dopa is infused, the GH response can be enhanced by the addition of a dopa-decarboxylase inhibitor; this shows that dopaminergic receptor sites *within* the blood-brain barrier also play a role in control of GH secretion. Furthermore, supporting this conclusion are the findings that GH secretion induced by gamma-aminobutyric acid (GABA) is blocked by pimozide, a centrally active dopamine receptor blocker, but not by domperidone (Cavagnini *et al.*, 1980). Apomorphine in low doses produces penile erection, yawning, and sedation in healthy men (Schlatter & Lal, 1972), and these effects are blocked by pimozide (Lal, Guyda, & Bikadoroff, 1977). Similar results have been reported in animals (Meren *et al.*, 1979) and can be blocked by neuroleptics. Therefore, these behavioral effects of apomorphine appear centrally mediated; as expected, domperidone does *not* block them (Corsini, Del Zompo, Gessa, & Mangoni, 1979), but does block the apomorphine-dependent GH secretion, as is consistent with an action of domperidone outside the blood-brain barrier (Lal *et al.*, 1982). Finally, domperidone does not decrease the antiparkinsonian effect of apomorphine (Corsini *et al.*, 1979) or bromocryptine (Agid, Pollak, Bonnet, Signoret, & Lhermitte, 1979), giving further support to the action of domperidone from outside the blood-brain barrier.

The alpha-adrenergic receptor blocker phentolamine was reported to inhibit GH response to insulin-induced hypoglycemia (Blackard & Heidingsfelder, 1968). Clonidine, an alpha-adrenergic receptor agonist, was shown to increase GH release, further confirming the effect of the noradrenergic system in the control of GH secretion (Lal, Tolis, Martin, Brown, & Guyda, 1975).

Clonidine is considered to release GH due to stimulation of postsynaptic alpha-2-adrenergic receptors. Several reports have noted that the ability of clonidine to release GH is blunted in unmedicated depressed patients compared to healthy controls and schizophrenics (Charney, Heninger, & Sternberg, 1982; Checkley, Slade, & Shur, 1981; Matussek *et al.*, 1980). This further suggests that in depressed patients these adrenergic receptors are insensitive. Electrophysiological and behavioral studies in animals suggest that alpha-adrenergic receptors are made supersensitive with chronic antidepressant treatment (Menkes & Aghajanian, 1981).

Desipramine (DMI) is a tricyclic antidepressant that after a single dose demonstrates increased release of norepinephrine and relatively specific and pronounced inhibition of reuptake of released norepinephrine. Hence it follows that DMI treatment should antagonize the expected sedative and hypotensive effects of clonidine; this does occur (Dadkar, Dohadwalla, & Bhattacharya, 1978; Pelayo, Dubocovich, & Zanger, 1980). After DMI treatment for 1 week, the endocrine effects of clonidine are transiently enhanced, so that GH release increases strikingly with clonidine administration. This apparent paradox may be due to the difference in reaction of norepinephrine systems in the hypothalamus controlling neuroendocrine secretion, compared to norepinephrine systems in the cerebral cortex. In fact, it has been shown that clonidine reduces norepinephrine release in the cortex, but enhances norepinephrine release in the hypothalamus (Glass, Checkley, Shur, & Dawling, 1982; Medgett, McCulloch, & Rand, 1978). Therefore, the effect of clonidine on releasing norepinephrine in the hypothalamus would be additive to that of DMI and would result in the observed increase in GH release from the pituitary. This change in GH response after DMI treatment for 1 week is probably not related to clinical change, since the increased response is somewhat attenuated after 3 weeks of DMI treatment, when clinical response would be expected to be increasing. Also, prior observations have shown that

GH response to clonidine did not increase in depressed patients tested 24 hours after the 7th treatment in a course of ECT (Slade & Checkley, 1980). However, subsequent studies in subhuman primates (baboons) showed that ECT was associated with enhancement of GH response to clonidine 1, 7, and 15 days after a course of 7 administrations of ECT (McWilliam, Meldrum, & Checkley, 1981). McWilliam *et al.* (1981) also reported that the absence of post-ECT augmentation of noradrenergic response in humans may relate to an effect of anesthesia on the time course of the development of this phenomenon.

It has been previously reported that GH response to clonidine is impaired in depressed patients (Checkley *et al.*, 1981; Matussek *et al.*, 1980). No comments have been made regarding a possible correlation of the enhanced GH response to clonidine after 1 week of treatment with DMI and subsequent final clinical outcome. If there is an association of enhanced GH response and its putative pathophysiology of increased noradrenergic function and treatment response, then clonidine stimulation of GH release may be a useful tool for predicting treatment outcome to DMI or other forthcoming and more specific "noradrenergic" antidepressant drugs.

The hypothesis that the postsynaptic alpha-2-adrenergic responsiveness is enhanced by chronic antidepressant treatment in man is not supported by recent work (Charney *et al.*, 1982; Siever, Uhde, Insel, Roy, & Murphy, 1982), which found no alteration in the pretreatment lack of GH response to clonidine after treatment with DMI, amitriptyline, or the selective monoamine oxidase-A (MAO-A) inhibitor, clorgyline, for a period of 3-6 weeks, Therapeutic responders were not different from nonresponders in terms of this lack of GH response to clonidine. Checkley and coworkers (1981), on the other hand, reported increased GH response to clonidine in depressed patients after chronic DMI treatment; more studies are needed to explain this discrepancy, as well as the reported lack of GH response to clonidine in depressed patients. Moreover, further study is needed to confirm the stimulated GH response's specificity and sensitivity for depression, and the possibility that assessment of this response would relate to clinically important measures (e.g., outcome, etc.).

In light of the foregoing conflicting data, the GH response of depressed patients to amphetamine has also been examined (Langer *et al.*, 1976), coincident with the concept of CNS monoamine disturbance in depression and monoamine control of GH secretion. It was observed that i.v. amphetamine sulfate produced a lesser GH response in 9 "endogenous" depressed patients than in normals, schizophrenics, and alcoholics (whose response was similar to that of normals). In contrast, 10 "reactive" depressed patients showed increased GH release to amphetamine. Amphetamine crosses the blood-brain barrier, and its effects on GH secretion are probably the result of multiple actions. Amphetamine is considered to release neuronal stored norepinephrine (Blackard & Heidingsfelder, 1968; Lai *et al.*, 1975); in addition, it probably releases dopamine, inhibits neuronal reputake of norepinephrine, perhaps inhibits MAO metabolism, and produces a direct noradrenergic agonist effect. In turn, these catecholaminergic neurons regulate GH-releasing factor and GH-inhibitory hormone, somatostatin. The normal GH response of schizophrenic patients to single doses of amphetamine does not necessarily argue against the dopamine hypothesis for the pathogenesis of schizophrenia, because the dopaminergic neuron in the hypothalamic tuberoinfundibular area that might be contributing to the control of GH release could be normal in schizophrenics, while dopaminergic systems elsewhere in the brain are abnormal and produce abnormal behavior.

It is probable that some of the behavioral effects of amphetamine are caused by serotonergic system activation. It has been shown in rats, at least (Sloviter, Drust, & Connor, 1978), that the side-to-side head weaving, forepaw padding, and splayed hindlimbs characteristic of intense serotonergic receptor activity are also produced by amphetamine. Prior treatment with alpha-methylparatyrosine to deplete catecholamines does not alter this post-amphetamine serotonergic syndrome, but 5-HTP depletion with parachlorophenylalanine prevents the appearance of the syndrome. Imura, Nakai, and Yoshimi (1973) showed that oral 5-HTP (150 mg) resulted in increased GH release. This again demonstrates the complexity of GH release by adding the importance of metabolic factors, such as amino acid (protein) ingestion, glucose level, prior circulating GH level, and so forth. The increase in GH was not considered stress-related in the studies of Imura *et al.*, because the eight normal healthy male volunteers did not report nausea with this oral dose of 5-HTP. Garver *et al.* (1975) found that the serotonin system, like the noradrenergic system, caused increased plasma GH levels. Further evidence of the role of serotonin systems in the control of GH secretion came from the work of Bivens, Lebovitz, and Feldman (1973), who showed that GH secretion was inhibited by the serotonin antagonists cyproheptadine and methysergide.

Finkelstein, Roffwarg, Boyar, Kream, and Hellman (1972) reported age-related changes in the 24-hour spontaneous secretion of GH, and it is now recognized that the major secretion of GH occurs early after sleep onset and often during slow-wave sleep (Honda *et al.*, 1969; Sassin *et al.*, 1969). It has also been reported that fasting (preinsulin) GH levels are significantly inversely related to age (Koslow *et al.*, 1982). Halbreich, Asnis, Halpern, Tabrizi, and Sachar (1980) reported in regard to a small number of cases (7 normal young men and 7 normal postmenopausal females) that GH response was greater in the younger healthy men. They also reported that recalculation of the prior data from Langer *et al.* (1976) showed that the GH responses were lower in their older normals (more than 39 years of age) as compared to the younger normals (less than 30 years of age). This is consistent with reported age-related decreases in brain CNS catecholamines (dopamine and norepinephrine) and increases in MAO activity (Robinson, 1975).

Basal GH levels are not altered in depressed patients compared to normals. This is a further argument for *other* abnormalities of GH release being important in the pathophysiology of the depression. It can be seen that the assessment of normal GH secretion by various stimuli can be extremely complicated, especially without complete knowledge of control of the system. Thus, the use of GH response to various agents is difficult to interpret except on an empirical basis. The empirical approach requires attention to sufficient numbers of patients who have been carefully screened for variables that might affect GH response as an integral part of that patient population.

THYROTROPIN-RELEASING HORMONE RESPONSE

In the past 10-15 years, the clinical use of thyrotropin-releasing hormone (TRH) has become widespread in endocrinology to assess thyroid status and function (Hershman, 1974). The tripeptide structure of TRH was first identified some 15 years ago, and the widespread distribution of TRH was first described inside (Jackson & Reichlin, 1974; A. Winokur & Utiger, 1974) and then outside (Morley, Garvin, Pekary, & Hershman, 1977) the tissues of the mammalian CNS. TRH is a releasing factor for anterior pituitary thyroid-stimulating hormone (TSH), but also for PRL and under certain conditions GH (Maeda *et al.*, 1975). In addition, many behavioral effects of TRH have been reported in animals (Nemeroff & Prange, 1978) and in humans (Prange, Loosen, & Nemeroff, 1979; Snyder & Utiger, 1972), though these are controversial and their clinical significance remains uncertain. In clinical endocrinology, the safe and relatively side-effect-free TRH test can be accomplished, with the subsequent serum TSH concentrations describing a picture characteristic of high, normal, or low thyroid function. This is especially true when the TSH concentrations are taken in association with other appropriate thyroid function tests (e.g., serum thyroxin, triiodothyronine, etc.).

The diminished TSH response to TRH that has been repetitively reported in some psychiatric patients during the past dozen years is *not* associated with abnormal thyroid function tests or clinical evidence of thyroid disease. No endocrine explanation for the findings of low or "blunted" TSH response has been identified in these psychiatric patients. A number of factors have been identified that will produce blunted TSH response to administered TRH in normal healthy controls, including increasing age; starvation; increased glucocorticoids (exogenous or endogenous, as in Cushing syndrome); thyroactive hormones; repeated administration of TRH; and administration of somatostatin, neurotensin, or dopamine. There is also a gender effect: Males have decreased TSH response compared to females.

Prange, along with Loosen, has worked very extensively since 1972 to characterize the TSH response to TRH in psychiatric patients (see Loosen & Prange, 1982). He notes that of the more than 40 studies to date, all but a handful have reported data consistent with their initial study (Prange, Wilson, Lara, Alltop, & Breese, 1972); in that study, 3 of 10 depressed patients had reduced TSH response to TRH in the absence of any endocrine or general health explanation for the finding. The response is not specific to depression, since it has also been reported in alcoholics during and after withdrawal and in alcoholics who have been dry for some years. Blunted TSH response has not been reported in schizophrenic patients and is probably normal in manics when they are off lithium. On lithium, manics may show enhanced TSH response, which is probably secondary to the tendency of lithium to induce hypothyroidism. However, some recent studies have reported blunted TSH response in small numbers of manic patients (Gold, Pottash, Extein, Martin, *et al.*, 1981; Kirkegaard, Bjorum, Cohn, & Lauridsen, 1978). A number of studies in anorexia nervosa have also reported low TSH responses, even in normal-weight anorexia nervosa patients. Prange *et al.* (1972) have reported that 0 of 73 normal men and women aged 20 to 70 years had TSH responses lower than 5.6 mIU/ml after i.v. administration of 0.5 mg TRH over a 1-minute interval. Test-retest data are very limited, but Prange has reported that in the 3 patients with blunted TSH response that he restudied, all remained blunted whether depressed or recovered on subsequent testing.

However, it is fair to say that no large population of psychiatric patients has been studied, with the exception of depressed patients. Hence the question of specificity still remains. Within the depressed populations studied by a variety of investigators, it seems evident that the age of the depressed patients, severity of depression, or prior medication history are not associated with blunted TSH response. Length of illness may be related (Takahashi, Kondo, & Yoshimura, 1974b), but more prospective data are obviously needed.

There are conflicting reports on the incidence of TSH blunting in primary vs secondary depression. TSH blunting generally is not associated with plasma cortisol elevation in depressed patients, though it is certainly clear that pronounced or chronic glucocorticoid excess is very frequently associated with blunted TSH response to TRH (Nicoloff, Fisher, & Appleman, 1979). Prange *et al.* (1972) reported that in a small sample of unipolar depressed females, TSH blunting was associated with plasma contisol elevation. However, another group of investigators found that only 30 of their unipolar depressed patients showed both TSH blunting and cortisol nonsuppression on the dexamethasone suppression test (DST), though 64% of patients showed TSH blunting alone and 50% showed dexamethasone nonsuppression alone (Extein, Pottash, & Gold, 1981). Also, alcoholic patients with TSH blunting did not show increased plasma cortisol concentration (Loosen, Prange, & Wilson, 1979). More work is needed to resolve the question of TSH blunting and its relationship to hypothalamic-pituitary-adrenocortical (HYPAC) activity in depressed patients.

It is now apparent that in some depressed patients with TSH blunting, the phenomena is unchanged when they recover. However, reports on state or trait association of TSH blunting are about equally divided. Linkowsky, Brauman, and Mendlewicz (1981) have recently pointed up the need to control for menstrual status and possibly subtype of depression in these studies. They found normalization of TSH blunting after recovery from depression in *premenopausal* depressed *bipolar* patients, but not in *postmenopausal* depressed *unipolar* patients.

The relationship between purported measures of central noradrenergic function (urinary MHPG) and TSH response to TRH has been examined in light of the CNS monoamine regulation of TRH release. In fact, though, it appears that the reasoning for examination of relationships is tenuous at our present state of knowledge. For example, we are unable to measure the endogenous secretion of TRH directly, and the levels of plasma TSH are normal in those individuals with blunted TSH response to exogenous TRH. Nevertheless, patients ($n = 7$) with blunted TSH response had significantly higher mean 24-hour urinary MHPG excretion than patients ($n = 13$) with normal TSH response (K. L. Davis *et al.*, 1981), and blunted responses did not correlate with plasma cortisol concentration or DST response. In another study, blunted TSH responses were found in 18 of 54 and "augmented" responses in 8 of 54 primary unipolar endogenous depressives; TSH response was "normal" (i.e., between 7 and 23 μg/ml) in all 19 nondepressed patients (Targum, Byrnes, & Sullivan, 1982). Agren and Wide (1982) reported that TSH response correlated with body height, that it was state-dependent, and that there was a significant negative correlation of TSH response to urinary free cortisol excretion.

A number of studies have reported that blunted TSH response is characteristic of unipolar depression, but is not found in bipolar, dysthymic, or secondary depressives (Sternbach *et al.*, 1983). Sternbach *et al.* also found a significant positive correlation between TSH response to TRH and urinary MHPG in men, but not in women. This is in contrast to the earlier report of K. L. Davis *et al.*, though these two groups of investigators used different cutoff criteria for definition of blunted TSH response.

In summary, it is evident that the blunted TSH response to administered TRH does exist in some depressed patients. Loosen and Prange (1982) place the incidence at about 25% of depressed patients. However, relatively few data are available regrading the incidence in other psychiatric categories, and the relationship of the abnormality to state or trait is still not clearly or decisively settled. The question of test-retest reproducibility is very important, and this has barely been addressed at all.

What are the implications of this abnormal TSH response when it is present? Clearly, the physiological control mechanism for TRH release in the hypothalamus is complicated to the point that one is hard put at this time to construct meaningful inferences or hypotheses about the neurotransmitter controls from the measurement of the pituitary TSH response to exogenous TRH. Loosen and Prange (1982) suggest as a working hypothesis that in patients with TSH blunting there is a preceding initial period of endogenous TRH hypersecretion. This initially results in TSH hypersecretion and perhaps in transient thyroid gland hyperactivity. The subsequent stage (apparently quickly developed, because of the lack of history of clinical hyperthyroidism) is one of pituitary receptor down-regulation and return to normal TSH and thyroid function. Obviously, until endogenous TRH levels or turnover can be assessed, we cannot adequately test this hypothesis.

Kirkegaard, Faber, Hummer, and Rogowski (1979) reported elevated cerebrospinal fluid (CSF) TRH concentrations in 15 patients with primary depression, but found no relationship between these TRH levels and the TSH response to administered TRH (i.e., they were not blunted). It has been shown that chronic long-term treatment with low doses of TRH results in loss of TSH diurnal rhythm (Spencer, Greenstadt, Wheeler, Kletzky, & Nicoloff, 1980). It has also been reported that unipolar depressed patients (but not bipolar) showed a reduced mean 24-hour serum TSH and absence of the normal nocturnal rise (Golstein, van Cauter, Linkowski, Vanhaelst, & Mendlewicz, 1980). The disruption of normal TSH diurnal rhythm after long-term TRH administration may only reflect feedback inhibition of the endogenous hypothalamic-pituitary-thyroid axis, and not a permanent state of abnormality. The finding of abnormal TSH levels in unipolar adpressed patients may be only a secondary state-related defect in the thyroid axis. Follow-up studies on both these patient populations would be revealing and important. Loosen and Prange (1982) note that if one accepts the hypothesis of an initially increased central TRH secretion, then it would be consistent with current knowledge of the monoamine control of TRH to postulate increased noradrenergic and/or decreased serotonergic activity in the hypothalamus. There is at least some agreement with the latter in the permissive hypothesis of affective disorders (Prange *et al.*, 1974).

Recent evidence (Agren & Wide, 1982; Maas *et al.*, in press; Stokes, Frazer, & Casper, 1981) supports the idea of increased noradrenergic function in depression instead of the more usually considered central noradrenergic depletion. In addition, a hyperdopaminergic state, if present, could produce inhibition of TSH response, not by altering endogenous TRH but by interfering with pituitary release of TSH (Bruuow *et al.*, 1977; Thorner *et al.*, 1978). Loosen and Prange (1982) also suggest that since TRH releases pituitary PRL as well as TSH, and since dopamine is the classical inhibitor of PRL secretion, then a study of the simultaneous release of PRL and TSH should provide evidence for a hyperdopaminergic state if both pituitary hormones show a blunted response to administered TRH.

Results in a number of studies to date on exactly this point are conflicting, and no clear answer is now available. Birkhaeuser *et al.* (1980) did show that a dopamine antagonist (metaclopramide) restored the blunted TSH response to administered TRH in depressed patients. They suggest that depressed patients who are TSH blunters would show an enhanced TSH response after conventional neuroleptic treatment, with the resultant dopaminergic blockade. They also note that excess brain neurotensin has been reported capable of inhibiting TSH response to TRH. Further, and more interestingly, GH-inhibitory factor or somatostatin can inhibit TSH release and at the same time could explain the inhibition of the pituitary GH release observed during insulin hypoglycemia in unipolar depressed patients (Gruen *et al.*, 1975). However, GH release inhibition is not confirmed during insulin hypoglycemia by other more extensive studies (Koslow *et al.*, 1982).

PROLACTIN

PRL secretion is thought to be controlled by at least two neurotransmitter systems in the CNS of humans (Boyd & Reichlin, 1978). Serotonergic input is considered to be stimulatory and dopamine tonically inhibitory to PRL secretion. Further complicating the picture of PRL control is the evidence for opiate agonists' and antagonists' having a regulatory role in PRL (and also cortisol) release (Gold *et al.*, 1980; Tolis, Hickett & Guyda, 1975). Basal PRL levels have variously been reported as unchanged (Meltzer, Piyakalmala, Schyre, & Fang, 1977) or increased as compared with normals or the same depressed patients after recovery (Carroll, 1978). Basal PRL levels were normal in patients with dementia of the Alzheimer type or multi-infarct dementia, suggesting that the dopaminergic neurons involved in PRL regulation are not severely affected in dementia (Balldin *et al.*, 1983).

Asnis, Nathan, Halbreich, Halpern, and Sachar (1980), however, reporting on 19 medically healthy depressed inpatients (15 of whom were women), found a slight *increase* in basal PRL levels in 17 of the 19 patients after recovery from depression and while on various tricyclic antidepressant drugs that have little-known dopamincrgic blocking effect. The basal PRL levels were all in the normal range — both the relatively lower levels during depression, and the slightly higher levels after recovery. Lower basal PRL levels were also reported by Judd *et al.* (1982) in depressives as compared to normals or other psychiatric patients. Previous reports have reported increases in serum PRL after treatment with the serotonergic drug clomipramine. However, it should be noted that the daughter metabolite has a more mixed and less serotonergic action.

PRL is classically released by neuroleptic blockade of dopaminergic receptors in the tuberoinfundibular area, and the PRL response has been shown to parallel the clinical potency of the neuroleptic drug, which potency in turn is thought to depend upon neuroleptic blockade of dopaminergic receptors in the mesolimbic dopaminergic system. Reserpine, unlike the neuroleptics, does not block *postsynaptic* dopaminergic receptors but depletes *presynaptic* dopamine, as well as norepinephrine and serotonin. Asnis, Sachar, Halbreich, Ostrow, *et al.* (1981) reported that reserpine was more potent than equal doses of haloperidol in releasing PRL; they also noted that preliminary studies in schizophrenics showed that some patients respond to as little as 3-6 mg of oral reserpine a day, which is less than the therapeutic dose of haloperidol.

Extein *et al.* (1980) showed that the PRL response to the opiate agonist morphine was "blunted" in depressed patients with major affective disorder, but not in normals. Similar data were reported in 50% of a group of 16 depressed patients studied by Judd *et al.* (1982). They point out that this blunted PRL response has been observed in depressed patients whith two different stimuli, TRH and opiate agonists (morphine and methadone), and that the blunted PRL response has been reported primarily in depressed patients and not in manic or schizophrenic patients thus far. They suggest that it could be considered a possible marker for depression, but are careful to note that the blunted PRL response observed in two of their normal controls raises further question about the specificity of this response. The data on PRL response to opiate agonists are consistent with the hypothesis that opioid peptide systems have important interrelationships with neuroendocrine regulation and possibly with the pathophysiology of affective disorders.

Meltzer, Fang, Tricou, Robertson, and Piyaka (1982) have recently found an association between dexamethasone nonsuppression of cortisol and coincident nonsuppression of plasma PRL in depressed patients. Dexamethasone inhibition of insulin-hypoglycemia-induced PRL release had been previously reported in nondepressed subjects (Copinschi *et al.*, 1975; Osterman, Fagius, & Wide, 1977; Sowers, Carlson, Brautbar, & Hershman, 1977). Kijne *et al.* (1982) had also shown that the 2-mg DST lowered basal TSH levels during the next day. These investigators also suggest that the multiple types of neuroendocrine dysfunction described thus far in depressed patients may argue for a widespread (reversible?) disruption of neuroendocrine regulation in depressive illness.

In conclusion, then, one can say that the data to date on basal PRL levels and PRL release after various stimuli are not tremendously persuasive; further careful evaluation is needed. In particular, the specificity of response in different diagnostic groups and subclassifications needs further attention. This is not an easy task or necessarily the most exciting one, but it will create a necessary information pool. The PRL studies are at a relatively early stage in their development, and attention to questions of test-retest reproducibility is essential to answering the questions of specificity and sensitivity of the test results. Very few data are currently available. Attention to individual investigations, normal values will be of importance. Appropriate within-investigsation control populations, matched for important varibles known to affect PRL basal levels and response to stimuli, will be required before reasonable conclusions can be obtained about the potential usefulness of PRL testing. The data regarding basal levels constitute another problem. Resting nonstimulated PRL levels are, like GH levels, low, and assay precision is thus pushed to its limit to delineate differences clearly. Therefore, demonstration of assay sensitivity and reproducibility are needed from each investigation.

THE HYPAC SYSTEM

Introduction

Over the past 60 years, increasing evidence has accumlated that demonstrates the involvement of the CNS and especially the hypothalamus in the activation of the pituitary and adrenal cortex. The importance of an intact hypothalamus and hypothalamic-pituitary portal capillary system for normal adrenocortical function was demonstrated by the work of Harris (1955), building on the earlier work of Scharrer and Scharrer (1940). This portal system allows transport of hypothalamic factors to the anterior pituitary, inducing release of adrenocorticotropic hormone (ACTH) into the systemic circulation. The releasing substance for the HYPAC system has now been identified, at least in sheep, as a 41-amino-acid peptide — a remarkably larger and more complex releasing factor than the tripeptide TRH. It is now well appreciated that stressful life events characterized by the unfamiliar or novel are associated with relatively transient and generally modest increases in plasma corticosteroids in most individuals. It is of interest that the increase in HYPAC activity noted in psychiatric patients in general tends to be more protracted and greater than that observed as a result of contrived laboratory "stress" situations, novelty effects, or anticipatory events. HYPAC activation in psychiatric patients was initially conceived of as a nonspecific effect of emotional arousal, activation, and stress, not as a phenomenon related to depression per se. By the mid-1960s (Stokes, 1966), sufficient evidence had accumulated, although in a small number of depressed patients, to suggest that perhaps relatively pronounced HYPAC activation was common in depression.

The extent of the abnormality of HYPAC function in depression was not generally appreciated, even though for many years psychic stress had been recognized by some clinical and basic scientists as an activator of the HYPAC system. It is interesting that in 1968 an international symposium on HYPAC function (James & Landon, 1968) did not contain a single paper on the effect of psychological events on that system, even though other reports on elevated HYPAC function in depression and abnormal DST had been made before that meeting. The first extensive studies demonstrating profound abnormalities of this system in larger numbers of psychiatric patients were generally met with considerable skepticism about the importance of these findings to biological psychiatry. Most investigators then considered these events to be the result of nonspecific stress of psychosis, novelty effects, hospitalization, and study. While these can be important factors that need to be controlled for, the state of HYPAC hyperactivity frequently observed in depressed patients cannot be explained by these phenomena.

Although there is some disagreement about the specificity of the findings of HYPAC hyperfunction, it is clear that the elevated plasma cortisol levels, increased cortisol secretion, abnormal circadian rhythm (Sachar, Hellman, *et al.*, 1973; Stokes, 1972), and dexamethasone nonsuppression are more frequent in severe depression than in other diagnostic categories (Carroll *et al.*, 1981; Stokes *et al.*, 1984; Stokes, Stoll, Mattson, & Sollod, 1976). It is also clear that the abnormal circadian rhythm persists for up to 2 months in hospitalized depressed patients with major affective disorder when not treated with effective antidepressant medications or treatments (Stokes, 1972).

A number of means are available for detecting HYPAC system hyperfunction. Ideally, one would like to be able to measure the activity of this system directly at all levels. This would of course include direct measurements of monoaminergic and peptidergic systems in the CNS influencing the secretion of corticotropin-releasing factor (CRF), as well as the measurement of CRF itself. In addition, one would like to be able to measure ACTH and cortisol in the macrocirculation; both of these measurements are now possible and have been done.

Since 1970 we know that the circadian rhythm of cortisol secretion is not a nice, smooth sine wave, as it might have been envisioned prior to that time. The work of Hellman *et al.* (1970) demonstrated that cortisol is secreted in episodic bursts through the circadian cycle of HYPAC activity, with large infrequent bursts between about 0500 hours and 1000 hours and then a gradual decrease in frequency and duration, to a low point and perhaps complete inactivity from about 2200 hours until about 0300 or 0400 hours. It has been shown by a number of investigators since then that in patients with increased HYPAC activity, as in Cushing syndrome and in some depressions, the episodes of cortisol secretion are more frequent and of longer duration, in varying degree from patient to patient, throughout the circadian cycle. This results in a relatively flat circadian rhythm and elevated mean plasma cortisol levels with higher than normal peak values.

The increased plasma cortisol concentration of such patients can exceed the binding capacity of the specific alpha-2 binding globulin present in the plasma. This globulin normally binds about 98% of circulating plasma cortisol. Consequently, more "free" or non-protein-bound cortisol is present in the plasma and enters extracellular fluid to perfuse the cells of all the organs of the body, including the CNS. This free cortisol is considered the biologically active fraction. Simultaneously, of course, increased free cortisol is presented to the kidney and is excreted in the urine as urinary free cortisol, where it can be measured as an integrated function over the 24 hours of HYPAC activity. In addition, plasma cortisol can be measured in the CSF, where it is largely non-protein-bound.

It has long been known from work in endocrinology that evidence of HYPAC hyperactivity is not necessarily associated with abnormal resistance to glucocorticoid-induced negative feedback (the basis of the DST). In fact, if HYPAC hyperactivity and dexamethasone nonsuppression were invariably linked, predexamethasone measures of HYPAC function could be substituted for the DST itself, obviating the necessity for the DST. The DST has proved a particularly useful measure of HYPAC function in psychiatry and in clinical endocrinology because of its simplicity compared to other measures of HYPAC function abnormality identified in depressives, such as an abnormal diurnal rhythm, adrenal hypersecretion, exaggerated pulsatile release of cortisol, and elevated urinary free cortisol.

Effect of Drugs on HYPAC Function

Certain factors have been recognized as important to control for in assessing the activity of the HYPAC system in regard to depression. It is clear that certain drugs can affect the apparent activity of the system. In particular, sedatives, estrogens, and anticonvulsants must be considered, since the effects of these compounds on HYPAC function measures may remain for days or weeks (Health and Public Policy Committee, American College of Physicians, 1984).

It is not clear that antidepressant drugs or neuroleptic drugs affect HYPAC function directly, although as the depressed mood is lost the increased HYPAC function tends to return toward normal (Greden *et al.*, 1980; Yerevanian *et al.*, 1983). The data to date suggest that the acute administration of either neuroleptic or antidepressant drugs is probably not associated with HYPAC dysfunction.

Effect of Age on HYPAC Function

Age has recently been identified as another factor that may influence HYPAC function — in particular, dexamethasone nonsuppression (Asnis, Sachar, Halbreich, Nathan, *et al.*, 1981). This report found a "surprising" relationship between age and cortisol hypersecretion in a population of 25 patients with endogenous depressive disorder. Hypersecretion, as measured by increased mean 24-hour plasma cortisol value compared to normals, occurred mainly in those patients over 50 years of age. The studies included a 24-hour multiple sampling of plasma cortisol levels obtaining a sample every 30 minutes by indwelling catheter (48 samples per patient). This was followed by a 2-mg DST with predexamethasone cortisol level at 1600 hours. Mean 24-hour and all other pre- and postdexamethasone plasma cortisol values correlated with age. The investigators found, using the conservative postdexamethasone cortisol criterion of 6 μg/dl proposed by Carroll *et al.* (1981), that all their dexamethasone-nonsuppressing patients were over 50 years of age. If the criterion cutoff was reduced to 3 μg/dl cortisol, only 1 of 10 patients under 50 years of age were nonsuppressing. These investigators postulated that the reported decrease in brain norepinephrine found in increasing age might allow HYPAC disinhibition, especially if a further functional norepinephrine deficit occurred during the course of depressive illness. However, Carroll *et al.* (1981) did not find any significant relationship between age and DST result in their group of 215 melancholic patients, although both Carroll *et al.* and Schlesser, Winokur, and Sherman (1979) noted that their depressed patients with dexamethasone nonsuppression were older than those patients who suppressed.

Tourigny-Rivard and Raskind (1981) subsequently investigated the effect of age on DST response in normal subjects further because of the reported increased resting corticosteroid levels observed in aged rats (Landfield, Waymire, & Lynch, 1978) and the increased dexamethasone nonsuppression reported in aged vs young rats (Riegle & Hess, 1972). However, Tourigny-Rivard and Raskind found no difference in the resting or postdexamethasone (1 mg) plasma cortisol concentration in 10 healthy elderly (mean age 75.3 years) versus 19 healthy young (mean age 29.9 years) men, or in their rate of recovery from dexamethasone suppression. Spar and La Rue (1983) found that in 44 hospitalized elderly depressed patients with major depression, dexamethasone nonsuppressors were slightly but not significantly older than the suppressors. The frequency of dexamethasone nonsuppression was relatively high in this population (60%) in the entire sample).

A recent study (Stokes *et al.*, 1984) showed that in 132 depressed patients with major affective disorder, all eight measures of HYPAC function examined were higher (5 measures significantly so) in depressed patients older than 50 years of age, compared to those under 50 years. The overall trend was one of higher plasma cortisol levels with increasing age in depressed patients. A unique finding derived from the age-matched cohort of 80 healthy controls was the absence of significant correlations of age with any HYPAC measure in the normals. Georgotas, Stokes, Krakowski, Fanelli, and Cooper (1984) have reported that elderly depressives have a greater incidence of dexamethasone nonsuppression, and Alexopoulos *et al.* (1984) have reported additional similar data. Furthermore, these latter authors have recalculated the dexamethasone nonsuppression data in Carroll *et al.*'s 215 melancholic patients and have found that dexamethasone nonsuppression was significantly more frequent in those over age 65 compared to those under 65. Lastly, Rubinow, Post, Savard, and Gold (1984) have found that age and depression interact to produce severe cognitive impairment, and they postulate that the depression-related cortisol hypersecretion may contribute to this cognitive dysfunction.

At this juncture, then, it appears that there is a distinct interaction between age and depression, with resultant increased HYPAC function. Hence age must be taken into account in studies of this neuroendorine axis in the future, either by statistical correction or preferably by the use of age-matched control subjects.

Effect of Weight and Weight Loss

Absolute (total) steroid production is increased in obesity, though production as measured by amount per unit of lean body mass (mg cortisol/g creatinine/

day) is weight-invariant (Strain, Zumoff, Strain, Levin, & Fukushima, 1980). Weight loss in anorexia nervosa and in patients with severe protein caloric malnutrition is frequently associated with dexamethasone nonsuppression and disturbances in circadian rhythm (Doerr, Fichter, Pirke, & Lund, 1980; Smith, Bledsoe, & Chhetri, 1975). It had earlier been shown in rats that inversion of food and water access from the normal night hours to daytime hours was associated with a parallel 12-hour shift in the circadian peak of plasma corticosterone and in A.M.-P.M. ratios of hippocampal norepinephrine and serotonin levels; this continued even when normal day-night lighting patterns were resumed. Thus, altered food intake, disrupted sleep-wake pattern, and associated changes in brain amine content may be contibutory to the abnormal HYPAC rhythm in depression.

Weight loss associated with diminished appetite is a prominent and characteristic symptom of depressed patients with major affective disorder. Therefore, Berger, Pirke, Doerr, Krieg, and von Zerssen (1983) compared the DST results of depressed patients with and without weight loss to normal volunteers during weight loss. About half the depressives with weight loss (7 to 13) and a smaller percentage of normals (9 to 24), but very few depressives without weight loss (2 of 30), had dexamethasone (1.5 mg) nonsuppression. The weight loss was slightly greater in the normal volunteers (mean 1.53 kg/week) than in the depressed patients (0.91 kg/week) with weight loss. All were within +30% to −20% of ideal body weight; hence underweight was not thought to account for the dexamethasone nonsuppression, and mood ratings did not change during weight loss for the normals. Kline and Beeber (1983) found a poor relationship between dexamethasone nonsuppression and a diagnosis of melancholia. Since weight loss is both a physiological stressor and a *Diagnostic and Statistical Manual of Mental Disorders*, third edition (DSM-III), criterion for melancholia, they retrospectively examined the relationship of dexamethasone nonsuppression to *reported* weight loss. Among patients with dexamethasone nonsuppression, 10 of 14 had reported weight loss. Among depressed patients with dexamethasone suppression, only 3 of 13 had reported weight loss ($p < .05$).

Galvao-Teles, Graves, Burke, Fotherby, and Fraser (1976) found highly significant increases in nighttime plasma free cortisol in obese patients who fasted from 7 to 11 days, and Neuwirth, Philip, and Bondy (1964) reported significant elevation in early A.M. plasma cortisol concentration in 3 normal volunteers who fasted for 1 week (mean weight loss 6.3 kg). Therefore, Edelstein, Roy-Byrne, Fawzy, and Dornfeld (1983) studied 18 depression-free, healthy, obese subjects before and after a protein-sparing fast. All subjects showed 1-mg dexamethasone suppression before a mean weight loss of 13.5 kg during an 8- to 12-week diet (320 kcal/day). Those who became dexamethasone nonsuppressors ($n = 5$, 27.5%) lost a significantly greater percentage of body weight than the persistent dexamethasone suppressors (17.6% vs. 14.5%). Lastly, data from 132 depressed patients with major affective disorder in the National Institute of Mental Health (NIMH) Collaborative Program on the Psychobiology of Depression (Stokes *et al.*, 1984) revealed modest significant negative correlations of body weight with HYPAC measures. Three of the 8 dexamethsone-nonsuppressing normals were over 50 years of age, though no correlation was found in the age-matched control group ($n = 80$). The depressed patients with reported weight loss of more than 4.5 kg had higher *pre*-DST urinary free cortisol levels than patients with no weight loss.

Thus, in summary, it appears that the presence of weight loss and perhaps of low body weight per se in depressed patients can predispose them to dexamethasone nonsuppression. Hence low body weight and weight loss must be controlled for when assessing HYPAC function in depressed patients. Here, again, the requirement for matched normal controls is essential. Differences between normal controls and depressed patients with weight loss are suggested by the data above, though both can develop dexamethasone nonsuppression during weight loss.

Physostigmine Stimulation of HYPAC Function

In 1974, Janowsky, Khaled, and Davis showed that i.v. physostigmine (an acetylcholinesterase inhibitor) was associated with decreases in speech and spontaneous behavior, slowed thoughts, sedation, and occasional nausea. These findings have been replicated since then (K. L. Davis, Hollister, Overall, Johnson, & Train, 1976), and evidence for stimulation of HYPAC function has been presented (B. M. Davis & Davis, 1979). Risch, Cohen, Janowsky, Kalin, and Murphy (1980) found that in normal volunteers physostigmine produced significantly increased plasma cortisol and beta-endorphin immunoreactivity, as well as alterations in mood, cognition, and behavior. Nausea and vomiting developed in three of nine volunteers. The investigators found a correlation between plasma beta-endorphin activity (but not cortisol levels or nausea) and depressive symptoms. They postulated that a cholinergically mediated beta-endorphin pathway is implicated in affective responses, especially depression. Carroll *et al.* (1978) showed that in normal subjects escape from dexamethasone suppression could be induced by physostigmine. B. M. Davis and Davis (1980) reported that in subjects not pretreated with dexamethasone, physostigmine increased plasma cortisol. However, interpretation of these studies is difficult, since all were associated with some aversive, stressful side effects in at least some of the subjects.

A further study was therefore undertaken by Doerr and Berger (1983). They pointed out that Sachar *et al.*'s (1976) earlier study had shown that physostigmine in normal volunteers increased the plasma levels of cortisol, PRL, and GH. However, after blockade of the unpleasant side effects with methscopolamine, a peripherally acting anticholinergic, the response of all three hormones to physostigmine administration was abolished. This is consistent with the lack of convincing evidence that in humans PRL secretion is specially stimulated by cholinergic CNS mechanisms; also, in animals it is generally considered that PRL release is inhibited by cholinergic mechanisms. Paradoxically, however, PRL is also lowered by atropine administration (Vijayan & McCann, 1980). In addition, it has been shown by Benkert, Klein, Hofschuster, and Seibold (1981) that the anticholinergic drug biperiden releases cortisol and increases plasma PRL levels without changing GH, luteinizing hormone (LH), follicle-stimulting hormone (FSH), or TSH levels. Doerr and Berger (1983) found that physostigmine administration was associated with HYPAC stimulation and increased plasma cortisol concentration or escape from dexamethasone suppression in their subjects pretreated with methscopolamine, but they ascribed the stimulation to stress responses or mood changes that occurred in their subjects. They pointed out that subjects studied by essentially all other investigators also had mood changes and/or aversive side effects. Consequently, Doerr and Berger could not dissociate a direct HYPAC activation by physostigmine stimulation of central cholinergic pathways from a stress response, and they concluded that the HYPAC axis was more responsive to stress stimuli and mood changes than to pharmacological interventions.

In conclusion, it appears that studies aimed at probing a possible cholinergic mechanism in modulation of HYPAC function in humans will require a more subtle and specific tool than that provided by physostigmine.

D-Amphetamine Stimulation of HYPAC Function

D-Amphetamine stimulation of the HYPAC system in humans was studied by Sachar *et al.* (1980) because of their earlier studies in monkeys that showed an amphetamine-induced fall in plasma cortisol concentration even after administration of pimozide, a dopaminergic blocker. This suggested that the apparent HYPAC inhibition might be secondary to the noradrenergic effects of amphetamines, and not to the alterations in dopaminergic pathways in the CNS that might occur secondary to amphetamine. Amphetamine was also of interest, because in normal subjects and in some depressed patients it produces a change in mood and behavior. Those depressed patients who experience euphoria and an antidepressant effect following amphetamine administration are reported to respond well to treatment with imipramine (Fawcett & Siomopoulos, 1971; van Kammen & Murphy, 1978). Sachar *et al.* (1980) found that D-amphetamine sulfate given intravenously produced a prompt decrease in plasma cortisol concentration in 10 depressed patients, while 10 saline control tests showed no change. In contrast, 5 healthy individuals given amphetamine showed *increased* plasma cortisol after i.v. amphetamine. These investigators suggested that amphetamine may transiently correct a CNS noradrenergic deficit that results in HYPAC disinhibition and overactivity in some depressed patients. The increased plasma cortisol levels in the normal subjects after D-amphetamine administration could not be explained.

Halbreich, Sachar, Asnis, Nathan, and Halpern (1981) reported that there was a diurnal variation in response to D-amphetamine administration in depressed patients, but not in normal controls. Depressed patients (13 of 18) tended to have a decrease in plasma cortisol level, especially when tested in the evening, while normals had an increase in plasma cortisol, no change, or a minimal decrease 60 minutes following amphetamine. In a small study (n = 18) of depressed patients, Ettigi *et al.* (1983) found that 11 of the 18 were dexamethasone nonsuppressors and that 13 of the 18 had a positive euphoric response to amphetamine, but these two tests did not correlate.

The response of the HYPAC system to noradrenergic agonists and antagonists is of interest because of the CNS noradrenergic control mechanism modulating HYPAC function. Further studies with amphetamine, and (we may hope) more specific noradrenergic-acting drugs, should be performed. It is important to note that activation of the HYPAC system has been reported in rats after peripheral infusion of epinephrine in doses that do not exceed the normal upper level of plasma epinephrine concentration (Mezey, Reisine, Palkovits, Brownstein, & Axelrod, 1983). These findings, if verified, complicate enormously the interpretation of at least the mechanism of action of D-amphetamine and similar substances, since peripheral receptors may be implicated in the hormone response. Specifically, the release of ACTH and cortisol after administration of D-amphetamine may occur in a manner analogous to that suggested for dopaminergic alteration of PRL release via receptors on the pituitary gland. The number of subjects studied is still small in regard to D-amphetamine, and the same concerns remain regarding sensitivity, specificity, test-retest reproducibility, and so on, as discussed in regard to PRL studies.

HYPAC Relationships to Insulin Hypoglycemia

An earlier section of this chapter (see "Growth hormone," above) has discussed the long-recognized resistance to insulin-induced hypoglycemia in depressed patients (Heninger, Mueller, & Davis, 1975; Wright, Jacisin, Radin, & Bell, 1978). This was confirmed again by Nathan, Sachar, Asnis, Halbreich, and Halpern (1981), who reported that multiple afternoon and evening plasma cortisol levels were higher in insulin-resistant than in insulin-sensitive depressed patients. They also confirmed again that resistance to insulin-induced hypoglycemia disappeared with recovery from depression. No investigator has reported any relationship of the resistance to insulin hypoglycemia with age, basal growth hormone levels, or nutritional state (Koslow *et al.*, 1982). A provocative report has very recently appeared showing that a substantial portion (about half) of patients with certain (genetically determined) subtypes of depression (G. Winokur, Cadoret, Dorzab, & Baker, 1971) displayed relative insulin resistance *even in the recovered phase of depression*. Recovered bipolar patients also showed resistance to insuin hypoglycemia when well in 50% of instances. All these recovered patients who were studied had normal plasma cortisol and urinary free cortisol and were studied for at least 10 days while off all medications. Most of these patients were dexamethasone nonsuppressors during the acutely depressed phase of their prior illness. These data were obtained on a relatively small number of patients, some of them mildly obese (<20% above ideal body weight). This study warrants repetition to see whether insulin resistance is associated with bipolar and FPDD unipolar patients while in remission, thus providing a useful trait-related marker for depressive illness or at least subtypes thereof.

Sensitivity and Specificity of HYPAC Abnormalities in Depression

For some years most investigators (though not all; see Amsterdam, Winokur, Caroff, & Conn, 1982) have reported an increased incidence of HYPAC hyperfunction, especially dexamethasone nonsuppression, in depressed patients as compared to other diagnostic categories (Stokes, Pick, Stoll, & Nunn, 1975). In the past few years reports have appeared suggesting a higher degree of specificity of increased HYPAC function for depression, particularly the endogenous subtype. Two of these reports have involved large numbers of patients and found very good specificity (Carroll *et al.*, 1981; Schlesser, Winokur, & Sherman, 1980). Carroll *et al.* also reported that only 4% of normal controls had dexamethasone nonsuppression. In contrast, a very recent report involving 246 subjects, including 132 depressives with primary major affective disorder and 80 age-matched control subjects (Stokes *et al.*, 1984), found that dexamethasone nonsuppression had less positive predictive value for major diagnostic category than some recent prior reports had suggested. This resulted from the finding of a high incidence of dexamethasone nonsuppression in manic patients (50%) and a greater incidence of dexamethasone nonsuppression in controls (10%) than previously reported using a single 0800-hours postdexamethasone cortisol sample. If dexamethasone nonsuppression was defined as any postdexamethasone plasma cortisol sample > 5 μg/dl, then the frequency of nonsuppression increased to 33%, making specificity and positive predictive value decrease.

A recent large study in Britain (Coppen *et al.*, 1983) is in agreement with these data, as are smaller studies such as that of Amsterdam *et al.* (1982). Coppen and coworkers found dexamethasone nonsuppression in 43.4% of neurotic depressed patients, 43.8% of patients with other neuroses, 46.7% of patients with senile dementia (all had significantly greater nonsuppression than the controls, $p < .001$), and 21.7% of schizophrenics. There were 9 to 79 dexamethasone nonsuppressors among healthy controls (11.4%). This study reported a high incidence (70%) of dexamethasone nonsuppression in major affective disorder, and 81% of their patients classified as endogenous by the Newcastle Scale had dexamethasone nonsuppression. Schlesser *et al.* (1980) reported that none of their subjects (48 schizophrenics and 61 manic patients) showed dexamethasone nonsuppression, and W. A. Brown, Johnston, and Mayfield (1979) reported that none of their eight schizophrenics were dexamethasone-resistant. In contrast, we (Stokes *et al.*, 1975) had previously reported 17% dexamethasone nonsuppression in schizophrenics, similar to the proportion found recently by Coppen *et al.* (1983). In addition, Graham *et al.* (1982) reported than 42% of 50 manic patients were dexamethasone-nonsuppressing, according to a plasma cortisol criterion of any postdexamethasone level above 6 μg/dl. These investigators used three post-DST plasma cortisol samples. In addition, Dewan, Pandurangi, Boucher, Levy, and Major (1982) found that 6 of 20 chronic schizophrenics had nonsuppression on the DST. Most of these reports gave no information on presence or absence of depressive symptoms at the time of the DST. Five of the hypomanic nonsuppressing patients reported in the NIMH Collaborative Program had mixed manic and depressive symptoms. This admixture of depressed and hypomanic symptomatology may explain the lack of significant difference between dexamethasone nonsuppression in manics vs the total depressed populations (unipolar and bipolar) in that study. However, some of the nonsuppressing hypomanic patients did *not* have mixed symptoms and were so-called "pure manics."

Haier and Keitner (1982) studied 119 psychiatric inpatients with a variety of diagnoses who underwent a DST within 1 week of admission to the hospital and during the acute phase of their illnesses. Of these patients, 49 received a 2-mg DST and 70 received a 1-mg DST. The age, sex, and distribution of major depression did not differ significantly between groups. Choice of dosage was by chance. As reported previously by Carroll *et al.* (1981), Haier and Keitner also found the sensitivity of the 2-mg test to be slightly lower than the 1-mg test. On the 1-mg test, there was approximately 50% nonsuppression (16 to 33) in the diagnostic category of major depression; however, nonsuppression also occurred in 2 of 2 with atypical depression, 1 of 2 with schizoaffective disorder, 2 of 2 with bipolar disorder, 3 of 10 with personality disorders, 4 of 9 with alcohol *and* substance abuse, and 2 of 2 with organic brain syndrome (DSM-III diagnoses).

Haier and Keitner concluded from this relative nonspecificity that their findings were consonant with their clinical experience that the DST is less likely to overlap (be associated) with a diagnostic subtype of an affective disorder (e.g., melancholia), but is more likely to define a broader but biologically homogeneous group of affective disorders that cuts across current classificatory systems. A number of investigators have recently voiced the same sentiment, reminiscent of the way the DST was originally viewed 15-20 years ago. It is interesting to note in the work of Coryell (1982), in which he studied HYPAC axis abnormality and the response to ECT in 42 patients, that about half of the patients were dexamethasone nonsuppressors ($n = 21$) and that over 80% of patients in both suppressing and nonsuppressing groups had melancholia. In other words, the incidence of melancholia was the same and was unrelated to DST status. It is also noteworthy that Coryell comments that the nonsuppressors were significantly older (53.3 ± 16.5 years of age) than the suppressors (36.1 ± 12.6). Hamilton Rating Scale for Depression (HRSD) scores were essentially identical for the two groups at 23 (mean and median). Dexamethasone nonsuppression was not associated with endogenous subtype, and the same was essentially true for primary versus secondary depression.

Targum, Wheadon, Chastek, McCabe, and Advani (1982) have found the DST useful in separating depressed from nondepressed alcoholic patients. Dexamethasone nonsuppression or escape was observed in 9 to 14 clinically depressed alcoholic patients after withdrawal and in 0 of 14 nondepressed alcoholic patients. Other investigators have not confirmed this, however (Marks & Wright, 1977).

Regarding subtypes of depression, Schlesser *et al.* (1980) found remarkable specificity of dexamethasone nonsuppression for primary depression and for family history subtype or unipolar depression (familial pure depressive disorder). This finding has been replicated in several small reports (W. A. Brown & Shuey, 1980; Coryell, Gaffney, & Burkhardt, 1982), although not in another such report (Amsterdam *et al.*, 1982) or in the large study of Coppen *et al.* (1983). Schlesser *et al.* also reported a much higher incidence of nonsuppression in bipolar than in unipolar depressed patients. In 41 primary depressed patients, Holden (1983) found a high association between the Newcastle Scale (a scale for the differential diagnosis of endogenous vs. neurotic depressions) and dexamethasone nonsuppression, but no *healthy* control subjects were studied.

Mendlewicz, Charles, and Franckson (1982) described high sensitivity of the DST (79%) to both primary unipolar and bipolar depression, with diagnostic confidence of 82%. However, only 18 healthy controls were studied in Mendlewicz *et al.*'s work. They also reported 81% nonsuppression in psychotic patients and 37% in nonpsychotic individuals. They found no association between dexamethasone nonsuppression and any familial genetic subgroup of affective disorder, in contrast to that reported by Schlesser *et al.* (1980). In addition, this study did not replicate Schlesser *et al.*'s report of increased dexamethasone nonsuppression in bipolar depressed patients. Rothschild, Schatzberg, Rosenbaum, Stahl, and Cole (1982) described 34 psychotic patients with various diagnoses. The psychotic depressed patients had significantly higher postdexamethasone plasma cortisol values than other psychotic patients.

Thus controversy remains regarding the diagnostic specificity of the DST (and other measures of HYPAC function) for major diagnostic categories and for nosological subtypes. All HYPAC measures appear less specific than recently suggested.

Healthy Controls and Frequency of Sampling in the DST

Most prior studies have not included healthy controls, and this may be a significant flaw. Only one study has obtained age-matched controls who have undergone in parallel the same extensive diagnostic and investigative procedures that were carried out with the study pateints (Stokes *et al.*, 1984). The significantly higher incidence of dexamethasone nonsuppression observed in this study (10%, 8 of 77) in control subjects may be related to the fact that these subjects were age- and sex-matched and went through a battery of testing procedures similar to those performed on the patients.

Some investigators used only one postdexamethasone plasma cortisol sample for controls (McHardy-Young, Harris, Lessoff & Lyne, 1967), and few used multiple samples. Some used a 2-mg DST (Carroll *et al.*, 1981) and this may have contributed to the lower incidence of nonsuppression observed in their healthy controls, since a significant decrease in nonsuppression (17%) was observed in depressed outpatients given 2 mg vs those given 1 mg dexamethasone (49% dexamethasone-nonsuppressing) by the same authors. Hallstrom *et al.* (1983) studied 80 women, half aged 38 and half aged 50, as part of an ongoing population study. Of the 80 subjects, 15 (19%) showed dexamethasone nonsuppression, and 5 of these persisted in nonsuppression when retested 3 months later; 4 of these 5 persisted when tested a third time 6 months later. No other study has done repeat DSTs on normals. The reproducibility of the DST results was poor (15 of 80 down to 4 of 80) in this normal population. The medical exclusion criteria proposed by Carroll *et al.* (1981) did not substantially change these nonsuppression findings when they were applied.

Nuller and Ostroumova (1980) reported a 9% incidence of nonsuppression in 85 healthy controls, while Gold, Pottash, Extein, and Sweeney (1981) found only a 4% incidence in 25 normal subjects. Tourigny-Rivard and Raskind (1981) found a 5% incidence (1 of 20) in nonsuppressing healthy controls. Rush *et al.* (1982), studying 23 healthy, normal, drug-free volunteers (all under 50 years of age), found only 4% dexamethasone nonsuppression after a 1-mg dose; however, after a 0.75-mg dose, 6 of 23 or 26.1% were nonsuppressing. This demonstrates the presence of a dexamethasone dose response.

The importance of the dexamethasone dose response and its relationship to the DST result is underscored by Holsboer, Haack, Gerken, and Vecsei's (1984) recent work. They found a strong relationship between dexamethasone response and and the plasma level of dexamethasone 17 hours after a 1-mg DST in depressed patients. This contrasts with earlier work by Carroll *et al.* (1980), but is consistent with the original observations of Miekle, Lagerquist, and Tyler (1975), who looked at pituitary-adrenal suppressibility and dexamethasone levels in Cushing syndrome. Thus, plasma dexamethasone levels appear to be an important determinant of DST response, though more work is needed to confirm this suggestion. With the exception of Carroll *et al.*'s (1981) study, and the NIMH Collaborative Program, very few elderly controls have been examined.

HYPAC as a Predictor of Treatment Outcome

The identification of a pretreatment finding that would allow the prediction of treatment outcome of depressed patients would obviously be helpful to patients and treating physicians alike. This would, in addition, perhaps provide some further insight into the pathophysiology or pathogenesis of depression. It was suggested some years ago that the DST might provide such information (McLeod, 1972). In a study of 70 patients, half were dexamethasone nonsuppressors, and about two-thirds of that subgroup did not respond to tricyclic antidepressant treatment and required ECT. Only one-third of the suppressor group required ECT.

More recently, the reverse has been suggested (W. A. Brown *et al.*, 1979; Coryell, 1982). Coryell found that 21 of 42 patients with pretreatment dexamethasone nonsuppression show *better* treatment response according to global rating (but not HRSD score) at discharge. The author correctly commented that this disrepancy underscores the necessity of appreciating outcome measure variability in any study of response prediction. Spar and La Rue (1983) very recently studied 42 elderly depressed patients. Of these, 27 were dexamethasone nonsuppressors, but clinically they were not significantly different from the suppressors ($n = 17$), except for being slightly older and rating their mood as "more disturbed" than did the suppressors. However, the dexamethasone nonsuppressors did significantly less well on tricyclic antidepressant treatment and required larger doses. A number of smaller studies have similarly been reported, with conflicting results. To date, no clear evidence of pretreatment DST prediction of final outcome has been published.

HYPAC Function as a Predictor of Improvement during Treatment and Potential for Relapse

The DST has been considered a state-related variable, because most patients with dexamethasone nonsuppression during the acute illness have been considered to revert to normally suppressing status as the depression remits. However, until very recently this has received relatively little systematic attention. Beginning in 1980, a small number of papers have now appeared addressing this subject. Thus far, the numbers of patients studied have been small, and treatment modality and study design have been variable. However, encouraging results are evident, even though no final conclusions can be reached at this time. Greden *et al.* (1980) showed that reversion of the DST from nonsuppression to suppression might be a useful laboratory index of recovery from clinical depression, and this was reinforced by a subsequent publication from the same group that showed serial decrease in dexamethasone nonsuppression among unipolar depressed patients undergoing a course of ECT (Albala, Greden, Tarika, & Carroll, 1981). Subsequently, Holsboer, Liebl, and Hofschuster (1982) followed 23 patients during treatment and observed that the DST reversion from nonsuppression to suppression generally heralded the clinical improvement of a patient by about a 2-week lead. Furthermore, in a few cases, clinical worsening was again *preceded* by reversion of the DST to nonsuppressing status. Out of this has come the hope that repeated DSTs during treatment would be a useful additional means of monitoring therapeutic progress and perhaps of predicting treatment outcome (maybe even in the long term).

Studies are currently in progress as to the possible association of DST status with relapse potential at discharge after adequate treatment. Logically, if the DST is a reliable state-related phenomenon, the nonsuppressing status should disappear as a patient recovers from depression. If the DST does not revert to normal suppression, then are we dealing with a useful subclinical laboratory indicator of potential relapse, or is this persistent nonsuppression part of the low incidence of nonsuppression found in supposedly normal populations? Could this persistent dexamethasone nonsuppression be a manifestation of a trait characteristic in a particular subgroup of depressed patients?

One recent small study provides some interesting and striking data worth noting. Yerevanian *et al.* (1983) studied 14 patients with primary major affective disorder, depressed endogenous type, who showed dexamethasone nonsuppression on admission. When these patients were considered clinically ready for discharge, the DST indicated nonsuppression in 10 of the 14, or 71%. Subsequently, 2 of these 10 nonsuppressing patients committed suicide within 5 days of discharge; another committed suicide 8 months later, after a prolonged and stormy course of hypomania. Three more of the discharge nonsuppressors were readmitted within 3 weeks with a diagnosis of major affective disorder, depressed type. Two of these were dexamethasone nonsuppressors again on readmission. Two other patients who were discharged continued to meet Research Diagnostic Criteria (RDC) for minor depressive disorder at 2- and 4-month follow-ups and were working only part-time. One other patient stated that she felt well and had returned to work, but on examination she appeared clearly depressed, and her husband noted that she was not back to her usual baseline. In contrast, three of the four dexamethasone suppressors at discharge were doing well and were back to baseline functioning. One had persistent characterological depression but was otherwise well and working.

The data obviously need further study, although they are certainly interesting. The DST could have a role in the clinical decision regarding discharge from the hospital, and could be identifying a subgroup of depressives with chronic poor functioning and prognosis. However, the number of patients studied by Yerevanian *et al.* was very small, and replication and extension of this study are urgently indicated. It is difficult to conceive just from consideration of one's clinical experience that this is a representative sample of outcome, especially if one takes the available overall incidence or sensitivity of dexamethasone nonsuppression in depressed patients with major affective disorder as about 50% This would indicate that one-half of the patients seen clinically would follow the terrible course outlined above.

ADRENOCORTICOTROPIC HORMONE

It is apparent in considering the functional steps in the HYPAC axis that measures of ACTH might prove useful in our attempts to understand affective illness. Since the disturbance in HYPAC function certainly does include the pituitary and the CNS, measurements of ACTH activity at the very least would provide another measure of the function of the HYPAC axis. In addition, it is possible that ACTH secretion in disturbances of HYPAC function in depression could be qualitatively as well as quantitatively abnormal. No data exist to support the possibility of qualitatively abnormal ACTH secretion in depressed populations. Furthermore, it seems very unlikely, due to the episodic nature of depression and the associated HYPAC abnormality, which appears to be state-related rather than permanently present. However, there is evidence that ACTH has behavioral effects in animals and perhaps in humans. There is also evidence that pituitary ACTH release and adrenocortical steroidogenesis are not always tied closely together in an output-and-feedback type of oscillatory movement. It has been suggested that, especially in states of physiological perturbation, other stimuli of adrenocortical steroidogenesis may work with ACTH stimulation (Al-dujaili, Williams, Edwards, Salacinski, & Lowry, 1982; Pederson & Brownie, 1980). There is a diurnal variation in ACTH response (Kaneko, Kaneko, Shinsako, & Dallman, 1981). It has also been shown that, contrary to the usual current concepts, beta-endorphin and ACTH control mechanisms may not always provide for concurrent parallel release or suppression of these two peptides. Administration of dexamethasone to monkeys or humans decreases plasma cortisol (and presumably ACTH), but not beta-endorphin (Kalin, Risch, Cohen, Insel, & Murphy, 1980).

Since it has been demonstrated that plasma cortisol concentrations do not always fluctuate in direct relationship to ACTH concentrations in plasma (Holaday, Martinez, & Natelson, 1977; Krieger & Allen, 1975), it cannot be assumed that the cortisol abnormalities that are frequently present in depressed patients reflect only hypothalamic or pitutary abnormalities. Fang,

Tricou, Robertson, and Meltzer (1981) reported that ACTH levels were not associated with concurrent plasma cortisol levels. They also noted that ACTH levels in postdexamethasone plasma specimens did not account for nonsuppression of plasma cortisol. On the other hand, Reus, Joseph, and Dallman (1982) found that resistance to dexamethasone suppression of plasma cortisol in depressed patients was related to increased pituitary secretion of ACTH and heightened plasma ACTH levels. In another recent study, Kalin, Weiler, and Shelton (1982) studied 28 psychiatric inpatients, 17 of whom were dexamethasone suppressors and 11 of whom were nonsuppressors. Plasma ACTH data showed a lack of relationship between ACTH and cortisol concentrations in individual patient samples. The pattern of changing ACTH concentrations after dexamethasone was not consistent for nonsuppressors or suppressors. Furthermore, ACTH secretion was altered in cortisol nonsuppressors and was not closely tied to cortisol secretion. Obviously, further data are needed in regard to ACTH secretion.

CORTICOTROPIN-RELEASING FACTOR

Since the characterization of ovine CRF and its subsequent synthesis and availability for study, it has been shown that administered CRF is associated with a dose-related increase in ACTH and cortisol (Orth *et al.*, 1983). This has been demonstrated in monkeys and in humans. Orth *et al.* (1982) showed that in two patients with Cushing disease with pituitary microadenomas, the i.v. bolus administration of CRF was associated with variable, though increased, release of ACTH and cortisol as compared to that in normals. This hyperresponsiveness was absent after surgical microadenectomy. In a subsequent, more extensive study, Chrousos *et al.* (1984) showed that administration of a bolus i.v. injection of ovine CRF caused an increase in the already elevated levels of ACTH and cortisol in all 13 patients with Cushing disease (pituitary microadenoma). Successful surgical treatment of the Cushing syndrome with removal of the pituitary adenoma was associated with prompt (without 1 week) normalization or near-normalization of ACTH and cortisol responses to the CRF stimulus. On the other hand, patients ($n = 6$) with ectopic ACTH syndrome who also had high basal plasma cortisol concentrations and high concentrations of ACTH showed on ACTH or cortisol response to CRF injection, consistent with the expected pituitary suppression. Patients ($n = 3$) with Cushing syndrome secondary to an adrenal tumor, with the expected excessive plasma cortisol and undetectable plasma levels of ACTH, had no ACTH or cortisol response to infused CRF. Consequently, the administration of CRF may provide a useful means of differentiating pituitary from ectopic or primary adrenal causes of Cushing syndrome. Further experience with CRF may lead to the ability to segregate various subgroups of depressed patients with and without HYPAC hyperfunction. Gold *et al.*

(1984) showed apparent down-regulation of pituitary CRF receptors, as evidenced by decreased cortisol response to CRF in depressed patients as compared to normals. This finding supports the concept of a CNS abnormality in depression with increased HYPAC activity, as compared to the pituitary disorder evident in classical Cushing disease. The work of Amsterdam, (Winokun, Abelman, Luchi, and Rickels (1983), showing heightened adrenocortical response to administered ACTH in depressed patients compared to normals, suggests that circulating ACTH is greater in these patients and is consistent with Gold *et al.*'s finding of decreased pituitary ACTH increment following CRF administration.

CONCLUSION

The current state of neuroendocrine measurement of depression is encouraging to those of us involved in psychoneuroendocrinology from a clinical or research viewpoint. The increase in publications in this field since the mid-1970s is a reflection of the intense research interest and the potential clinical utility that may ensue. However, even after 25 years of increasingly productive effort, we are still largely involved in the period of characterization of neuroendocrine responses within and between various psychiatric syndromes and populations. This is not surprising and should not dismay those of us working in the areas of clinical or *in vivo* animal investigation in neuroendocrinology.

Current endocrinology took many years to develop from its original emergence at about the beginning of the 20th century as a clinical discipline relating symptoms and signs to pathological tissue findings at autopsy or operation. The subsequent interval of development, starting before World War I, was an era of indirect biological measurements of hormonal concentrations and activity. These indirect observations of the purported physiological effects of hormones were pursued through procedures such as the glucose tolerance test for assessing adequacy of insulin responses (and, we now know, many other hormone responses) involved in metabolizing a load of administered glucose, or bioassays such as the rabbit ovarian follicle maturation test for detecting pregnancy via the presence of gonadotropins in the urine of pregnant women. This period was a long one, but began to fade in the 1930s when the first biological "wet chemistry" tests appeared for direct spectrophotometric measurement of steroid hormones via chromogenic compounds produced from hormones or their metabolites.

After World War II came an explosion of techniques in endocrinology that have been increasingly employed in psychoneuroendocrine research. A pinnacle during this interval was the development of direct chemical measurement of biogenic amines and hormones in tissue fluids. These techniques have evolved further and now allow for repeated hormonal analyses within individuals and for multiple analyses across populations. In consequence, the questions of sensitivity-specificity and state-trait relatedness of the hormonal meaures can be and are being addressed experimentally. As yet, we have made less progress in understanding the meaning and the potential function (or dysfunction) of the hormonal changes we have been observing and characterizing in depressed patients. There is little doubt in my mind that investigation of such hormonal changes is necessary to increase our understanding of the biological aspects of depression.

It may well be that certain hormones play a role in the pathogenesis of at least selected kinds of depression. The evidence that pharmacological doses of glucocorticoids, as seen in Cushing syndrome or steroid hormone therapy, can produce remarkable affect changes in humans is impressive. Recently, glucocorticoids have been shown to bind selectively to certain limbic system neurons in animals. This, combined with the knowledge that steroid hormones can alter the activation of selected sited on the genome, all make it likely that hormonal changes may be more than epiphenomena or coincidental covariants of other underlying mechanisms that modify mood or cognition. For example, these glucocorticoid hormones could, via their genomic effect, alter the production of synthetic or degradative enzymes involved in biogenic amine production or degradation, or could, via their effect on the cell membrane, alter amine receptor function. Furthermore, the evidence that peptides such as ACTH (or analogues thereof) and vasopressin can alter behavior and learning in animals (de Wied, Witter, & Greven, 1975; Niesink & van Ree, 1983) and perhaps in humans (Kastin, Plotnikoff, Hall, & Schally, 1975) implicates neuroendocrine activity further as a potential modifier of CNS control of memory and expression.

Thus, it is becoming clearer that the classic endocrine function of hormones appears to be only one of their multiple potentials. We have much to learn about many other peptides that until recently were considered gut hormones but that have now been identified in the brain and can affect such specific behaviors as feeding (Vale & Brown, 1979). Recent data implicate the CNS opioid systems in the functioning of these peptidergic pathways (Niesink & van Ree, 1983). The intimate connections between neuroendocrine function and CNS aminergic transmission need further clarification. We know that the specialized neurons with their locus in the hypothalamus that elaborate and secrete CRF are modified in their secretory activity by inputs from noradrenergic, serotonergic, and perhaps cholinergic and opioid pathways as well. It is possible that a feedback system is operative between the aminergic and other transmission systems controlling CRF secretion and the hormones it release — ACTH, or partially degradated peptide fragments of ACTH, and cortisol.

Although the field of psychoneuroendocrinology has made remarkable progress in the last 20 years, many avenues of investigation remain to be fully explored and characterized in the future. Especially important are multisteroid analyses of repetitive plasma, urine, and cerebrospinal fluid samples in sick and recovered psychiatric populations, including various diagnostic categories and carefully matched healthy normal controls. Coincidental measurements of biogenic amines and their metabolites are needed, along with measures of other putative CNS neuroransmitters as their measurements become available. Careful assessment of the psychopathology and demographic characteristics of populations must be included. Ongoing attention to assay precision and to sensitivity and specificity of the association of biochemical measurements to behavior is paramount, with appropriate attention to test-retest reliability. Overall, the future looks encouraging for a fuller understanding of the "psychoendocrine profile" of affective states, especially of depression.

References

Agid, Y., Pollak, P., Bonnet, A. M., Signoret, J. L., & Lhermitte, F. (1979). Bromocriptine associated with a peripheral dopamine blocking agent in treatment of Parkinson's disease. *Lancet, 1*, 570-572.

Agren, H., & Wide, L. (1982) Patterns of depression reflected in pituitary-thyroid and pituitary-adrenal changes. *Psychoneuroendocrinology, 7*, 309-327.

Albala, A. A., Greden, J. F., Tarika, J., & Carroll, B. J. (1981). Changes in serial dexamethasone suppression tests in unipolar depressives receiving electroconvulsive treatment. *Biological Psychiatry, 16*, 551-560.

Al-dujaili, E. A. S., Williams, B. C., Edwards, C. R. W., Salacinski, P., & Lowry, P. J. (1982). Human γ-melanotropin precursor potentiates corticotropin-induced adrenal steroidogenesis by stimulating mRNA synthesis. *Biochemistry Journal, 204*, 301-305.

Alexopoulos, G. C., Young, R. C., Kocsis, J. H. Brockner, N., Butler, T. A., & Stokes, P. E. (1984). Dexamethasone suppression test in geriatric depression. *Biological Psychiatry, 19*, 1567-1571.

Amsterdam, J. D., Winokur, A., Caroff, S. N., & Conn, J. (1982). The dexamethasone suppression test in outpatients with primary affective disorder and healthy control subjects. *American Journal of Psychiatry, 139*, 287-291.

Asnis, G. M., Nathan, R. S., Halbreich, U., Halpern, F. S., & Sachar, E. J. (1980). Prolactin changes in major depressive disorders. *American Journal of Psychiatry, 137*, 1117-1118.

Asnis, G. M., Sachar, E. J., Halbriech, U., Nathan, R. S., Novacenko, H., & Ostrow, L. C. (1981). Cortisol secretion in relation to age in major depression. *Psychosomatic Medicine, 43*, 235-242.

Asnis, G. M., Sachar, E. J., Halbriech, U., Ostrow, L. C., Nathan, R. S., & Halpern, F. S. (1981). The prolactin stimulating potency of reserpine in man. *Psychiatry Research, 5*, 39-45.

Balldin, J., Gottfries, C.-G., Karlsson, I., Linstedt, G., Langstrom, G., & Walinder, J. (1983). Dexamethasone suppression test and serum prolactin in dementia disorders. *British Journal of Psychiatry, 143*, 277-281.

Benkert, O., Klein, H. E., Hofschuster, E., & Seibold, C. (1981). Effect of the anticholinergic drug biperiden on pituitary hormones and cortisol. *Psychoneuroendocrinology, 6*, 231-238.

Berger, M., Pirke, K.-M., Doerr, P., Krieg, C., & von Zerssen, D. (1983). Influence of weight loss on the dexamethasone suppression test. *Archives of General Psychiatry, 40*, 585-586.

Birkhaeuser, M. H., Staubb, J. J., Grani, I., Girard, J., Noelpp, B., & Good, G. (1980). control of TSH response to TRH in depressive illness. In *Abstracts of the XI International Congress of the International Society of Psychoneuroendocrinology, Florence, Italy, June 16-20, 1980* (p. 61).

Bivens, C. H., Lebovitz, H. E., & Feldman, J. M. (1973). Inhibition of hypoglycemia-induced growth hormone secretion by the serotonin antagonists cyproheptadine and methysergide. *New England Journal of Medicine, 289*, 236-239.

Blackdard, W. G., & Heidingsfelder, S. A. (1968). Adrenergic receptor control mechanism for growth hormone secretion. *Journal of Clinical Investigation, 47*, 1407-1414.

Boyd, A. E., Lebovitz, H., & Pfieffer, B. (1970) Stimulation of growth hormone secretion by L-dopa. *New England Journal of Medicine, 283*, 1425-1429.

Boyd, A. E., & Reichlin, S. (1978). Neural control of growth hormone secretion in man. *Psychoneuroendocrinology, 3*, 113-130.

Brown, G. M., Seeman, P., & Lee, T. (1976). Dopamine/neuroleptic receptors in basal hypothalamus and pituitary. *Endocrinology, 99*, 1407-1410.

Brown, G. M., Seggie, J. A., Chambers, J. W., & Ettigi, P. G. (1978). Psychoendocrinology and growth hormone: A review. *Psychoneuroendocrinology, 3*, 131-153.

Brown, W. A., Johnston, R., & Mayfield, D. (1979). The 24 hour dexamethasone suppression test in a clinical setting: Relationship to diagnosis, symptoms and response to treatment. *American Journal of Psychiatry, 136*, 543-547.

Brown, W. A., & Shuey, I. (1980). Response to dexamethasone and subtype of depression. *Archives of General Psychiatry, 37*, 747-751.

Burrow, G. N., May, P. B., Spaulding, S. W., & Donabedian, R. K. (1977). TRH and dopamine interactions affecting pituitary hormone secretion. *Journal of Clinical Endocrinology and Metabolism, 45*, 65-72.

Caron, M. G., Beaulieu, M., Raymond, V., Gagne, B., Drouin, J., Lefkowitz, J., & Labrie, F. (1978). Dopaminergic receptors in the anterior pituitary gland. *Journal of Biological Chemistry, 253*, 2224-2253.

Carroll, B. J. (1978). Neuroendocrine function in psychiatric disorders. In M. A. Lipton, A. Dimascio, & K. F. Killam (Eds.), *Psychopharmacology: A generation of progress* (pp. 487-497). New York: Raven Press.

Carroll, B. J., Feinberg, M., Greden, J. F., Tarika, J., Albala, A., Haskett, R., James, N. M., Kronfol, Z., Lohr, N., Steiner, M., de Vigne, J. P., & Young, E. (1981). A specific laboratory test for the diagnosis of melancholia: Standardization, validation and clinical utility. *Archives of General Psychiatry, 38*, 15-22.

Carroll, B. J., Greden, J. F., Rubin, R. T., Haskett, R., Feinberg, M., & Schteingart, D. (1978). neurotransmitter mechanism of neuroendocrine disturbance in depression. *Acta Endocrinologica, 220* (Suppl.), 14.

Carroll, B. J., Schroeder, K., Mukhopadhyay, S., Greden, J. F., Feinberg, M., Ritchie, J., & Tarika, J. (1980). Plasma dexamethasone concentrations and cortisol suppression response in patients with endogenous depression. *Journal of Clinical Endocrinology and Metabolism, 51*, 433-437.

Casper, R. C., Davis, J. M., Pandey, G., Garver, D. L., & Dekirmenjian, H. (1977). Neuroendocrine and amine studies in affective illness. *Psychoneuroendocrinology, 2*, 105-113.

Cavagnini, F., Benetti, G., Invitti, C., Ramella, G., Pinto, M., Lazza, M., Dubini, A., Marelli, A., & Muller, E. E. (1980). Effect of gamma-aminobutyric acid on growth hormone and prolactin secretion in man: Influence of pimozide and domperidone. *Journal of Clinical Endocrinology and Metabolism, 51*, 789-792.

Charney, D. S., Heninger, G. R., & Sternberg, D. E. (1982). Failure of chronic antidepressant treatment to alter growth hormone response to clonidine. *Psychiatry Research, 7*, 135-138.

Checkley, S. A., Slade, A. P., & Shur, E. (1981). Growth hormone and other responses to clonidine in patients with endogenous depression. *British Journal of Psychiatry, 138*, 51-55.

Christie, J. E., Whalley, L. J., Brown, N. S., & Dick, H. (1982). Effect of ECT on the neuroendocrine response to apomorphine in severely depressed patients. *British Journal of Psychiatry, 140*, 268—273.

Chrousos, G. P., Schulte, H. M., Oldfield, E. H., Gold, P. W., Cutler, G. B., & Loriaux, D. L. (1984). The corticotropin-releasing factor test: An aid in the evaluation of patients with Cushing's syndrome. *New England Journal of Medicine, 310*, 622-626.

Copinschi, G., L'Hermite, M., LeClerq, R., Golstein, J., Vanhaelst, L., Virasoro, E., & Robyn, C. (1975). Effect of glucocorticoids on pituitary hormonal responses to hypoglycemia: Inhibition of prolaction release. *Journal of Clinical Endocrinology and Metabolism, 40*, 442-449.

Coppen, A., Abou-Saleh, M., Milln, P., Metcalfe, M., Harwood, J., & Bailey, J. (1983). Dexamethasone suppression test in depression and other psychiatric illness. *British Journal of Psychiatry, 142*, 498-504.

Corsini, G. V., Del Zompo, M., Gessa, G. L., & Mangoni, A. (1979). Therapeutic efficacy of apomorphine combined with an extracerebral inhibitor of dopamine receptors in Parkinson's disease. *Lancet, 1*, 954-956.

Coryell, W. (1982). Hypothalamic-pituitary-adrenal axis abnormality and ECT response. *Psychiatry Research, 6*, 283-291.

Coryell, W., Gaffney, G., & Burkhardt, P. E. (1982). DSE-III melancholia and the primary-secondary distinction: A comparison of concurrent validity by means of the dexamethasone suppression test. *American Journal of Psychiatry, 139*, 120-122.

Dadkar, N. K., Dohadwalla, A. N., & Bhattacharya, B. K. (1978). Role of peripheral vascular resistance and reactivity in the interaction between clonidine and imipramine in spontaneously hypertensive rats. *Journal of Pharmacy and Pharmacology, 30*, 580.

Davis, B. M., & Davis, K. L. (1979). Acetylcholine and anterior pituitary secretion. In K. L. Davis & P. A. Berger (Eds.), *Brain acetylcholine and neuropsychiatric disease* (pp. 445-458). New York: Plenum.

Davis, B. M., & Davis, K. L. (1980). Cholinergic mechanism and anterior pituitary hormone secretion. *Biological Psychiatry, 15*, 303-310.

Davis, K. L., Hollister, L. E., Overall, J., Johnson, A., & Train, K. (1976). Physostigmine: Effects on cognition and affect in normal subjects. *Psychopharmacology, 51*, 23-27.

Davis, K. L., Hollister, L. E., Mathe, A. A., Davis, B. M., Rothpearl, A. B., Faull, K. F., Hsieh, J. Y. K., Barchas, J. D., & Berger, P. A. (1981). Neuroendocrine and neurochemical measurements in depression. *American Journal of Psychiatry, 138*, 1555-1562.

Dewan, M. J., Pandurangi, A. K., Boucher, M. L., Levy, B. F., & Major, L. F. (1982). Abnormal dexamethasone suppression test results in chronic schizophrenic patients. *American Journal of Psychiatry, 139*, 1501-1503.

de Wied, D., Witter, A., & Greven, H. M. (1975). Behaviorally active ACTH analogues. *Biochemical Pharmacology, 24*, 1463-1468.

Doerr, P., & Berger, M. (1983). Physostigmine-induced escape from dexamethasone suppression in normal adults. *Biological Psychiatry, 18*, 261-268.

Doerr, P., Fichter, M., Pirke, K. M., & Lund, R. (1980). Relation between weight gain and hypothalamic pituitary adrenal function in patients with anorexia nervosa. *Journal of Steroid Biochemistry, 13*, 529-537.

Edelstein, C. K., Roy-Byrne, P., Fawzy, F. I., & Dornfeld, L. (1983). Effects of weight loss on the dexamethasone suppression test. *American Journal of Psychiatry, 140*, 338-341.

Ettigi, P. G., Hyaes, P. E., Narasimhachari, N., Hamer, R. M., Goldberg, S., & Secord, G. J. (1983). D-amphetamine response and dexamethasone suppression test as predictors of treatment outcome in unipolar depression. *Biological Psychiatry, 18*, 499-504.

Extein, I., Pottash, A. L. C., & Gold, M. S. (1981). Relationship of thyrotropin-releasing hormone test and dexamethasone test abnormalities in unipolar depression. *Psychiatry Research, 4*, 49-53.

Extein, I., Pottash, A. L. C., Gold, M. S., Sweeney, D. R., Martin, D. M., & Goodwin, F. K. (1980). Deficient prolactin response to morphine in depressed patients. *American Journal of Psychiatry, 137*, 845-846.

Fang, V. S., Tricou, B. J., Robertson, A., & Meltzer, H. Y. (1981). Plasma ACTH and cortisol levels in depressed patients: Relation to dexamethasone suppression. *Life Sciences, 29*, 931-938.

Fawcett, J., & Siomopoulos, V. (1971). Dextroamphetamine response as a possible predictor of improvement with tricyclic therapy in depression. *Archives of General Psychiatry, 25*, 247-255.

Finkrelstein, J. W., Roffwarg, H. P., Boyar, R. M., Kream, J., & Hellman, L. (1972). Age related change in the twenty-four hour spontaneous secretion of growth hormone. *Journal of Clinical Endocrinology and Metabolism, 35*, 665-670.

Frazer, A. (1975). Adrenergic responses in depression: Implications for a receptor deficit. In J. Mendels (Ed.), *The psychobiology of depression* (pp. 7-26). New York: Spectrum.

Galvao-Teles, A., Graves, L., Burke, C. W., Fotherby, K., & Fraser, R. (1976). Free cortisol in obesity; Effect of fasting. *Acta Endocrinologica, 81*, 321-329.

Garver, D. L., Pandey, G. N., Dekirmenjian, H., & DeLeon-Jones, F. (1975). Growth hormone and catecholamines in affective disease. *American Journal of Psychiatry, 132*, 1149-1154.

Georgotas, A., Stokes, P., Krakowski, M., Fanelli, C., & Cooper, T. (1984). Hypothalamic-pituitary-adrenocortical function in geriatric depression: Diagnostic and treatment implications. *Biological Psychiatry, 19*, 685-693.

Glass, I. B., Checkley, S. A., Shur, E., & Dawling, S. (1982). The effect of desipramine upon central adrenergic function in depressed patients. *British Journal of Psychiatry, 141*, 372-376.

Gold, P. W., Chrousos, G., Kellner, C., Post, R., Roy, A., Augerinos, P., Schulte, H., Oldfield, E., & Loriaux, D. L. (1984). Psychiatric implications of basic and clinic studies with corticotropin-releasing factor. *American Journal of Psychiatry, 141*, 619-627.

Gold, P. W., Extein, I., Pickar, D., Rebar, R., Ross, R., & Goodwin, F. K. (1980). Suppression of plasma cortisol in depressed patients by acute intravenous methadone infusion. *American Journal of Psychiatry, 137*, 862-863.

Gold, M. S., Pottash, L. C., Extein, I., Martin, D. M., Howard, E., Mueller, E. A., & Sweeney, D. R. (1981). The TRH test in the diagnosis of major and minor depression. *Psychoneuroendocrinology, 6*, 159-169.

Gold, M. S., Pottash, A. L. C., Extein, I., & Sweeney, D. R. (1981). Diagnosis of depression in the 1980s. *Journal of the American Medical Association, 245*, 1562-1564.

Golstein, J., van Cauter, E., Linkowski, P., Vanhaelst, L., & Mendlewicz, J. (1980). TSH nyctohemeral pattern in primary depression: Differences between unipolar and bipolar women. *Life Sciences, 27*, 1695-1703.

Graham, P. M., Booth, J., Gianfranco, B., Galenhase, S., Myers, C. M., Teoch, C. L., & Cox, L. S. (1982). The dexamethasone suppression test in mania. *Journal of Affective Disorders, 4*, 201-211.

Greden, J. J., Albala, A. A., Haskett, R. F., James, N. M., Goodman, L., Steiner, M., & Carroll, B. J. (1980). Normalization of dexamethasone suppression test: A laboratory index of recovery from endogenous depression. *Biological Psychiatry, 15*, 449-458.

Greenwood, F., Landon, J., & Stamp, T. (1966). The plasma sugar, free fatty acid, cortisol and growth hormone response to insulin: I. In control subjects. *Journal of Clinical Investigation, 45*, 429-436.

Gregoire, F., Brauman, H., de Buck, R., & Corvilain, J. (1977). Hormone release in depressed patients before and after recovery. *Psychoneuroendocrinology, 2*, 303-312.

Gruen, P. H., Sachar, E. J., Altman, N., & Sassin, J. (1975). Growth hormone responses to hypoglycemia in postmenopausal depressed women. *Archives of General Psychiatry, 32*, 31-33.

Gruen, P. H., Sachar, E. J., Langer, G., Altman, N., Leiffer, M., Frantz, A., & Halpern, F. S. (1978). Prolactin responses to neuroleptics in normal and schizophrenic subjects. *Archives of General Psychiatry, 35*, 108-116.

Haier, R. J., & Keitner, G. I. (1982). Sensitivity and specificity of 1 and 2 mg dexamethasone suppression tests. *Psychiatry Research, 7*, 271-276.

Halbriech, U., Asnis, G. M., Halpern, F., Tabrizi, M. A., & Sachar, E. J. (1980). Diurnal growth hormone response to dextroamphetamine in normal young men and post-menopausal women. *Psychoneuroendocrinology, 5*, 339-344.

Halbreich, U., Sachar, E. J., Asnis, G. M., Nathan, S., & Halpern, F. (1981). Studies of cortrisol diurnal rhythm and cortisol response to D-amphetamine in depressive patients. *Psychopharmacology Bulletin, 17(3)*, 114-116.

Hallstrom, T., Samuelsson, S., Balldin, J., Walinder, J., Bengtsson, C., Nystrom, E., Andersch, B., Linstedt, G., & Lundberg, P. (1983). Abnormal dexamethasone suppression test in normal females. *British Journal of Psychiatry, 42*, 489-497.

Harris, G. W. (1955). *The pituitary gland*. London: Edward Arnold.

Health and Public Policy Committee, American College of Physicians. (1984). The dexamethasone suppression test for the detection, diagnosis, and management of depression. *Annals of Internal Medicine, 100*, 307-308.

Hellman, L., Nakado, F., Curti, J., Kream, J., Roffwarg, H., Ellman, S., Fukushima, D. K., & Gallagher, T. F. (1970). Cortisol is secreted episodically by normal man. *Journal of Clinical Endocrinology and Metabolism, 30*, 411-422.

Heninger, G. R., Mueller, P. S., & Davis, L. S. (1975). Depressive symptoms and the glucose tolerance test and insulin tolerance test. *Journal of Nervous and Mental Disease, 161*, 421-432.

Hershman, J. M. (1974). Clinical application of thyrotropin releasing hormone. *New England Journal of Medicine, 290*, 886-890.

Holaday, J. W., Martinez, H. M., & Natelson, B. H. (1977). Synchronized ultradian cortisol rhythms in monkeys: Persistence during corticotropin infusion. *Science, 198*, 56-58.

Holden, N. I. (1983). Depression and the Newcastle Scale: Their relationship to the dexamethasone suppression test. *British Journal of Psychiatry, 142*, 505-507.

Holsboer, F., Liebl, R., & Hofschuster, E. (1982). Repeated dexamethasone suppression test during depressive illness. *Journal of Affective Disorders, 4*, 93-101.

Holsboer, F., Haack, D., Gerken, A., & Vecsei, P. (1984). Plasma dexamethasone concentrations and differential suppression response of cortisol and corticosterone in depressives and controls. *Biological Psychiatry, 19*, 281-291.

Honda, Y., Takahashi, K., Azumi, K., Irie, M., Sakuma, M., Tsushima, T., & Shizume, K. (1969). Growth hormone secretion during noctural sleep in normal subjects. *Journal of Clinical Endocrinology and Metabolism, 29*, 20-29.

Imura, H., Nakai, Y., & Yoshimi, T. (1973). Effect of 5-hydroxytrytophan (5-HTP) on growth hormone and ACTH release in man. *Journal of Clinical Endocrinology and Metabolism, 36*, 204-206.

Jackson, I. M. D., & Reichlin, S. (1974). Thyrotropin releasing hormone (TRH): Distribution in hypothalamic and extrahypothalamic brain tissues of mammalian and submannalian chordates. *Endocrinology, 96*, 854-862.

James, V. H. T., & Landon, J. (Eds.). (1968). *The investigation of hypothalamic-pituitary-adrenal function*. Cambridge, England: Cambridge University Press.

Janowsky, D. S., Khaled, M. K., & Davis, J. M. (1974). Acetylcholine and depression. *Psychosomatic Medicine, 36*, 248-257.

Judd, L. L., Risch, C., Parker, D. C., Janwsky, D. S., Segal, D. S., & Huey, L. Y. (1982). Blunted prolactin response: A neuroendocrine abnormality manifested by depressed patients. *Archives of General Psychiatry, 39*, 1413-1416.

Kalin, N. H., Risch, S. C., Cohen, R. M., Insel, T., & Murphy, D. L. (1980). Dexamethasone fails to suppress βendorphin plasma concentrations in humans and rhesus monkeys. *Science, 209*, 827-828.

Kalin, N. H., Weiler, S. J., & Shelton, S. E. (1982). Plasma ACTH and cortisol concentrations before and after dexamethasone. *Psychiatry Research, 7*, 87-92.

Kaneko, M., Kaneko, K., Shinsako, J., & Dallman, M. F. (1981). Adrenal sensitivity to adrenocorticotropin varies diurnally. *Endocrinology, 109*, 70-75.

Kaptein, E. M., Kletzky, O. A., Spencer, C. A., & Nicoloff, J. T. (1980). Effects of prolonged dopamine infusion on anterior pituitary function in normal males. *Journal of Clinical Endocrinology and Metabolism, 51*, 488-491.

Kastin, A. J., Plotnikoff, N. P., Hall, R., & Schally, A. V. (1975). Hypothalamic hormones and the central nervous system. In M. Motta, P. G. Crosignani, & L. Martini (Eds.), *Hypothalamic hormones: Chemistry, physiology, pharmacology and clinical uses*. New York: Academic Press.

Kijne, B., Aggernaes, H., Fog-Moller, F., Andersen, H. H., Nissen, J., Kirkegaard, C., & Bjorum, N. (1982). Circadian variation of serum thyrotropin in endogenous depression. *Psychiatry Research, 6*, 277-282.

Kirkegaard, C., Bjorum, N., Cohn, D., & Lauridsen, U. (1978). TRH stimulation test in manic depressive disease. *Archives of General Psychiatry, 35*, 1017-1023.

Kirekegaard, C., Faber, J., Hummer, L., & Rogowski, P. (1979). Increased levels of TRH in cerebrospinal fluid from patients with endogenous depression. *Psychoneuroendocrinology, 4*, 227-235.

Kline, M. D., & Beeber, A. R. (1983). Weight loss and the dexamethasone suppression test. *Archives of General Psychiatry, 40*, 1034-1035.

Koslow, S. H., Stokes, P. E., Mendels, J., Ramsey, A., & Casper, R. (1982). Insulin tolerance test: Human growth hormone response and insulin resistance in primary unipolar depressed, bipolar depressed and control subjects. *Psychological Medicine, 12*, 45-55.

Krieger, D. T., & Allen, W. (1975). Relationship of bioassayable and immunoassayable plasma ACTH and cortisol concentrations in normal subjects and in patients with Cushing's disease. *Journal of Clinical Endocrinology and Metabolism, 40*, 675-687.

Laduron, P. M., & Leysen, J. E. (1979). Domperidone a specific in vitro antagonist, devoid of in vivo central dopaminergic activity. *Biochemical Pharmacology, 28*, 2161-2165.

Lal, S., de la Vega, C. E., Sourkes, T. L., & Friesen, H. G. (1972). Effect of apomorphine on human growth hormone secretion. *Lancet, 2*, 661.

Lal, S., Guyda, H., & Bikadoroff, S. (1977). Effect of methysergide and pimozide on apomorphine-induced growth hormone secretion in man. *Journal of Clinical Endocrinology and Metabolism, 44*, 766-770.

Lal, S, Nair, N. P. V., Iskander, H. L., Etienne, P., Wood, P. L., Schwartz, G., & Guyda, H. (1982). Effect of domperidone on apomorphine-induced growth hormone secretion in normal men. *Journal of Neural Transmission, 54*, 75-84.

Lal, S., Tolis, G., Martin, J. B., Brown, G. M., & Guyda, H. (1975). Effect of clonindine on growth hormone, prolactin, luteinizing hormone, follicle stimulating hormone and thyroid stimulating hormone in the serum of normal men. *Journal of Clinical Endocrinology and Metabolism, 41*, 827-831.

Landfield, P. W., Waymire, J. C., & Lynch, G. (1978). Hippocampal aging and adrenocorticoids: Quantitative correlations. *Science, 202*, 1098-1101.

Langer, G., Heinze, G., Reim, B., & Matussek, N. (1976). Reduced growth hormone responses to amphetamine in "endogenous" depressive patients: Studies in normal, "reactive" and "endogenous" depressive, schizophrenic, and chronic alcoholic subjects. *Archives of General Psychiatry, 33*, 1471-1475.

Leebaw, W. F., Lee, L. A., & Woolf, P. D. (1978). Dopamine affects basal and augmented pituitary hormone secretion. *Journal of Clinical Endocrinology and Metabolism, 47*, 480-487.

Linkowsky, P., Brauman, H., & Mendlewicz, J. (1981). Thyrotrophin response to TRH in unipolar and bipolar affective illness. *Journal of Affective Disorders, 3*, 9-16.

Loosen, P. T., & Prange, A. J., Jr. (1982). Serum thyrotropin response to thyrotropin-releasing hormone in psychiatric patients: A review. *American Journal of Psychiatry, 139*, 405-415.

Loosen, P. T., Prange, A. J., Jr., & Wilson, I. C. (1979). TRH (protirelin) in depressed alcoholic men: Behavioral changes and endocrine responses. *Archives of General Psychiatry, 36*, 540-547.

Maas, J. W., Koslow, S. H., Frazer, A., Davis, J., Katz, M., Berman, N., Gibbons, R., & Stokes, P. E. (in press). Catecholamine metabolism and diposition in healthy and depressed subjects. *Archives of General Psychiatry.*

Maeda, K., Kato, Y., Ohgo, S., Chihara, K., Yashimoto, Y., Yamaguchi, N., Kuromaru, S., & Imura, H. (1975). Growth hormone and prolactin release after injection of thyrotropin releasing hormone in patients with depression. *Journal of Clinical Endocrinology and Metabolism, 40,* 501-505.

Marks, V., & Wright, J. W. (1977). Endocrinological and metabolic effects of alcohol. *Proceedings of the Royal Society of Medicine, 70,* 337-344.

Matussek, N., Ackenheil, M., Hippius, H., Muller, F., Shroder, H.-T., Schultes, H., & Wasilewski, D. (1980). Effects of clonidine on growth hormone release in psychiatric patients and controls. *Psychiatry Research, 2,* 25-36.

McHardy-Young, S., Harris, P., Lessoff, M., & Lyne, C. (1967). Single dose dexamethasone suppression for Cushing's syndrome. *British Medical Journal, 1,* 740-744.

McLeod, W. R. (1972). Poor response to antidepressants and dexamethasone nonsuppression. In B. Davies, B. J. Carroll, & R. M. Mowbray (Eds.), *Depressive illness: Some research studies* (pp. 202-208). Springfield, IL: Charles C. Thomas.

McWilliam, J. R., Meldrum, B. S., & Checkley, S. A. (1981). Enhanced growth hormone response to clonidine after repeated electroconvulsive shock in a primate species. *Psychoneuroendocrinology, 6,* 77-79.

Medgett, I. C., McCulloch, M. W., & Rand, M. J. (1978). Partial agonist of clonidine on pre-junctional and post-junctional alpha adrenoreceptors. *Naunyn-Schmiedebergs Archives of Pharmacology, 304,* 215-221.

Meltzer, H. Y., Fang, V. S., Tricou, B. J., Robertson, A., & Piyaka, S. K. (1982). Effect of dexamethasone on plasma prolactin and cortisol levels in psychiatric patients. *American Journal of Psychiatry, 139,* 763-768.

Meltzer, H. Y., Piyakalmala, S., Schyre, P., & Fang, V. S. (1977). Lack of effect of tricyclic antidepressants on serum prolactin levels. *Psychopharmacology, 51,* 185-187.

Mendels, J., Frazer, A., & Carroll, B. (1974). Growth hormone response in depression. *American Journal of Psychiatry, 131,* 1154-1155.

Mendelson, W. B., Jacobs, L. S., Sitaram, N., Wyatt, R. J., & Gillin, J. C. (1978). Methscopalamine inhibition of sleep related growth hormone secretion. *Journal of Clinical Investigation, 61,* 1683-1690.

Mendlewicz, J., Charles, G., & Franckson, J. M. (1982). The dexamethasone suppression test in affective disorder: Relationship to clinical and genetic subgroups. *British Journal of Psychiatry, 141,* 464-470.

Menkes, D. B., & Aghajanian, G. K. (1981). Alpha-1-adrenoceptor-mediated responses in the lateral geniculate nucleus are enhanced by chronic antidepressant treatment. *European Journal of Pharmacology, 74,* 27-35.

Meren, G. P., Scarnati, E., Paglietti, E., Quarantotti, B. P., Chessa, P., Di Chiara, G., & Gessa, G. L. (1979). Sleep induced by low doses of apomorphine in rats. *Electroencephalography and Clinical Neurophysiology, 46,* 214-219.

Merimee, T. J., & Fineberg, S. E. (1971). Studies of the sex based differences of human growth hormone secretion. *Journal of Clinical Endocrinology and Metabolism, 33,* 896-902.

Mezey, E., Reisine, T. D., Palkovits, M., Brownstein, M. J., & Axelrod, J. (1983). Direct stimulation of β_2-adrenergic receptors in rat anterior pituitary induces the release of adrenocorticotropin in vivo. *Proceedings of the National Academy of Sciences USA, 80,* 6728-6731.

Miekle, A. W., Lagerquist, L. G., & Tyler, F. H. (1975). Apparently normal pituitary-adrenal suppressibility in Cushing's syndrome: Dexamethasone metabolism and plasma levels. *Journal of Laboratory and Clinical Medicine, 86,* 472-478.

Morley, J. E., Garvin, T. J., Pekary, A. E., & Hershman, J. M. Thyrotropin releasing hormone in the gastrointestinal tract. *Biochemical and Biophysics Research Communications, 79,* 314-318.

Mueller, P. S., Heninger, G. R., & McDonald, R. K. (1969). Insulin tolerance test in depression. *Archives of General Psychiatry, 21*, 587-594.

Mueller, P. S., Heninger, G. R., & McDonald, P. K. (1972). Studies on glucose utilization and insulin sensitivity in affective disorders. In T. A. Williams, M. M. Katz, & J. A. Shield (Eds.), *Recent advances in the psychobiology of the depressive illnesses* (DHEW Publication No. PHS 70-9053, pp. 235-248). Washington, DC: U.S. Government Printing Office.

Nathan, S., Sachar, E. J., Asnis, G. M., Halbreich, U., & Halpern, F. (1981). Relative insulin insensitivity and cortisol secretion in depressed patients. *Psychiatry Research, 4*, 291-300.

Nemeroff, C. B., & Prange, A. J., Jr. (1978). Peptides and psychoneuroendocrinology. *Archives of General Psychiatry, 35*, 999-1010.

Neuwirth, R. S., Philip, B. A., & Bondy, P. K. (1964). The effect of prolonged starvation on adrenal cortical function. *Yale Journal of Biological Medicine, 36*, 445-454.

Nicoloff, J. T., Fisher, D. A., & Appleman, M. D. (1979). The role of glucocorticoids in the regulation of thyroid function in man. *Journal of Clinical Investigation, 49*, 1922-1929.

Niesink, R. J. M., & van Ree, J. M. (1983). Normalizing effect of an adrenocorticotropic hormone (4-9) analog ORG 2766 on disturbed social behavior in rats. *Science, 221*, 960-962.

Nuller, J. L., & Ostroumova, M. N. (1980). Resistance to inhibiting effect of dexamethasone in patients with endogenous depression. *Acta Psychiatrica Scandinavica, 61*, 169-177.

Orth, D. N., DeBold, C. R., DeChreney, G. S., Jackson, R. V., Alexander, A. N., Rivier, C., Speiss, J., & Vale, W. (1982). Pituitary microadenomas causing Cushing's disease response to corticotropin release factor. *Journal of Clinical Endocrinology and Metabolism, 55*, 1017-1019.

Orth, D. N., Jackson, R. V. DeCherney, G. S., DeBold, C. R., Alexander, A. N., Island, D. P., Rivier, J., Rivier, C., Spiess, J., & Vale, W. (1983). Effect of synthetic ovine corticotropin-releasing factor: Dose response of plasma adrenocrticotripin and cortisol. *Journal of Clinical Investigation, 71*, 587-595.

Osterman, P. O., Fagius, J., & Wide, L. (1977). Prolactin levels in the insulin tolerance test with and without pretreatment with dexamethasone. *Acta Endocrinologica, 84*, 237-245.

Pedersen, R. C., & Brownie, A. C. (1980). Adrenocortical response to corticotropin is potentiated by part of the amino-terminal region of pro-corticotropin/endorphin. *Proceedings of the National Academy of Sciences USA, 77*, 2239-2243.

Pelayo, F., Dubocovich, M. L., & Zanger, S. Z. (1980). Inhibition of neuronal uptake reduces the presynaptic effects of clonindine but not of a alpha-methylnoradrenaline on the stimulation-evoked release of 3-H-noradrenaline from rat occipital cortex slices. *European Journal of Pharmacology, 64*, 143-155.

Prange, A. J., Jr., Loosen, P. T., & Nemeroff, C. B. Peptides application to research in nervous and mental disorders. In S. Fielding (Ed.) *New frontiers of psychotropic drug research*. Mt. Kisco, NY: Futura.

Prange, A. J., Jr., Wilson, I. C., Lara, P. P., Alltop, L. B., & Breese, G. R. (1972). Effects of thyrotropin releasing hormone in depression. *Lancet, 2*, 999-1002.

Prange, A. J., Jr., Wilson, I. C., Lynn, C. W., Alltop, L. B., Stikeleather, R. A., & Raliegh, N. C. (1974). L-tryptophan in mania: Contribution to permissive hypothesis of affective disorders. *Archives of General Psychiatry, 30*, 56-62.

Raiti, S., Davis, W. T., & Blizzard, R. M. (1967). A comparison of the effects of insulin hypoglycemia and arginine infusion on release of human growth hormone. *Lancet, 2*, 1182-1183.

Reus, V. I., Joseph, M. S., & Dallman, M. F. (1982). ACTH levels after the dexamethasone suppression test in depression. *New England Journal of Medicine, 306*. 238-239.

Riegle, G. D., & Hess, G. D. (1972). Chronic and acute dexamethasone suppression of stress activation of the adrenal cortex in young and aged rats. *Neuroendocrinology, 9*, 175-187.

Risch, S. C., Cohen, R. M., Janowsky, D. S., Kalin, N. H., & Murphy, D. L. (1980). Mood and behavioral effects of physostigmine on humans are accompanied by elevations in plasma β-endorphin and cortisol. *Science, 209*, 1545-1546.

Robinson, D. S. (1975). Changes in monoamine oxidase and monoamines with human development and aging. *Federation Proceedings, 34*, 103-107.

Roth, J., Glick, S. M., Yallow, R. S., & Berson, S. A. (1963). Hypoglycemia: A potent stimulus for secretion of growth hormones. *Science, 140*, 987-988.

Rothschild, A. J., Schatzberg, A. F., Rosenbaum, A. H., Stahl, J. B., & Cole, J. O. (1982). The dexamethasone suppression test as a discriminator among subtypes of psychotic patients. *British Journal of Psychiatry, 141*, 471-474.

Rubinow, D. R., Post, R. M., Savard, R., & Gold, P. W. (1984). Cortisol hypersecretion and cognitive impairment in depression. *Archives of General Psychiatry, 41*, 279-283.

Rush, A. J., Schlesser, M. A., Giles, D. E., Crowley, G. T., Fairchild, C., & Altshuler, K. Z. (1982). The effect of dosage on the dexamethasone suppression test in normal controls. *Psychiatry Research, 7*, 277-285.

Sachar, E. J., Altman, N., Gruen, P. H., Glassman, A., Halpern, F. S., & Sassin, J. (1975). Human growth hormone response to levodopa: Relation to menopause, depression, and plasma dopa concentration. *Archives of General Psychiatry, 32*, 502-503.

Sachar, E. J., Asnis, G., Nathan, S., Halbreich, U., Tabrizi, M. A., & Halpern, F. S. (1980) Dextroamphetamine and cortisol in depression. *Archives of General Psychiatry, 37*, 755-757.

Sachar, E. J., Finkelstein, J., & Hellman, L. (1971). Growth hormone responses in depressive illness. *Archives of General Psychiatry, 25*, 263-269.

Sachar, E. J., Frantz, A. G., Altman, N., & Sassin, J. (1973). Growth hormone and prolactin in unipolar and bipolar depressed patients: Responses to hypoglycemia and L-dopa. *American Journal of Psychiatry, 130*, 1362-1367.

Sachar, E. J., Gruen, P. H., Altman, N., Halpern, F. S., & Frantz, A. G. (1976). Use of neuroendocrine techniques in psychopharmacological research, In E. J. Sachar (Ed.), *Hormones, behavior, and psychopathology* (pp. 161-176). New York: Raven Press.

Sachar, E. J., Hellman, L., Roffwarg, H. P., Halpern, F., Fukushima, D. K., & Gallagher, T. F. (1973) Disrupted 24 hour pattern of cortisol secretion in psychotic depression. *Archives of General Psychiatry, 28*, 19-25.

Sachar, E. J., Mushrush, G., Perlow, M., Weitzman, E. D., & Sassin, J. (1972). Growth hormone responses to L-dopa in depressed patients. *Science, 178*, 1304-1305.

Sassin, J. F., Parker, D. C., Mace, R. W., Gotlin, R. W., Johnson, L. C., & Rossman, L. G. (1969). Human growth hormone release: Relation to slow wave sleep and sleep waking cycles. *Science, 165*, 513-515.

Schlatter, E. K. E., & Lal, S. (1972). Treatment of alcoholism using Dent's oral apomorphine method. *Quarterly Journal of Studies on Alcohol, 33*, 430-436.

Schlesser, M. A., Winokur, G., & Sherman, B. M. (1979). Genetic subtypes of unipolar primary depressive illness distinguished by hypothalamic-pituitary-adrenal activity. *Lancet, 1*, 739-741.

Schlesser, M. A., Winokur, G., & Sherman, B. M. (1980). Hypothalamic-pituitary-adrenal axis activity in depressive illness. *Archives of General Psychiatry, 37*, 737-743.

Siever, L. J., Uhde, T. W., Insel, T. R., Roy, B. F., & Murphy, D. L. (1982). Growth hormone respone to clonidine unchanged by chronic clorgyline treatment. *Psychiatry Research, 7*, 139-144.

Slade, A. P., & Checkley, S. A. (1980). A neuroendocrine study of the mechanism of action of ECT. *British Journal of Psychiatry, 137*, 217-222.

Sloviter, R. S., Drust, E. G., & Connor, J. D. (1978). Evidence that serotonin mediates some behavioral effects of amphetamine. *Journal of Pharmacology and Experimental Therapeutics, 206*, 348-352.

Smith, S. R., Bledsoe, T., & Chhetri, M. K. (1975). Cortisol metabolism and the pituitary adrenal axis in adults with protein-calorie malnutrition. *Journal of Clinical Endocrinology and Metabolism, 40*, 43-52.

Snyder, P. J., & Utiger, R. D. (1972). Response to thyrotropin releasing hormone (TRH) in normal man. *Journal of Clinical Endocrinology and Metabolism, 34*, 380-385.

Sowers, J. R., Carlson, H. E., Brautbar, N., & Hershman, J. (1977). Effect of dexamethasone on prolactin and TSH responses to TRH and metoclopramide. *Journal of Clinical Endocrinology and Metabolism, 44*, 237-241.

Spar, J. E., & La Rue, A. (1983). Major depression in the elderly: DSM-III criteria and the dexamethasone suppression test as predictors of treatment and response. *American Journal of Psychiatry, 140*, 844-847.

Spencer, C. A., Greenstadt, M. A., Wheeler, W. S., Kletzky, O. A., & Nicoloff, J. T. (1980). The influence of long term low dose thyrotropin releasing hormone infusions on serum thyrotropin and prolactin concentrations in man. *Journal of Clinical Endocrinology and Metabolism, 51*, 771-775.

Spitz, R., & Wolf, K. (1946). Anaclitic depression. *Psychoanalytic Study of the Child, 2*, 313-342.

Sternbach, H. A., Kirstein, L., Pottash, A. L. C. Gold, M. S., Extein, I., & Sweeney, D. R. (1983). The TRH test and urinary MHPG in unipolar depression. *Journal of Affective Disorders, 5*, 233-237.

Stokes, P. E. (1966). Pituitary suppression in psychiatric patients. In *Program of the 48th Meeting of the Endocrine Society, Chicago, Illinois* (p. 101).

Stokes, P. E. (1972). Studies on the control of adrencortical function in depression. In T. Williams, M. Katz, & J. A. Shield (Eds.), *Recent advances in the psychobiology of the depressive illnesses* (DHEW Publication No. PHS 70-9053, pp. 199-220). Washington, DC: U.S. Government Printing Office.

Stokes, P. E., Frazer, A., & Casper, R. (1981). Unexpected neuroendocrine-transmitter relationships. *Psychopharamacology Bulletin, 17* (1), 72-75.

Stokes, P. E., Pick, G. R., Stoll, P. M., & Nunn, W. D. (1975). Pituitary-adrenal function in depressed patients: Resistance to dexamethasone suppression. *Journal of Psychiatric Research, 12*, 271-281.

Stokes, P. E., Stoll., P., Koslow, S. H., Maas, J. W., Davis, J. M., Swann, A. C., & Robins, E. (1984). Pretreatment DST and hypthalamic-pituitary-adrenocortical function in depressed patients and comparison groups: A multicenter study. *Archives of General Psychiatry, 41*, 257-267.

Stokes, P. E., Stoll, P. M., Mattson, M., & Sollod, R. N. (1976). Diagnosis and psychopathology in psychiatric patients resistant to dexamethasone. In E. Sachar (Ed.), *Hormones, behavior and psychopathology* (pp. 225-229). New York: Raven Press.

Strain, G. W., Zumoff, B., Strain, J. J., Levin, J., & Fukushima, D. K. (1980). Cortisol production in obesity. *Metabolism, 29*, 980-985.

Takahashi, S., Kondo, H., & Yoshimura, M. (1974a). Growth hormone responses to administration of L-5-hydroxytryptophan in manic depressive psychoses. In N. Hatotani (Ed.), *Psychoneuroendocrinology: Workshop Conference of the International Society for Psychoneuroendocrinology, Mieken, 1973* (pp. 32-38). Basel: S. Karger.

Takahashi, S., Kondo, H., & Yoshimura, M. (1974b). Thyrotropin responses to TRH in depressive illness: Relation to clinical subtypes and prolonged duration of depressive episode. *Folia Psychiatrica Neurologica Japonica, 28*, 355-365.

Targum, S. D., Byrnes, S., & Sullivan, A. C. (1982). The TRH stimulation test in subtypes of unipolar depression. *Jpournal of Affective Disorders, 4*, 29-34.

Targum, S. D., Wheadon, D., Chastek, C. T., McCabe, W. J., & Advani, M. T. (1982). Dysregulation of hypothalamic-pituitary-adrenal axis function in depressed alcoholic patients. *Journal of Affective Disorders, 4*, 347-353.

Thorner, M. O., Ryan, S. M., Wass, J. A. H., Jones, J., Bouloux, P., Williams, S., & Besser, G. M. (1978). Effect of the dopamine agonist, lergotrile mesylate, on circulating anterior pituitary hormones in man. *Journal of Clinical Endocrinology and Metabolism, 47*, 372-378.

Tourigny-Rivard, M.-F. & Raskind, D. (1981). The dexamethasone suppression test in an elderly population. *Biological Psychiatry, 16*, 1177-1184.

Vale, W., & Brown, M. (1979). Neurobiology of peptides. In F. O. Schmitt & F. G. Worden (Eds.) *The neurosciences: Fourth study program* (pp. 1027-1042). Cambridge, MA: MIT Press.

van Kammen, D. P., & Murphy, D. L. (1978). Prediction of imipramine antidepressant response by a one day D-amphetamine trial. *American Journal of Psychiatry, 135*, 1179-1184.

Vijayan, E., & McCann, S. M. (1980). Effect of blockade of dopaminergic receptors on acetylcholine (ach)-induced alterations of plasma gonadotropins and prolactin in conscious ovariectomized rats. *Brain Research Bulletin, 5*, 23-29.

Winokur, A., & Utiger, R. (1974). TRH: Regional distribution in the rat brain. *Science, 185*, 265-267.

Winokur, G., Cadoret, R., Dorzab, J., & Baker, M. (1971). Depressive disease — a genetic study. *Archives of General Psychiatry, 24*, 135-144.

Wislocki, G. B., & King, L. (1936). The permeability od the hypophysis and hypothalamus to vital dyes, with a study of the hypophyseal vascular supply. *American Journal of Anatomy, 58*, 421-472.

Wright, J. H., Jacisin, J. J., Radin, N. S., & Bell, R. A. (1978). Glucose metabolism in unipolar depression. *British Journal of Psychiatry, 132*, 386-393.

Yerevanian, B. I., Olafsdottir, H., Milanese, E., Russotto, J., Mallon, P. Baciewicz, G., & Sagi, E. (1983). Normalization of the dexamethasone suppression test at discharge from hospital: Its prognostic value. *Journal of Affective Disorders, 5*, 191-197.

SECTION III

Behavioral and Psychological Measurement

CHAPTER 7

The Measurement of Behavioral Aspects of Depression

LYNN P. REHM
University of Houston

INTRODUCTION

This chapter consists of two parts. The first provides a behavioral perspective on assessment of depression generally, and the second part reviews specific measures of behavioral aspects of depression. The first part describes various dimensions of assessment. The goal of this initial section is to provide a basis for critiquing existing instruments and pointing to areas that are deficient in current practice. In addition, the discussion of the dimensions of assessment has implications for the nature of our conceptions of depression. Traditional clinical conceptions of depression, theories of the nature of depression, and clinical descriptions of the entity all take on contrasting shapes when viewed within the dimensional space suggested by assessment concerns. These dimensions thus define the focus and limits of the second part of the chapter. What is usually referred to as "behavioral assessment" falls into particular areas of the full assessment space. Behavioral assessments derived from observations of interviews or therapy, from analogue situations, from marital interactions, from ward observations, and from activity monitoring are reviewed.

BEHAVIORAL PERSPECTIVE ON ASSESSMENT

Assessment from a behavioral perspective has become a growing topic in and of itself. The proliferation of texts and the publication of two journals attest to the growth in interest generated by behavioral assessment. Much of this conceptualization employs the idea of domains of generalization (cf. Cone, 1977). The assumption is that all assessment is concerned with sampling and generalization across a variety of dimensions. Generalization theory has become an important way of conceptualizing psychometric development. For the purposes of this chapter, domains of generalization can be considered as various dimensions of a multidimensional assessment space. The system to be described is an adaptation of Cone's (1978) Behavioral Assessment Grid. The concept of a syndrome such as depression implies that many aspects of a person's behavior are deviant from norms in the population. The syndrome is said to exist when these behaviors are concurrently displayed. Depression encompasses many behaviors, as reflected in lists of clinical symptoms, diagnostic criteria, and items on depression scales. In part, depression is characterized by the wide range of behaviors affected. The behavioral manifestations of depression can be said to generalize broadly across domains of behavior in the person's repetoire. The behavioral responses (e.g., symptoms, test items) associated with depression can be categorized in many ways. One of the basic dimensions of assessment stressed from a behavioral perspective has to do with the response mode.

Response Mode

Behavioral assessment has traditionally distinguished among three modes of the depressive response: verbal/cognitive, somatic, and overt/motor (Lang, 1968). It is a basic tenet of behaviorism that psychology as a science should concern itself with observables. We are limited in our ability to assess a human being to what we can observe about the person. A behavioral approach to assessment stresses the sampling of observables as the essential nature of the assessment process. Assumptions of equivalence, groupings of symptoms, higher-order inferences, and abstractions all need to keep this essential feature in mind.

Verbal/Cognitive Mode

The first category of behavior that we can observe about a person is verbal behavior. We attempt to understand the subjective experience of the person through what the person can convey to us verbally through speech or writing in structured or unstructured formats. Cognitive behavior includes descriptions of experience, complaints, attitudes, beliefs, evaluations, inferences, and processes. Cognitive symptoms of depression are many and complex. Typically cited in clinical descriptions are pessimism, hopelessness, helplessness, low self-esteem, guilt, and thoughts of death and suicide. Certain theories of depression view cognitive symptoms as the primary symptoms of depression. For instance, Beck (Beck, Rush, Shaw, & Emery, 1979) views the essential features of depression in terms of the cognitive triad of negative view of self, future, and world. Seligman, in his reformulated learned helplessness theory (Abramson, Seligman, & Teasdale, 1978), posits a depressive attributional style as the core factor in depression. Inferences and conclusions that individuals habitually draw about the causes of events in their lives interact with stressful events to produce depression, according to this theory.

Typical assessment instruments evaluate cognitive aspects of depression in terms of the content of statements about oneself (i.e., experiences, complaints, beliefs, evaluations, and inferences about oneself). Verbal/cognitive behavior is most typically assessed by paper-and-pencil questionnaires, but may also be observed directly over a period of time or elicited in an interview format. For the most part, verbal behavior is assessed for its content, but occasionally speech is viewed as a form of overt behavior and paralinguistic features of speech (tone, volume, reaction time, rate, etc.) are assessed. Verbal/cognitive symptomatology may also be inferred by the observer, as in the scoring of projective story content. Cognitive processes can be assessed as well. The person may complain of problems in concentration or memory, and these functions may be assessed by observations of the person's behavior on various tasks. Overt behavioral performance is used to assess concentration, memory performance, processing speed, and so on. It is important to distinguish between a subjective complaint of memory difficulties and a direct observation of memory performance. Depressed persons may exaggerate performance deficits, and this negative bias is itself an important symptom of depression.

Verbal/cognitive aspects of depressive behavior may also be the targets of intervention. Beck's cognitive therapy in particular targets specific cognitive distortions as the focus of intervention, and Seligman's model (e.g., Seligman, 1981) suggests a variety of cognitive interventions.

Somatic Mode

The clinical syndrome of depression involves a number of somatic or neurovegetative signs and symptoms. These are held to be particularly important clinically and may be the defining features of certain subtypes of depression (e.g., endogenous or melancholic). A variety of somatic symptoms and changes can be directly observed in depression (e.g., weight loss). For most symptoms, however, we rely on the accuracy of patients' observation of their own behavior (e.g., constipation). Studies in depressive psychopathology have included physiological assessment of depressed individuals, and a number of dimensions of physiology suggest promising lines for assessment. For example, Schwartz's work (Schwartz, Fair, Salt, Mandel, & Klerman, 1976) with facial electromyogram (EMG) recording and the work of Kupfer and Foster (1972) and others on sleep electroencephalograms (EEGs) and rapid eye movement (REM) recordings, have been provocative. Somatic assessment also includes evaluation of biochemical changes. Current theories of depression include a variety of biochemical theories focusing on biogenic amines and other biochemical variables. Assessment of biochemistry is becoming an important diagnostic tool; biochemical assays are used to titrate the level of interventions via drugs; and assessment of the efficacy of drugs is also aided by biochemical assessment.

Overt/Motor Mode

We can assess depression by observation of the overt/motoric behavior of the person. The depressed person displays a sad demeanor, weeping, head hanging, frowning, and slowness of speech and of gait. Among the primary symptoms of depression are retardation or agitation. The motoric behavior of depressed persons is affected in a wide range of areas, including work, family, recreation, social life, and so on. In each instance, behavior is typically reduced quantitatively and may be changed qualitatively. Overt behavior has been the focus of behavioral theories of depression. Ferster (1973), in a seminal paper on the behavioral analysis of depression, argues that the prime datum of depression should be response rate. That is, a lowered rate of behavior in a variety of domains or response classes should be the identifying factor in the assessment of depression. Peter Lewinsohn and his colleagues (e.g., Lewinsohn, Biglan, & Zeiss, 1976) have developed a means of assessing activity level in the form of their Pleasant Events Schedule. The rate or frequency of these behaviors becomes the target of therapeutic intervention. Behavioral assessment often makes the differentiation between behavioral excesses and behavioral deficits. Certain behaviors increase in frequency with depression, and others decrease in frequency. Weeping, sad demeanor behaviors, complaining, sleeping, and the like may increase, while social and work behavior may decrease.

An important aspect of overt behavior in depression is interpersonal behavior. Clinical accounts of depression often identify themes in the interpersonal relationships of depressed persons. Interpersonal anger (often poorly expressed), dependency, irritability, and conflict often typify the interpersonal relationships of the depressed person. The work of Coyne (1976) and others suggests that the behavior of depressed persons has a negative effect on others in interpersonal interactions. Individuals who interact with a depressed person find the experience aversive and do not wish further contact with the person. Identifying the specific behaviors that produce these themes and these effects on others has become an important topic of research. Interpersonal aspects of depression are becoming more a focus of research, theory, and therapy.

From a behavioral perspective, these three response modes encompass the domains available to us for observation. The symptomatology of depression ranges across these domains broadly. Depression is complex and multivariate. Symptomatology within each of these domains covaries imperfectly, and verbal/cognitive, somatic, and overt/motor behavioral assessment data are necessary to map out the domain of depression.

Clarification of Terms

This tripartite division of response modes is at variance with some other systems for categorizing behavior. Some specific terms need to be defined and elaborated in this system. First, among these is the term "affect." In many systems, "affect" is held to be a different domain from verbal/cognitive, somatic, or overt/motor behavior. From the behavioral prospective, "affect" is defined within these three domains. We infer affect — for instance, anxiety — from a person's verbal/cognitive behavior, from somatic assessments, and from observations of overt/motor behavior. Inferences of anger, elation, or depression are similarly made from observations in these three areas. In a practical sense, we often ask patients, relatives, clinicians, or others to make direct assessment of affect (e.g., degree of anxiety, degree of depression or sadness). From a behavioral perspective, what is being asked is for a summary inference intergrating data on verbal/cognitive, somatic, and overt/motor behavior. For a person to say that he or she feels depressed is to give an integrated summary of his or her somatic, verbal/cognitive, and overt/motor state. People respond in an integrated and often idosyncratic fashion to situations, and they learn to label an integrated response with an emotional term, but it should be considered an inference summarizing across response modes.

The term "motivation" can be described in a similar fashion. "Motivation" is an abstract construct that has verbal/cognitive, somatic, and overt/motor references. An inference of reduced motivation results from and summarizes behaviors from these three domains. A verbal report of reduced enjoyment of food, a reduced rate and frequency of eating, and loss of weight, taken together, indicate a reduced level of motivation with regard to eating. All of this is implied in the summary statement that the person has a motivational deficit in this area.

The term "symptom" also needs to be clarified. What are usually referred to as "symptoms" are a variety of simple to complex responses, as seen within this system. Some symptoms may reflect single behaviors within one response mode. For instance, pessimism as a symptom of depression is clearly a cognitive behavior. Other symptoms may be much more complex, with verbal/cognitive, somatic, and overt/motor components. Loss of motivation as described above would be an example of this. Other symptoms may involve very complex behaviors. An example would be "suicidality," which would have cognitive components (e.g., recurring thoughts of death, suicidal planning, wishes to be dead, hopelessness about the future) as well as overt behavioral components (e.g., the history of suicide attempts, suicidal communications to others, and overt steps taken to prepare for suicidal attempts). Symptoms are often assumed to represent a single domain when in fact they are complex and involve multiple domains. For example, somatic complaints may also reflect cognitive symptomatology in terms of hypochondriacal concerns, helplessness, and negative interpretations of events. They may have behavioral components as well, such as interpersonal dependence, help-seeking behavior, and so on. Many primary symptoms such as sleep disturbance or loss of libido can be analyzed into verbal/cognitive, somatic, and overt/motor components.

Items on assessment instruments (questionnaires, clinical interviews, behavioral checklists) may, like symptoms, reflect behaviors within one domain or complex combinations across multiple domains of behavioral expression. Instruments vary in the degree to which they draw from these various domains. This is also true of descriptions of depressive psychopathology. Different descriptions weigh behaviors in these various domains differently.

Level of Inference

Within these three domains, assessment can be discussed in terms of levels of inference. All assessment is an abstraction about a domain of behavior. We abstract in terms of generalized dimensions, and we abstract in terms of samples from a domain of potential observations. An important consideration here is the level of inference. Low levels of inference would include direct counts of the rates of certain classes of behavior (e.g., speech rate, frequency of smiling, amount of time spent out of bed). In contrast, many forms of assessment of depression involve a high level of inference. These would include ratings of degree of depression, bizarreness of behavior, inappropriateness of guilt, or loss of insight. This is clearly a dimension and many different degrees of level of inference may be involved in different types of instruments.

Level of inference is often highly correlated with the nature of the instrument. Direct observational assessments tend to involve lower levels of inference. Clinical and diagnostic evaluations based on interviews more frequently tend to involve high levels of inference. Diagnoses may often involve inferences from multiple sources of data, including interview, history, and information from collateral sources. High- and low-level inference assessments tend to take different forms. Low-level inferences are more likely to involve assessments of the presence or absence of a behavior, frequency counts, duration, rate, or the like. Middle levels of inference may ask for true-false judgments or for presence or absence of more complex symptoms. Higher-level inferences often involve ratings of the degree or severity of relatively abstract symptoms. The same behavior may be assessed on different instruments with items of different levels of inference. Lack of comparability between instruments may in part be a function of the lack of comparability in item format and consequent level of inference. It is important to keep in mind that this is a domain of generalization. We expect generalization in the form of correspondence, correlation, or reliability between high- and low-level inference measures of the same construct. We have greater confidence in the validity of a construct if it covaries closely with specific behavioral instances. For example, a clinical rating of "agitation" should correspond to observational measures of specific inpatient ward behaviors such as pacing.

Psychometric Domains of Generalization

Within a behavioral perspective, response mode and level of inference are two descriptive dimensions and two domains of generalization. A clinical entity such as depression involves symptomatology in these domains, and this symptomatology can be interrelated or correlated. From the perspective of psychometrics, four other domains of generalization are important. They pertain to the reliability and validity (Cone, 1977) of instruments, but they also point to important aspects of our assumptions about the nature of the phenomena of depression. These four domains of generalization are rater, scorer, time, and place.

Rater generalization involves the classical problem of interrater reliability. When two observers view the same behavior, watch the same interview, or interview the same patient, we expect that they will come up with the same or similar ratings. Lack of interrater generalization would suggest that the dimensions of rating are vague or multidimensional, or that the raters are poorly trained or have idosyncratic views of the dimensions of the rating. Scorer generalization is the closely related idea that a test protocol produced by a single patient should yield the same score when different people do the scoring. This becomes an important issue in assessment methodologies involving higher-level inferences, such as projective techniques.

Time is an important domain of generalization when discussing depression. The psychometric consideration most closely associated with time is that of test-retest reliability. It is assumed that the clinical phenomena have some stability over time; that is, is assumed that a sample taken at one point will be closely related to a sample taken at another point in time relatively soon after the first measure. Stability is assumed to occur under constant conditions, though random factors may make contributions to a second measure. Assumptions of stability are basic to problems of measuring change. The assessment of change assumes that some known factor (e.g., psychotherapy or life events) may influence clinical phenomena in a particular direction, and that this change can be detected over and above the random factors that would otherwise produce relative stability. Another issue with regard to time is the size of the sampling period or time frame for an assessment. Assessments abstract or summarize over particular time periods. Differing instruments may assess over the entire period of a depressive episode, a specified time period (e.g., the past week, or an hour of observation) or particular points in time (e.g., how the person is feeling right now). Many instruments are vague about the specific time period to be sampled.

Clinical conceptions of the nature of depression and individual assessment instruments have implicit assumptions about sampling periods, and these in turn have implications for assessments of reliability and change. Depression is usually assumed to be a state rather than a trait factor. While there are certain traits that may be related to depression or to risk for depression, depression per se is seldom considered a trait. As a state, however, it is nevertheless usually considered to be relatively stable over fairly long periods. An episode of depression may last for days, weeks, months, or years. The criteria of the *Diagnostic and Statistical Manual of Mental Disorders*, third edition (DSM-III), for example, require a minimum of 2 weeks of continuous depression to qualify for an episode. This is much in contrast to other emotional disorders such as anxiety. An anxiety episode can be assessed in minutes or hours and occasionally in days. With the possible exception of rapidly cycling bipolar disorders, episodes of depression are considered in a much longer time frame. The depression literature does make a distinction between an episode of clinical depression and fluctuation in mood. Mood may vary from hour to hour or day to day. While the continuity between depressive mood and clinical depression is a topic of some debate, instruments meant to assess severity of depression may reflect variation in mood as well as level of clinical depression.

Particular types of assessment instruments have corresponding typical time samples and stability assumptions. The episode is the time sample period for some diagnostic assessment instruments for depression. Often, in such instances, symptomatology at the worst point of the episode is assessed. Such assessments are usually done for the purposes of case identification and are seldom considered for test-retest reliability assessment, despite the fact that there is an implicit assumption that within an episode symptomatology may vary in quality and quantity. Test-retest reliability is much more frequently considered relevant to measures of severity of depression. Such measures vary in their time frame assumptions. These measures are typically those used for assessment of change where the pace of assessment is usually in terms of weeks to months. A few measures have been specifically constructed for measuring mood. These usually assess a restricted domain of responses or symptoms — for example, self-referent adjectives on an adjective checklist or global ratings on a single high-inference scale. With such measures, day-to-day mood can be assessed, and occasionally even shorter time periods are used. Recent research on mood induction involves assessing changes in mood at points less than an hour apart within a particular induction session. Direct behavioral observations assessing such behaviors as activity level may specify short time periods for observation and then aggregate these data into a total or mean for days or weeks. Here empirical, temporal reliability becomes an important issue for choosing time periods and aggregation periods. Time frame is important to keep in mind when considering the purpose of an assessment and the comparability of one type of assessment to another.

The domain of place or situation is very important to certain kinds of assessment. Anxiety assessment, especially within the behavioral literature, has frequently taken on a very situational format. Self-report instruments, clinical interviews, and observations may survey situations or contrast anxiety-provoking versus non-anxiety-provoking stimulus configurations. Depression, in contrast, is assumed to be relatively nonsituational. People who are depressed are usually assumed to be depressed across situations in their daily lives. We do not usually assume that people will be depressed at home and nondepressed at work, or nondepressed with their family but depressed with friends.

This assumption is reflected in the relative nonsituationality of items on most measures of depression. Only a few instruments related to depression reflect situational assumptions. For example, some instruments that assess attributional style ask the individual what kinds of attribution of causality he or she would make for a variety of hypothetical situations. These situations make up the items of the test, and the frequency of depressive attributions becomes the score for depressive attributional style.

There are a variety of hints in the research literature for situational factors in the expression of depressive behavior. For example, Sacco and Hokanson (1978) found performance differences related to depression in public versus private settings. Mood measures and assessments of depressive behavior involving low-level inferences are appropriate to the detection of situational factors influencing depression. As with the domains of rater, scorer, and time, there are differing place assumptions and expectations for different instruments. It is important to be aware of these assumptions and their implications for our understanding of depressive phenomena.

Vantage of Assessment

Instruments typically assess depression from four different vantage points: (1) self, (2) observer, (3) clinician, and (4) mechanical. When we assess behavior, we may ask for the observations of the patient, a person who has the opportunity to observe the patient over a period of time, or an expert clinician, or we may employ some objective, mechanical means of assessment. These perspectives can be thought of as another domain of generalization. We assume that assessments from each of these perspectives will agree with one another. This domain of generalization is orthogonal to the other domains, although there is a tendency for instruments from each vantage to focus on certain domains of response, level of inference, and the like. For example, clinician scales often call for high levels of inference, and mechanical methods are useful only for a restricted range of responses.

Self-Report Vantage

Self-report instruments are the most frequently used form of assessment in psychological research. Numerous self-report scales for depression exist — for example, the Beck Depression Inventory (BDI; Beck, Ward, Mendelsohn, Mock, & Erbaugh, 1961); the Zung Self-Rating Depression Scale (SDS; Zung, 1965); the Minnesota Multiphasic Personality Inventory (MMPI) Depression (*D*) scale (Hathaway & McKinley, 1942); or the Depression scale on the Symptom Checklist — 90, revised (SCL-90R; Derogatis, 1977). These scales vary in their range and coverage of specific symptoms, but all cover behaviors from the verbal/cognitive, somatic, and overt/motor domains. Persons reporting on themselves are asked to report on their thoughts, attitudes, and beliefs, their physical state, and the nature of their recent behavior. Self-report techniques may have a special validity in evaluating verbal/cognitive symptomatology. Subjective data of all kinds are perhaps best assessed by self-report. These instruments vary in level of inference required, time frame assumptions, and the degree to which they tap the situational factors. Interrater reliability is irrelevant to self-report, but interscorer reliability may be important for certain kinds of instruments. The self-report techniques derive from the psychological tradition of personality assessment and tend to be typical of psychological research. These techniques usually yield a severity score derived from assessments of the extent and number of specific symptom items.

Observer Vantage

Observer scales include a variety of measures that are based on direct observation of the patient. Observers may include specially trained technicians, research assistants, and psychiatric nurses, as well as untrained observers such as spouses or significant persons in the patient's environment. Observations may be done in a variety of settings, including inpatient wards, patients, homes, therapy sessions, interviews, or specially structured situations. They vary considerably in the degree to which they are naturalistic observations versus observations in artificial situations. For the most part, these measures involve low to moderate levels of inference. The lowest levels of inference include specific behavior coding. These measures tend to stress the assessment of overt/motor responses, although they may involve some ratings of verbal/cognitive behavior or even somatic symptoms. Other scales involve moderate levels of inference, as in rating scales for use by family members or ward staff.

Behavioral coding systems have the problem of the validity of the codes. Are the specially coded behaviors correlated with other symptomatology of depression? Interrater reliability is very important with these measures. These measures usually use some form of time sampling, and questions arise as to the generality over the domain of time of the samples. Generalization across situation or place is also an important issue with these measures: For example, are measures taken on a ward predictive of the same measures taken at home? Does behavior in structured situations generalize to behavior in naturalistic situations? These techniques have special advantage and validity for evaluating overt/motor aspects of depression, and also for evaluating interpersonal behavior from the perspective of members of the person's social environment. The observers themselves may represent a sample of the patient's environment. These measures may be particularly useful for planning behavioral interventions and for tracking change in the patient's condition across time in an idiographic fashion.

Clinician Vantage

Many assessment devices have been constructed for use by expert clinicians. By and large, these derive from the psychiatric tradition of expert evaluation, with the additional element of quantification. In most cases, the data base is an interview with the patient. Instruments vary in their degree of structure, and some instruments suggest that judgments should be made from an integration of multiple interviews with the patient and collateral respondents. For the most part, these instruments involve relatively high levels of inference. They assume that judgments about complex and subtle psychiatric symptoms require expert inference and that the clinician's experience and skill will anchor these judgments.

These instruments have their own special problems with regard to psychometrics. The first problem has to do with the data source. Using an interview means that the clinician is relying on the patient's report of the patient's behavior and somatic symptomatology; the patient may add an element of distortion, independent of the questions of clinician reliability. Interrater reliability of clinicians is also a problem, for several reasons. Clinicians may have idiosyncratic biases. They may develop general impressions of patients that produce halo effects, and reliability may be spuriously increased by shared biases of clinicians on a particular research project or in a particular clinic. Also, whenever judgments are made on complex dimensions, different raters may stress or use different elements of the same dimension.

Mechanical Vantage

The ultimate in objectivity is to use mechanical means for assessment. In experimental studies, mechanical means have been used to evaluate verbal/cognitive, overt/motor, and physiological or somatic behavior. Voice volume and length of speeches can be mechanically recorded. Activity level and other measures of overt behavior can be evaluated mechanically. Physiological parameters may be recorded with the help of the physiograph, and biochemical assays may be derived via mechanical means. The objectivity of these measures is balanced by the intrusiveness and expense of the measuring devices and the limited behaviors that can be assessed by these methods. They also have their own problems of the validity of the response as it correlates with other aspects of depression. There are unreliabilities of mechanical scoring, problems of time and place sampling, and so on. Few measures of this sort are used with any regularity, but from a research perspective, we might expect growth in this form of assessment and the beginnings of their integration into clinical use.

The Assessment Space

The various domains of generalization that have been described above can be conceptualized as a large multidimensional assessment space. A portion of such a space is shown in Table 7-1. The table shows four domains of generalization: vantage, symptom, response mode, and level of inference. Within each of the vantages, one can conceptualize the same set of symptoms or responses, and these may be classified (S_1 through S_x) within the response domains of verbal/cognitive, overt/motor, or somatic. Summary judgments of the symptoms across domains may be called for by particular instruments. Within each of these response domains, items may be formulated to require high or low levels of inference.

This space could be expanded. The entire space could be repeated a number of times across, in columns representing different times of assessment. Similarly, the expanded space could be repeated vertically in rows representing different situations or places. Stacks of such superspaces could represent rater and scorer generalization or reliability. Even such an expanded space is not entirely complete. Any of the dimensions could be broken down further or

TABLE 7-1 Behavioral Assessment

		Verbal/cognitive		Overt/motor		Somatic		
Source	Symptom	Low	High	Low	High	Low	High	Summary
Self-report	S_1							
	S_2							
	S_3							
	.							
	.							
	.							
	S_x							
Observer	S_1							
	S_2							
	S_3							
	.							
	.							
	.							
	S_x							
Clinician	S_1							
	S_2							
	S_3							
	.							
	.							
	.							
	S_x							
Mechanical	S_1							
	S_2							
	S_3							
	.							
	.							
	.							
	S_x							

expanded with other categories, and additional dimensions could be imagined. For example, no mention has been made in this analysis of item format. The same symptom or response might yield a different score, depending upon the format of the item. Formats vary considerably. For instance, similar instruments could measure the same symptom by asking for a single severity rating, a degree of agreement with a statement, an estimate of frequency of the problem behavior, or the number of yes-no responses to a series of specific statements. Each of these methods may carry with it its own particular biases and may be a source of method variance.

Representing the assessment space in all of its dimensions can serve various functions for the clinician and the researcher. Importantly, the assessment space can be applied as a method of description. Any particular assessment instrument can be placed within the space to characterize its content, structure, and properties. Also, different scales can be readily compared. Such comparisons can be revealing. For example, Levitt and Lubin (1975) surveyed some 16 self-report instruments assessing depression and found them to cover a total of 54 different symptoms. Individual symptoms were tapped on from 2 to 16 of the different instruments. The lack of similarity in content between scales becomes more apparent when looked at systematically in terms of classes of responses. We (Barlow, Rokke, Carter, & Rehm, 1986) looked at the content of 12 depression scales — 6 self-report scales that measure depression only, 3 depression subscales from larger inventories, and 3 clinician rating scales. Trained raters classified each item into affective, verbal/cognitive, overt behavioral, and somatic. The results of this classification are shown in Table 7-2. It is immediately obvious that these well-known instruments vary considerably in the response domains that they cover and tend to emphasize. As an example, note the difference between the content loadings of the BDI and those of the Hamilton Rating Scale for Depression (HRSD; Hamilton, 1960). The BDI has a total of 73% verbal/cognitive and affective items and only 19% somatic items; the HRSD has 58% verbal/cognitive and affective items and 38% somatic items. The differential weighing here could well mean that research studies that select one or the other to screen or select subjects or to evaluate therapy outcome may be biasing the assessment in specific directions. Imagine an outcome study comparing a cognitive psychotherapy to a drug therapy. It is possible that the former might have a greater impact on verbal/cognitive symptoms and the latter might have a greater impact on somatic symptoms. Subjects selected on the basis of BDI or HRSD scores, and outcomes assessed by BDI or HRSD scores, might differentially favor one versus the other therapy modality.

It is important to stress that from a scientific point of view no specific domain, class of response, or vantage point is necessarily more valid than any other domain in the space. Such arguments for superiority of validity for particular domains occur frequently in the literature. Two examples should make this clear. First, different theorists have claimed that different response content domains have greater validity than other content domains. Cognitive

TABLE 7-2 Response Mode Content of Depression Scales

Scale	Total	Affective	Verbal/cognitive	Overt behavioral	Somatic	Misc.
BDI	21	2 (9%)	13.5 (64%)	1.5 (7%)	4 (19%)	0 (0%)
SDS	20	3 (15%)	8 (40%)	2.5 (12%)	6.5 (32%)	0 (0%)
SRQ-D	18	3 (17%)	5 (28%)	3 (16%)	5 (28%)	2 (11%)
Wakefield	12	4 (33%)	3 (25%)	1 (8%)	4 (33%)	0 (0%)
CES-D	20	6.5 (32%)	8 (40%)	2 (10%)	3.5 (17%)	0 (0%)
MDI	115	17 (15%)	76.5 (67%)	9.5 (8%)	12 (10%)	0 (0%)
MMPI *D*	60	5 (8%)	30 (50%)	9.5 (15%)	15.5 (26%)	0 (0%)
SCL-90R	13	2 (15%)	8 (61%)	1 (8%)	2 (15%)	0 (0%)
IPAT-D	40	7 (17%)	23.5 (59%)	3.5 (9%)	6 (15%)	0 (0%)
HRSD	23	1 (5%)	9 (43%)	2.5 (12%)	8 (38%)	0.5 (2%)
Wechsler	28	2 (7%)	13.5 (48%)	6.5 (24%)	6 (21%)	0 (0%)
Cronholm-Ottson	8	3 (37%)	3 (37%)	0 (0%)	2 (25%)	0 (0%)

Note. Abbreviations: BDI, Beck Depression Inventory; SDS, Zung Self-Rating Depression Scale; SRQ-D, Self-Rating Questionnaire for Depression; CES-D, Center for Epidemiologic Studies Depression Scale; MDI, Multiscore Depression Inventory; MMPI *D*, Minnesota Multiphasic Personality Inventory, Depression subscale; SCL-90R, Symptom Checklist — 90, revised; IPAT-D, Institute for Personality and Ability Testing Depression Scale; HRSD, Hamilton Rating Scale for Depression.

theories of depression tend to view and define depression in cognitive terms, and to postulate that certain cognitive characteristics and mechanisms are the essential or core aspects of depression that should be targeted for modification and remediation. Behavioral views of depression have postulated that particular features of overt/motor behavior are the defining characteristics of depression and should be the targets for intervention startegies. In a very similar way, biological theories have postulated that somatic factors may be the defining characteristics of depression and are the core factors requiring chemical intervention and modification. From the point of view of scientific assessment, these theoretical perspectives should not influence the desirability of assessing the full range of depressive behaviors across each of these response domains. It is important to avoid biases in scale selection that reflect biases in theory.

Second, vantage points have been subject to arguments for the superior validity of one domain versus another. Self-report, observer, clinician, and mechanical assessments each have a role to play in an overall assessment strategy. Indeed, each of these vantage domains may have its own special validity; that is, each may tap a separate, valid, and important source of variance. Traditionally, various sources of judgment lead us to define behavior as disordered or psychopathological. These sources include distress experienced by the individual, distress experienced by the person's interpersonal environment, expert detection of pathology according to agreed-upon criteria, and objective indices of deviance. These are precisely the vantage points represented by assessment instruments. Self-report instruments may have special validity in tapping the individual's subjective distress. Observer instruments applied by members of the person's social environment may tap that environment's interpersonal distress in dealing with the individual. Clinician measures objectify expert opinion according to specified criteria. Finally, mechanical measures provide us with objective assessment of deviance. Thus, each may be especially valid to a particular defining domain of abnormality. These domains may not agree perfectly, and disagreements may have important scientific implications. Clearly, we would not be satisfied with the outcome of a psychotherapy procedure or a drug therapy if it produced significant improvement from the vantage point of the patient but not from the vantage point of an expert clinician, or vice versa. If improvement occurred in both of these modalities but the family was still distressed and unable to deal with the person, the clinician would surely want to investigate the source of such distress.

A particular instance of this issue is the contrast between the psychiatric literature and the psychological literature in depression. The psychiatric literature tends to view the clinician vantage as the criterion measure of depression, whereas the psychological literature tends to view the self-report vantage as the criterion measure. Psychiatric tradition stresses expert clinical evaluation; psychological tradition stresses the development of psychometrically valid self-report scales. From a scientific point of view, each method has its own advantages and disadvantages. The contribution of method or vantage variance should always be recognized when evaluating the interrelationships among scales. For example, we should not make the error of concluding that self-report severity scales are less valid than clinician severity scales because they correlate less highly with psychiatric diagnosis. Psychiatric diagnosis is an instance of a particular type of clinician instrument. Thus the correlation between two clinician instruments, one a severity scale and one a dichotomous diagnostic decision, would be expected for purely psychometric reasons to be higher than the correlations between a self-report severity scale and a clinician's dichotomous diagnostic decision. It is theoretically quite possible to construct a self-report instrument that is a dichotomous diagnostic decision. In fact, some of the computerizations of structured diagnostic interviews may be leading exactly in that direction. In such instances, one would expect that a self-report severity scale would probably correlate more highly with the diagnosis than would a clinician severity scale.

It is one of the central tenets of this chapter that we ultimately can only develop assurance in the validity of our assessments of depression if we attend carefully to the parallel sampling and reliability of measures across the various domains of generalization. Instruments for measuring depression should be considered valid only if they have been demonstrated to tap various response domains and intercorrelated symptomatic behaviors reliably across time and place (or within particular important time spans or situations). It would be highly desirable to have parallel assessments across vantage of assessment. We would also be more sure of our instruments if assessments involving high-level inferences correlate with specific instances of the broader construct. The construct depression is assessed validly and reliably when generalization across the various domains is demonstrated and when various sources of method or domain variance are isolated.

ASSESSMENT OF BEHAVIORAL ASPECTS OF DEPRESSION

In its broadest sense, behavioral assessment encompasses all of the assessment space described above. In a narrower sense, however, behaviorally oriented researchers have made major contributions in specific areas of the assessment space. Much of the work on behavioral assessment has focused on the overt/motor response mode. Much of this research has focused on speech, where verbal content, paralinguistic features of speech, and nonverbal concomitants of speech are assessed. Behavioral assessment tends to be low in inference level. Behavior codes and time-sampling methodology have been behavioral contributions to the depression assessment literature. For the most part, behavioral assessment tends to stress the observer vantage, but has also made some interesting contributions to the self-report vantage with self-monitoring methods. Behavioral assessment tends to stress the importance of settings, and the present review is organized around setting formats.

It should be stressed that this is a selective review of an arbitrarily defined area. It should be clear that the term "behavioral" when applied to assessment does not have a very clear referent. Behavioral theory is not a single coherent position. It spans a range of positions from "radical" behavioral, to "neobehavioral," to "social learning," to "cognitive-behavioral" (cf. Wilson, 1978). Behavioral assessment has always stressed the use of multiple measures of constructs (e.g., Lang, 1968).Thus this review is taking a particular focus on assessment methods that may cover a portion of the assessment grid often given less attention by traditional perspectives. The measures reviewed here should be seen as parts of larger assessment strategies that expand our confidence in the validity, reliability, and generalizability of our results. Other contributions to the assessment of depression by behaviorally oriented researchers in the areas of self-report and physiological measurement are covered by other chapters in this book.

Observations in the Interview and in Therapy

Clinicians have traditionally seen patients in interview and therapy settings and have made clinical observations of the patient's behavior in these settings. Behavioral assessment has attempted to codify some of these typical behavioral observations. A number of studies, for instance, have looked at the differences between depressed and nondepressed subject samples on specific forms of behavior. In two early studies, Waxer (1974, 1976) had raters view silent videotapes of depressed and nondepressed psychiatric patients and asked them to comment on which of 10 body cues were most expressive of depression. A group of raters who were given no suggestions as to which areas of the body to observe achieved a correlation of 0.37 between their general impressions of depression and the subjects' MMPI D scores. The correlations for observers cued to the specific areas of the body increased to 0.60. Raters reported poor eye contact, downward contractions of the mouth, downward angling of the head, and lack of hand movement as the most prominent depression cues. Hinchliffe, Lancashire, and Roberts (1970, 1971) conducted studies comparing speech samples from depressive and control surgical patients. Depressives' speech was characterized by a lower rate, higher frequency of personal references, lower frequency of nonpersonal references, a higher number of "negators," and a higher number of expressions of feelings. There were no differences in length of pauses or use of value judgments. Depressed subjects were also found to show a reduced frequency and duration of eye contacts during the interview. Eye contact was found to increase as the patients recovered. Teasdale, Fogarty, and Williams (1980) focused on speech rate as a single measure of depression and found that short-term variations in depression were reflected in speech rates within subjects. Speech pause time was the focus of a study by Szabadi, Bradshaw, and Besson (1976). Four depressed patients and four normals were asked to count to 10, and voice prints were taken. Pause times were longer for depressed patients and they improved with time. This measure, however, did not correlate with other measures of motor response (e.g., tapping time) or with ratings of retardation. The small number of subjects may have precluded detecting such relationships.

Ranelli and Miller (1977) reported on a study of 17 psychiatric inpatients who were observed over the course of six weekly interviews on 23 movement and 4 paralinguistic variables. The design was blind as to the drug or placebo condition of the subjects and focused on the distinction between behavioral illustrators (i.e., hand and head movements that contribute to communication) versus adaptors (i.e., movements that are unrelated to or detract from communication). Overall, they found that all subjects tended to improve somewhat over time and showed more hand gestures and illustrators while initiating fewer utterances. Drug-treated subjects increased in behavioral adaptors, came to establish more eye contact, and showed fewer speech pauses.

A group of Swiss researchers (Fisch, Frey, & Hirsbrunner, 1983; Frey, Jorns, & Daw, 1980) have described a coding system whereby precise positions of the doctor's and the patient's head, trunk, shoulders, upper arms, hands, upper legs, feet, and chair position can be described on a total of 32 scales. Position changes are recorded at 0.5-second intervals during 3-minute segments of interviews. This time series recording allows for derived measures of mobility (percentage of time in motion), complexity (simultaneous movements), and dynamic activation (rapidity of movement onset and offset). All three of these measures were shown to increase with clinical improvement. Individual differences overshadowed depressed-nondepressed state differences. Interestingly, depressed states also had a strong influence on interviewers' behavior. Doctors showed less movement than patients and changed more with patient improvement, although doctor changes did not correlate strongly with patient changes.

Lewinsohn and his colleagues (Lewinsohn, Weinstein, & Alper, 1970; Libet & Lewinsohn, 1973; Libet, Lewinsohn, & Javorek, 1973) have employed a coding system for verbal behavior in group therapy and home situations that assesses the total number of behaviors emitted by and directed toward each individual, use of positive and negative reactions by each individual, interpersonal efficiency ratio (number of verbal behaviors directed toward an individual, relative to the number the individual emits), and the range of interactions with others. In general, interrater reliabilities were found to be satisfactory, but temporal stability was low for some of the variables. Libet and Lewinsohn (1973) found that the depressed subjects had lower total activity levels, were slower in responding to others, emitted fewer positive reactions to others, and had a more restricted interpersonal range. They did not differ on negative reactions, and there were no differences on interpersonal efficiency. Libet *et al.* (1973) compared therapy and home visit observations and found situational differences between the two settings. In therapy groups, depressed males were less verbally active and were slower in their reactions. They were also affected more by aversive reactions from others and elicited fewer positive reactions. Results for females were in the same direction but were nonsignificant. In home observations, depressed males emitted fewer verbal behaviors in total but initiated more actions. This reversal was attributed to less participation in ongoing conversations initiated by others. Depressed males were also more silent, were slower to respond, and elicited a lower rate of positive reinforcement. In an interesting clinical application of the coding methodology, Lewinsohn *et al.* (1970) gave patients in a therapy group weekly feedback on their behavior codes, and this material was used as a basis for a therapeutic discussion of the interpersonal skill and impact of each.

Lewinsohn and his colleagues have also assessed behavior using these and other codes and then targeted the specific behavior for therapeutic intervention. For example, Robinson and Lewinsohn (1973) targeted the slowed speech rate of a chronically depressed psychiatric patient for intervention. They demonstrated an ability to increase speech rate as measured in 30-second intervals by an observer. Lewinsohn and Atwood (1969) made home observations in the case of a 38-year-old depressed woman, and, on the basis of the coding of the verbal interactions, targeted increasing the family's verbal behavior toward the patient. Lewinsohn and Shaffer (1971) reported on three more cases where the use of home observations added valuable information to the formulation of behavioral therapy plan. Two other reports, one by Aiken and Parker (1965) and one by Ince (1972), demonstrated the possibility of using reinforcement procedures within therapy sessions to increase the frequency of specific verbal response classes, especially positive self-references.

In a series of outcome studies of a behavior therapy program for depression my colleagues and I have used a variety of behavior codes assessed in pretest and posttest clinical interviews and in first- and last-group therapy sessions as adjunct measures of depressive behavior and behavior change. Our intent was to identify behaviors that previous literature had suggested were symptomatic of or correlated with depression. We attempted to develop reliable methods of rating these behaviors, to assess the validity of the behaviors by comparisons with nondepressed samples and by correlations with other indices of depression, to assess the situational stability between interview and therapy of the measures, and to determine whether these measures changed over time following therapy.

Although the measures changed somewhat from study to study, four types of measures were used. These included, first, paralinguistic codes that involved quantitative aspects of speech behavior (e.g., duration, latency, etc.)

Paralinguistic measures included number of words in a transcript of a 5-minute interview sample, the number of speech disfluencies in a 5-minute sample, and some ratings of expressivity and loudness. A second set of codes quantified nonverbal behavior such as eye contact, which was timed, and smiles and arm movements, which were all counted as occurrences or nonoccurrences in either 5- or 10-second intervals on videotape. Third, we used some relatively simple content measures, such as the frequency of positive and negative references to self and to others. Finally, we also asked our raters to make global judgments of depression.

I review the results from three of our studies (Rehm, 1980). In the first study, we (Rehm, Fuchs, Roth, Kornblith, & Romano, 1979) compared a self-control program to an assertion skills program. One of the measures was a taped assertiveness situation test in which subjects were asked to respond to a situation and an initial statement on a tape as if they were actually in the assertiveness situation. These measures are parallel to some depression measures. In addition, at the beginning of the first and last therapy sessions, subjects were asked individually to say something about their current functioning. These statements were observed and used as the basis for behavior coding. The same group procedure was used in the second study (Rehm, *et al*, 1981). In this latter study, we also began videotaping pretest and posttest assessment interviews and using the tapes as a basis for behavioral observations. In the third study, we (Kornblith, Rehm, O'Hara, & Lamparski, 1983) used the interview and group interaction situations. Observations were made in 10-minute segments during the first and last sessions, from which the therapist excused herself and asked the participants of each group to interact among themselves.

The specific behavior codes used in these studies are shown in Table 7-3. Table 7-4 shows the reliabilities of these measures. Reliability indices included percent agreements, Spearman *R* correlations, and kappa coefficients. As can be seen from the table, reliability across raters was generally quite satisfactory for virtually all of these measures. The results on the validity of the measures, however, were not so encouraging. Table 7-5 presents the correlations of each of the behavior codes with self-report and clinician measures, including the BDI, the MMPI *D* scale, the HRSD, the Raskin Three-Item Scale (Raskin, Schulterbrandt, Reating, & Rice, 1967), and the Global Assessment Scale (GAS) (Spitzer, Gibbon, & Endicott, 1973). Viewed overall, these data suggest that these behavioral indices across subjects were unrelated to measures of depression from the other two vantages.

In another study, we compared subjects who were interviewed in the Rehm *et al.* (1979) study with a group of subjects who met Research Diagnostic Criteria (RDC) for major affective disorder but were excluded on the basis of RDC for bipolar disorder (either mania or hypomania), and with a group of matched normal women. Of the 11 measures taken in the interview, only loudness and latency discriminated depressed from nondepressed subjects,

TABLE 7-3 Behavior Codes

Type of measure		Study I		Study II		Study III	
		Taped situation	Group statement	Group statement	Interview	Interview	Group interaction
Paralinguistic	1.	Average duration	Duration first speech	Duration first speech	Duration 5 min.	Duration 5 min.	Duration first speech
	2.	Loudness	Loudness	Loudness	Loudness	Loudness	Loudness
	3.	Affect	Affect	Expressivity	Expressivity	Expressivity	Expressivity
	4.	Fluency	Fluency	Speech disruption	Speech disruption	Speech disruption	Speech disruption
	5.	Latency			Latency	Latency	Latency
	6.			Episode duration			Episode duration
	7.			Number of words	Number of words	Number of words	Number of words
	8.			Speech rate	Speech rate		
	9.			Disruption rate			
Nonverbal	10.		Eye contact	Duration of gaze	Duration of gaze	Duration of gaze	Duration of gaze
	11.				Smiles	Smiles	
	12.				Head movements	Head movements	
	13.				Body movements	Body movements	
	14.				Arm movements	Arm movements	
Content	15.		Positive self-references	Positive self-references			Positive self-references
	16.		Negative self-references	Negative self-references			Negative self-references
	17.		Positive references to others	Positive references to others			Positive references to others
	18.		Negative references to others	Negative references to others			Negative references to others
	19.	Compliances					
	20.	Requests					
	21.	Opinion					
Global	22.	Depression	Depression				
	23.	Assertion	Assertion				

TABLE 7-4 Reliabilities

Type of measure		Study I		Study II		Study III	
		Taped situation	Group statement	Group statement	Interview	Interview	Group interaction
Paralinguistic	1.			.99 (*r*)	.89-.92 (*r*)	86- 91 (*r*)	.99 (*r*)
	2.	99%	100%	.52 (*r*)	.72-.96 (*r*)	76- 97%	.82 (*r*)
	3.	95%	95%	.52 (*r*)	.56-.85 (*r*)	81- 95%	.91 (*r*)
	4.	96%	100%	.92 (*r*)		.95 (*r*)	.95 (*r*)
	5.				.66-.96 (*r*)	.86-.98 (*r*)	.97 (*r*)
	6.			.99 (*r*)			.99 (*r*)
	7.			.95 (*r*)	.97 (*r*)		.95 (*r*)
	8.				.95 (*r*)		
	9.			.98 (*r*)			
Nonverbal	10.		93%		.91-.92 (*r*)	.69-.83 (*r*)	.93 (*r*)
	11.				.93-.97 (κ)	84- 97%	
	12.				.70-.82 (κ)	85- 93%	
	13.				.75-.93 (κ)	86- 94%	
	14.				.84-.97 (κ)	87- 90%	
Content	15.		100%	.92 (*r*)			.95 (*r*)
	16.		98%	.96 (*r*)			.80 (*r*)
	17.		100%	.79 (*r*)			.82 (*r*)
	18.		100%	.96 (*r*)			.77 (*r*)
	19.	87%					
	20.	82%					
	21.	72%					
Global	22.		100%				
	23.	85%	98%				

TABLE 7-5 Correlations of Behavior Codes with Other Measures of Depression

		Study I				Study II					Study III				
		Taped situation		Group statement		Group statement					Interview				
Type of measure		BDI	MMPI *D*	BDI	MMPI *D*	BDI	MMPI *D*	HRSD	Raskin	GAS	BDI	MMPI *D*	HRSD	Raskin	GAS
Paralinguistic	1.	−.20	.09	.14	.27	−.09	−.10	.16	.15	−.06	−.26	−.08	.01	−.06	.06
	2.	.13	.31	.26	.01	−.33	−.06	.09	.05	.02	.05	.17	.20	−.04	.09
	3.	.14	.47	.15	.11	−.16	.16	.21	.07	.17	−.05	.05	−.05	−.14	.15
	4.	.39	.45	.49	.35	−.07	.17	.02	.12	−.38					
	5.	−.06	−.41								.04	.00	.05	.20	−.28
	6.					−.03	−.09	.08	.10	−.10					
	7.					−.09	−.07	.10	.09	.00					
	8.					−.33	.00	−.03	−.10	.11					
	9.					−.04	−.07	−.13	−.22	.02					
Nonverbal	10.			.11	.08	.02	−.24	−.06	.01	−.08	.22	.06	.13	−.11	.01
	11.										−.29	−.17	−.35	−.34	.37
	12.										−.30	−.02	−.09	−.02	.02
	13.										−.18	−.08	.04	−.24	.22
	14.										−.29	−.26	−.18	−.30	.28
Content	15.			−.27	−.05	.09	−.31	.09	.08	−.01					
	16.			.42	.38	.14	−.07	−.10	.16	.14					
	17.			.18	.19	.05	.03	−.05	.06	.28					
	18.			.16	.06	.00	−.29	−.06	.05	−.12					
	19.	.20	.35												
	20.	.28	−.15												
	21.	−.08	−.31												
Global	22.	.05	.14	−.35	−.46										
	23.	−.08	.14	.13	−.07										

with speech duration and number of smiles approaching significance. These four variables in a discriminant-function analysis were able to correctly classify 57% of the cases (Lamparski, Rehm, O'Hara, Kornblith, & Fitzgibbon, 1979). Finally, Table 7-6 shows the pretest-posttest reliability and situational stability of the various measures, as well as whether or not each measure improved significantly with therapy. As can be seen, pretest-posttest reliability was relatively poor, although the intervening therapy may have been expected to interfere with reliability over time. Indices of cross-situational reliability also indicated that these measures, although reliably assessed within situations, did not generalize across situations. Despite these limits, it is notable that quite a few of the measures did improve significantly with therapy, although some measures changed in directions opposite to predictions!

Taken together, we can draw some conclusions and some cautions from the data available on behavioral observations from interview and therapy situations. These measures can be defined, codified, and reliably rated. While the measures have face validity in assessing depression, correlations with traditional measures are not supportive of consensual validity. With some inconsistencies, a fair number of studies have shown that certain behavior codes can differentiate depressed and nondepressed subjects. Those studies that have used more than one situation have fairly consistently shown situational differences in behavior. This may relate in part to the specific characteristics of those situations. The demands of a dyadic interview are very different from the demands of a group therapy situation or an interaction with the family at home. Some codes applicable to the group situation (e.g., number of initiations) are scarcely applicable to the dyadic interview, where the expectation is that the interviewer will initiate the questions and the patient will only respond. The dyadic interview may also involve a great deal of close control of the verbal behavior of the patient, which is not so much the case in the group situation. While consistent individual differences have not been easily identified, it may be that the major place for measures in interviews and therapy is the idiographic measurement of persons across time. Normal individual differences may involve such a degree of variance that group differences may be difficult to obtain.

Ward Observations

Observations of inpatients on wards provide the possibility of much longer observational periods. Behavior on the ward, while it might not be entirely representative of behavior outside the hospital, may nevertheless be much more representative than behavior in the special situations of interview or therapy. Quite a few scales have been developed for assessing ward behavior (cf. Lyerly, 1975). Most of these scales are meant to be used by experienced clinicians. They are often based on interviews with inpatients and usually involve relatively high-level inference ratings of psychopathology. A few such

TABLE 7-6 Pretest-Posttest Reliability, Cross-Situation Correlations, and Significant Improvement after Therapy

		Study I			Study II					Study III	
		Taped situation		Group statement	Group statement			Interview		Interview	Group interaction
Type of measure		Cross-situation	Improvement	Improvement	Reliability	Cross-situation	Improvement	Reliability	Improvement	Improvement	Improvement
Paralinguistic	1.	.28	X		.29	−.10	X	.21		X	X
	2.	.10	X		.00	.05		.50			
	3.	−.18	X	X	.05	.20		.45	X		X
	4.	−.03	X		.30						
	5.							.56	X		
	6.				−.12	−.12	X				
	7.				.31	−.09					X
	8.				.56		X				
	9.				.51	.12					
Nonverbal	10.			X	−.18	.14	X	.56			
	11.							.24		X	
	12.							.17			
	13.							.50			
	14.							.46			
Content	15.			X	−.03		X				
	16.			X	−.19		X				X
	17.			X	−.23						
	18.				−.14						
	19.										
	20.										
	21.										
Global	22.	.04		X							
	23.	.03	X	X							

Note. An X in the "Improvement" columns indicates significant improvement.

scales, such as the Nurses' Observation Scale for Inpatient Evaluation (NOSIE-30; Honigfeld, Gillis, & Klett, 1966), the Psychotic Inpatient Profile (Lorr & Vestre, 1968), the Psychotic Reaction Profile (Lorr, 1961), and the Ward Behavior Inventory (Burdock & Hardesty, 1968), are based on direct observation of patients. They employ relatively low-level inferences and derive scales of depression or of dimensions closely related to depression (e.g., withdrawal or retardation). These measures all, however, require summary estimates across periods of time and for the most part do not have any specific validity data relevant to their use for assessing depression.

A series of studies by Kupfer and his colleagues (e.g., Kupfer, Detre, Foster, Tucker, & Delgado, 1972) describes an apparatus that permits 24-hour telemetric reporting of activity level of patients in inpatient settings. An electronic device is worn on a wrist or ankle band, and amount of movement can be recorded on a minute-by-minute basis. A reliability of 91.7% agreement was reported for five subjects wearing transmitters on two wrists, and a .73 correlational reliability was found between wrist and ankle transmitters. Weiss, Kupfer, Foster, and Delgado (1974) found differences between unipolar and bipolar depressives prior to drug treatments. Unipolars had higher levels of activity. No drug treatment effects were found, but clinically improved unipolars decreased in activity level. No significant correlations were obtained with self-rating depression items, but a correlation of .85 was found with self-rated anxiety. This is perhaps not surprising, in that the unipolar patients were apparently agitated before drug treatment. This assessment technique has the promise of being a definitive measure of psychomotor activity, but it needs additional psychometric evaluation to establish its place as a measure of depression.

Williams, Barlow, and Agras (1972) described a behavioral assessment procedure for coding the behavior of 10 depressed psychiatric inpatients. At randomly determined points during each half hour of the day from 8:00 A.M. to 4:00 P.M. a trained observer noted the presence or absence of four classes of behavior: (1) talking, (2) smiling, (3) motor activity, and (4) time out of room. Interrater reliability of 96% was reported. Analysis of correlations among the four behavioral measures across response classes yielded a Kendall coefficient of concordance of .70. Thus, the scores were summed and treated as a single severity index of depression. Validity comparisons with the BDI and the HRSD were made at 3-day intervals during the course of patients' hospitalizations. Mean within-subject correlations between the measures were as follows: BDI and HRSD, .82; HRSD and behavior index, .71; BDI and behavior index, .67. Thus these measures have demonstrated consensual validity for depression with a self-report and a clinician measure. Hersen, Eisler, Alford, and Agras (1973) used this behavior rating scale to assess improvement in three patients in a token economy ward. With single-subject reversal designs, improvement on the behavior index was demonstrated to occur when patients were under token reinforcement conditions; no self-report measures were taken. Another use of the scale was less successful. Williams, Barlow and Agras (1975) attempted to assess diurnal variation in depression in nine unipolar patients reporting such variation. Morning and evening observations did not indicate the predicted variation. This scale is promising as a direct observational scale that has some established validity for the idiographic measure of depression. These studies also show that it is possible to find consensual validity across measures of very different perspectives.

It should be noted that the measures reviewed to this point have all been conceptualized as general measures of depression and not as measures of behaviors to be targeted by behavioral intervention. One exception to this in an inpatient setting was a study by Reisinger (1972), who described a single-subject reversal design study on a token economy ward where the patient received token reinforcement and response cost for increases in smiling behavior and decreases in crying behavior, respectively. Interrater reliabilities of 90% for behavioral observations were obtained, and the behaviors were demonstrated to be under reinforcement control. The potential for a more specific connection between behaviors measured and targets for behavioral intervention exists, but has yet to be explored in the research literature. For example, Paul and Lentz (1977) have described an observational recording system for use on inpatient wards, which includes a Staff-Residents Interaction Chronograph and a Time-Sample Behavior Checklist. The first involves the coding of verbal content, and the second includes a variety of behavior codes relevant to the patients' location, position, awake-asleep status, facial expression, social orientation, concurrent activities, and "crazy" behaviors. This system allows both nomothetic and idiographic assessment of psychiatric patients' behavior and is used to select targets for intervention. While the measures were not designed specifically for the assessment of depression, some initial work with them indicates promising correlations with ratings of depression and retardation (Farrell & Mariotto, 1982; Mariotto & Paul, 1974). The utilization of a behavioral observation system tied directly to a behavioral intervention system should be the model for future research in this area.

Observations of Marital Interaction

Marital relationships have a particularly important bearing on depression, especially in women. Evidence from several epidemiological studies (cf. Radloff, 1975) suggest that among women, married women are more depressed, whereas among men, married and divorced men are least depressed. Weissman and Paykel (1974) found that marital and family conflict were the most frequently cited problem areas in the lives of depressed women in a community sample. In their study of vulnerability factors for depression, Brown and Harris (1978) found that for a sample of English women, having three or more children under the age of 14 at home and a lack of a confiding relationship with a member of the opposite sex were two important factors in depressive vulnerability. The growing evidence for the importance of marital factors in the development and maintenance of depression has recently been reviewed by Coyne, Kahn, and Gotlib (in press).

Only a few studies, however, have attempted to do direct observational assessment of the interaction between depressed individuals and their spouses. Viewing depression as failure to control one's interpersonal environment, McLean, Ogston, and Grauer (1973) randomly assigned 20 depressed outpatients and their spouses to either a behavioral marital therapy condition or a treatment-as-usual condition. As part of the outcome assessment, each couple made a 30-minute audiotape recording of a problem-oriented discussion at home. A second such recording was made at the conclusion of therapy. The tapes were coded according to a format adapted from the system used by Peter Lewinsohn. Positive and negative initiations and reactions were coded at 30-second intervals. Scores were derived reflecting proportion of negative interactions averaged for each taped session. Interscorer agreement was good. Couples in both groups made significantly more negative remarks in responding than in initiating statements. Couples in the experimental groups significantly decreased their use of negative reactions with therapy. Those in the comparison group did not. The experimental group also showed a significant decrease in negative actions and reactions taken together, in contrast to the comparison group.

Hinchliffe, Hooper, and Roberts (1978) coded the interactions of 20 depressed inpatients with their spouses and with an opposite-sex stranger while they were in the hospital, and then did a second observation of their interactions with their spouses after hospitalization. A control group of surgical patients and their spouses was also included. In comparison to the surgical patients and their spouses, the depression patients' interactions were initially characterized by greater tension and negative expressiveness. There were high levels of disruption, negative emotional outbursts, and incongruity between different channels of communication. It was notable that the marital interactions were much more pathological than the interactions between patients and strangers. After hospitalization, the interactions of male patients with their wives resembled those of surgical controls. The interactions of depressed women with their husbands showed little change from hospitalization to recovery.

In another study of depressed female inpatients and their spouses, Merikangas, Ranelli, and Kupfer (1979) audiotaped six weekly sessions over the course of patients' hospitalizations. Fifteen-minute segments of these interactions were audiotaped and coded for the relative influence of each spouse on a revealed-differences task where the frequency and duration of speech and joint speech (i.e., interruptions) was assessed. Motor activity was also assessed by wrist monitors. Over sessions, patients increased in their influence on the revealed-differences task, with decisions reflecting a more equal balance of power following therapy. There was also a decrease in joint speech or interruptions, and the motor activity of the patients who responded to medication increased.

A very extensive evaluation of the verbal behavior of couples with a depressed partner has been reported by a group working in a clinic in Berlin (Hautzinger, Linden, & Hoffman, 1982; Linden, Hautzinger, & Hoffman, 1983). A total of 26 distressed couples, 13 of whom had one partner with a major depressive disorder and 13 of whom had neither partner with a major depressive disorder, were tape-recorded over 312 minutes of conversation. Six independent observers rated each couple on 28 categories of verbal behavior. Behaviors coded included (1) nonverbal affects and mood expressions (2 categories); (2) self-related and self-centered verbalizations (7 categories); (3) interaction-related and partner-related verbalizations (9 categories); and (4) information and neutral categories (10 categories). Categories were coded with high reliability between raters. A discriminant function differentiated between depressed and nondepressed individuals. Depressed individuals were characterized by more negative self-evaluation, more verbalizations of negative well-being, more negative future orientation, and more agreements and positive statements about the partner and the relationship. Nondepressed individuals were higher on verbalizations of positive well-being, positive self-evaluation, positive and neutral future orientations, initiation of activity, and giving and asking for help.

Overall, the interactions between depressed couples were characterized as uneven, negative, and asymmetrical, in contrast to the positive, supportive, and reciprocal interactions of nondepressed (though distressed) couples. The Berlin group has drawn the conclusion that couples with one depressed partner may develop a pattern of interaction that is both reinforcing and aversive: The depressed person expresses negative feelings in self-evaluations; these are intermittently reinforced by positive and supportive statements from the spouse; the spouse is negatively reinforced by the cessation of the depressed partner's complaints; the aversive character of the depressed person's interactions produces avoidance behavior on the part of the spouse; and the interaction is stabilized in a system of aversive control and coercion.

The findings of these studies of marital interaction, though they are relatively few in number, appear to converge with some regularity. Research to date has not addressed the degree to which these aversive marital interactions cause depression or are mere concomitants or results of depression on the part of one of the spouses. There is evidence that relationships and interactions improve with therapy, but it is not clear that this is necessarily the function of a specific intervention. Assessment in this area could potentially be linked directly with treatment interventions. Various forms of marital therapy attempt to modify communication patterns in ways that would be compatible with the assessment procedures described here. The depression assessment and therapy literature could benefit from this bridge to the marital and family assessment and therapy literature.

Social Skills Assessments

A number of behavioral theorists have suggested that social skills deficits, especially in the area of assertion, may be central to depression and may represent potential targets for intervention. Wolpe (1971) and Lazarus (1974) have recommended assertion training for at least a subset of depressed clients. Lewinsohn (e.g., Lewinsohn *et al.*, 1976) has argued within his behavioral model that social skills deficits may be one of the ways in which depressed individuals may find themselves in a situation of loss or lack of response-contingent positive reinforcement. Assertion training has been a component of a number of complex behavioral therapy packages that have been used for the treatment of depression (e.g., McLean & Hakstian, 1979; Shaw, 1977; Taylor & Marshall, 1977).

Despite the theoretical and treatment interests in social skills in depression, relatively little empirical study has been given to the topic of social skills assessment. The Libet and Lewinsohn (1973) study of the behavior of college students with varying levels of depression in group interaction was interpreted in terms of social skills dimensions. Activity level, latency, interpersonal range, and rate of positive reactions were assumed to be measures of skill in obtaining positive reinforcement. Lewinsohn, Mischel, Chaplin, and Barton (1980) had depressed subjects, psychiatric controls, and normal controls in group interactions rate themselves and others with regard to social skills. Depressed subjects rated themselves and were rated by others as less socially competent. Self-ratings of depressed subjects improved with treatment. Interestingly, depressed subjects tended to be accurate in seeing themselves as others saw them, while normal subjects and psychiatric controls tended to see themselves more positively than they were seen by others. Posttreatment assessments of depressed subjects showed the same pattern as those of nondepressed subjects.

Kornblith (1977) studied college students who had scored high and low on a depression scale on a videotaped behavioral assertiveness task. Using assessment codes and criteria from the assertiveness literature, he found essentially no behavioral deficits associated with depression. In addition, he found no differences between depressed and nondepressed students in their abilities to decode social cues or in their evaluations of themselves and others on assertiveness dimensions. Thus, these results do not replicate the results above with regard to either behavioral deficits or self-evaluation. It should be noted, however, that the very mild level of depression studied may not be representative of the more severe depression studied in the Lewinsohn *et al.* (1980) research.

Another study using college students contributes a potentially valuable methodological point. Jacobson and Anderson (1982) observed mildly depressed and nondepressed college students in waiting-room interactions with a confederate. Depressed students made more negative self-statements but were not different from other students on an additional seven content codes. However, when conditional probabilities were taken into account, a predicted *sequence* difference was noted. Depressed subjects self-disclosed at inappropriate times in their interactions in comparison to normals, even though absolute frequencies were similar. The authors argue for the potential value of evaluating sequential characteristics of verbal behavior in studying interpersonal behavior in depression.

To date, two studies have assessed assertion training or social skills training as a primary modality for treating depression. As cited earlier, we (Rehm *et al.*, 1979) compared a self-control therapy program to assertion training. Subjects were randomly assigned to conditions, and assertiveness was assessed by an audiotaped behavioral assertiveness task. Assertiveness behavior codes of latency, duration, compliance, requests for new behavior, statements of opinion, loudness, appropriate affect, fluency, and overall depression were reliably coded. The two conditions validly influenced different targets. Subjects receiving assertion training were significantly more improved at posttest on duration of responses, number of requests for new behaviors, number of statements of opinion, loudness of response, fluency of response, and overall assertiveness. Interestingly, self-evaluation of the adequacy of response improved more for the self-control group, in which self-evaluative behavior had been specifically targeted. The self-control condition showed greater improvement on paper-and-pencil measures of self-control behavior. In addition, the self-control condition was significantly more improved on measures of depression.

Bellack, Hersen, and Himmelhoch (1981, 1983; Hersen, Bellack, Himmelhoch, & Thase, 1984) reported on a study that compared social skills training with amitriptyline and with placebo, to traditional psychotherapy with placebo, and to amitriptyline alone. In this study, a behavioral assertiveness test was used to assess specific dimensions of social skills. The deficient dimensions were used idiographically as the target behaviors for role-playing problems relevant to family/heterosexual situations, work, friends, or strangers. Results indicated positive outcome on a behavioral assertiveness test and on assessments of depression for the social skills training condition. Social skills subjects were more like normals on behavioral measures of social skills at posttest. All groups improved equally in depression.

The findings on social skills measures as they are usually assessed are somewhat inconsistent, but have not been very thoroughly researched. Again, the question can be raised as to whether social skills deficits are causes or mere concomitants of episodes of depression. Changes in social skill behavior have been shown with specific assertion or social skills interventions, and they have been used to identify the targets for intervention. Again, the depression therapy research field could benefit from a further adaptation of assessment and therapy intervention techniques from the well-developed literature on social skills training.

Activity Schedules

The methodology of self-monitoring has been one of the prominent developments in behavioral assessment. Self-monitoring can be seen as low-level inference recording of verbal/cognitive, overt/motor, or somatic responses by the subjects over the course of their daily life in their normal environment. Self-monitoring methods have been used in depression research for assessment, target selection, and evaluation of outcome.

The best-developed instruments psychometrically, and the most sophisticated methodology for assessing depression, have been developed by Peter Lewinsohn and his colleagues in the form of several events schedules. The Pleasant Events Schedule (PES), developed by MacPhillamy and Lewinsohn (1974), is based on Lewinsohn's model of depression, which assumes that depression is caused by a loss or lack of response-contingent positive reinforcement. The PES is intended to assess the amount of external positive reinforcement the individual receives. The instrument consists of 320 items generated from lists of positive events elicited from a variety of subjects. The instrument in used in two ways. First, it is used as a retrospective report of the last 30 days; second, it is used as a checklist for daily logs of ongoing behavior. When it is used as a retrospective instrument, respondents indicate how frequently each item occurred within the last 30 days on a 3-point scale (0 — "did not happen"; 1 — "happened a few times"; 2 — "happened 7 or more times"). Subjects then go through the list a second time indicating how pleasant or enjoyable each event was or potentially would be, again using a 3-point scale (0 — "not pleasant"; 1 — "somewhat pleasant"; 2 — "very pleasant"). Three scores are derived from these ratings. First, Activity Level is defined as the sum of the frequency ratings. Second, Reinforcement Potential is defined as the sum of the pleasantness ratings. Third, Obtained Reinforcement is defined as the sum of the cross-products of the frequency and pleasantness ratings for each item. Psychometric properties of the PES have been well evaluated (Lewinsohn, Youngren, & Grosscup, 1979). Internal-consistency alpha coefficents were found to be in the upper 0.90s, and test-retest reliabilities from 4 to 8 weeks were 0.85 for Activity Level, 0.66 for Reinforcement Potential, and 0.72 for Obtained Reinforcement. A similar instrument, entitled the Unpleasant Events Schedule (UES), was developed by Lewinsohn and Talkington (1979) to measure aversive events in the same fashion. A third schedule, the Interpersonal Events Schedule (IES), was developed by Youngren and Lewinsohn (1980) to assess interpersonal events related to assertiveness skills.

One of the theoretically and practically most interesting findings with these events schedules is that when they are used as a checklist for daily logs, daily events are found to correlate with daily measures of mood. Lewinsohn and Libet (1972) found consistent within-subject correlations between mood ratings and self-recording of engaging in pleasant events. No differences in the magnitude of correlations were found among depressed subjects, psychiatric controls, and normal controls. Lewinsohn and Graf (1973) found similar correlations between pleasant activities and mood. They also examined cross-lagged correlations between activity and mood for the day before or the day after. Cross-lagged coefficients were consistently lower, suggesting that there was not a day-to-day causal effect of prior activity or mood. In this study, depressed subjects were found to engage in fewer, less frequent pleasant events than nondepressed subjects. Lewinsohn and Amenson (1978) found correlations between mood and both pleasant and unpleasant events. I have replicated these findings (Rehm, 1978), using self-generated lists of events rather than the Lewinsohn events schedules. Within subjects, pleasant events correlated positively with mood, negative events correlated negatively, and these two lists of events essentially did not correlate at all with each other. The strongest correlations were the multiple correlations of positive and negative events with mood. This study also found no cross-lagged effects.

Research on the events schedules in depression has been summarized by Lewinsohn *et al.* (1979). Across studies, depressed subjects tend to score lower on frequency, pleasantness, and obtained reinforcement measures. PES and IES scores tend to improve with therapy, with greater improvement for the most improved patients. With regard to the UES, depressed subjects show higher aversiveness scores and higher cross-product scores. Experienced aversiveness decreases with clinical improvement. High rates of aversive events on the UES are associated with lower pleasantness ratings on the PES.

The self-monitoring literature suggests that self-monitoring of a category of events alone is likely to influence the frequency of those events. This was not true in one study (Hammen & Glass, 1975) with the PES, nor in another study (O'Hara & Rehm, 1979) with shortened versions of the PES and UES. Lewinsohn (1975) has pointed out that the subjects in these studies were not clinically depressed, that there was no demonstration of initial low level of activity, and that activities were not selected for being specifically mood-related.

Events schedules have been used extensively and articulate well with Lewinsohn's mode of therapy. Lewinsohn (1976; Lewinsohn *et al.* 1976) described a sequence where patients recorded events on the PES and mood for 30 days, and the derived data were then used to choose approximately 10 pleasant events, that became the targets for attempts to increase activity in the treatment program. Zeiss, Lewinsohn, and Munoz (1979) described a therapy study in which scores on the PES, the IES, and an additional measure, the Cognitive Events Schedule (CES; Lewinsohn, Larson, & Munoz, 1982) were assessed prior to treatment of depression in therapy modalities attempting either to increase activity, to increase social skills, or to change depressive cognitions. The results suggested that all three therapy conditions produced improvement but that the effects were not specific to the separately measured pleasant, interpersonal, and cognitive events. In a somewhat similar design, we

(Rehm, Kaslow, & Rabin, 1987) evaluated three forms of our self-control behavior therapy program for depression, aiming separately at behavioral, cognitive, and combined targets. Subjects were assessed initially on a shortened PES and a shortened CES. Again, results were positive and equivalent among conditions. There were no differences in improvement on the three measures, nor was there any interaction between initial deficits and therapy condition. Thus, the specificity of these deficits with regard to treatment modality has not been demonstrated.

It should be pointed out that self-monitoring methods have several uses in therapy programs for depression. Lewinsohn and his colleagues have used his events schedules primarily for target selection, both for selecting specific activities and for making some decisions between activity increase versus other treatment modules. Our self-control treatment program (Rehm, 1977, 1981) uses self-monitoring methods as a part of a therapy program. Throughout the program, subjects monitor daily mood and positive activities on a list of categories somewhat more general than the PES. These data are used session by session in the program. One element of the intervention is to try to increase participants' awareness of the positive activities in which they engage. Thus self-monitoring methodology is seen as an intervention per se. Later and throughout the course of the program, self-monitoring data are used as a measure of change and progress. Cognitive therapy makes use of self-monitoring methodologies as well. For example, Rush, Khatami, and Beck (1975) described case studies of cognitive therapy in which patients kept daily logs of specific behaviors to serve as a basis for correcting cognitive distortions of their experiences.

When seen in the general context of depression assessment, self-monitoring techniques can be seen as valid, low-level inference measures of the qualitities of daily activity. We (O'Hara & Rehm, 1979) found that it was indeed the quality of daily activities and not overt/motor activity per se that correlated with mood. As measures of specific forms of daily interpersonal behavior, self-monitoring methods have begun to demonstrate a potential for contribution to depression assessment.

CONCLUSION

The behavioral perspective on assessment highlights the breadth of the potential domains of assessment. Clinical and theoretical conceptions of depression tend to place the phenomena in a configuration within these dimensions. Certain assumptions are typically made, such as generality across response modes, generality across situations, and relative consistency across time. Existing instruments tend to tap the domain of depression rather narrowly. There are sampling differences between instruments, and they vary considerably in their typical level of inference. Overt behavioral phenomena, particularly interpersonal behavior, tend to be relatively neglected by traditional assessment instruments. Ideally an assessment methodology would represent various vantages in both low-level and high-level inferences in a parallel fashion across response modes.

Behavioral assessment tends to focus on low-level inferences, employing observational methodologies of assessing overt/motor and verbal/cognitive behavior. Various formats for assessment have been used. In general, the behavioral methodologies provide highly reliable coding. Attempts to measure depression generally with an array of specific depressive responses in interview, therapy, and home settings have resulted in findings of a mixed nature. Correlations with more traditional measures are low at best, and results tend to be highly situational and inconsistent in differentiating between depressed and nondepressed persons. A more idiographic approach might be more useful. The few studies available that have assessed depressive behaviors on inpatient wards are promising, particularly as they begin to articulate assessment dimensions with intervention targets. This tendency to use behavioral assessment for target selection or for selection of type of behavioral intervention shows some promise in the marital, social skills and activity-monitoring domains of assessment. Results of these latter assessment studies also raise some questions for earlier assumptions about the nature of depression. The behavioral assessment literature consistently points to situational factors in depression. Assessment of various behaviors in different settings and the correlation between mood and day-to-day events all suggest situational or environmental effects on level of depression. Variations of levels of depression as a function of activity across time question the practice of assessing level of depression across long time frames. In general, behavioral assessments suggest the potential for expanding the perspective of depression assessment. Their more systematic use may have a heuristic value in the study of depression.

It is difficult at this point to recommend specific instruments or specific coding schemes for regular use as part of an assessment battery. The primary recommendations that derive from this review have to do with overall assessment strategies for research and clinical purposes. Several of the points have been made above, but can be summarized here in terms of five specific recommendations:

1. Assessment methods from all vantages should give greater weight and attention to overt/motor response modes in assessing depression. Actual changes in such behavior should be examined, along with its cognitive and somatic concomitants. Interpersonal behavior should be given special attention, as current psychological models tend to be giving added emphasis to this aspect of depression.

2. Assessment methods should given greater attention to their assumptions of generality across time and place. There is little standardization or comparability in time frames of current instruments. Depressive affect may vary from day to day or hour to hour. Covariation of mood with place (situation

or event) may be important in the evaluation of the disorder and in treatment planning.

3. Assessment methodology for depression would benefit from greater attention to low-level inferences. Assessment in such areas as sleep, eating, sex, and work habits would benefit from anchoring in specific samplings of behavioral parameters (e.g., amount, frequency, duration, etc.). Patients' responses on questionnaires or in interviews may reflect depressive cognitive biases that may be minimized by the use of questions or recording involving more specific, low-level inferences. Instruments making use of low-level inferences may supplement ratings involving high-level inferences.

4. Assessment of depression would benefit from greater use of direct observational methodologies, including self-observation. This recommendation follows from the first three recommendations. Direct observation by trained observers adds a relatively objective perspective to an overall assessment battery. Mechanical recording, where feasible, may be the ultimate in objectivity. Ratings by significant others such as spouses or friends may add a perspective uniquely reflecting the person's social impact.

5. Overall, greater attention should be given to parallel sampling across vantages. Assessment from multiple perspectives greatly increases the generalizability of findings to domains of personal distress, social impact, expert opinion, and objective patterns of behavior. Parallel assessment would improve comparability and help to identify sources of inconsistency.

For specific assessment methods in the behavioral assessment of depression, the field needs to continue to develop and validate instruments. A promising strategy is adapting methods from other research domains (e.g., ward behavior scales, marital interaction, and social skills assessment). More adaptations could be made from the research literature on assessment of problems that are symptoms of depression (e.g., insomnia, sexual dysfunction, anorexia-obesity).

Given the current status of research, investigators might use the following direct observational methods. For interviews or assessments of therapy, content measures of positive and negative references to self and others appear useful. Paralinguistic measures of speech rate may be useful within subjects, and nonverbal measures of sad demeanor (head hanging, frowning) may contribute to generic measurement of depression. Ward evaluations could usefully adopt the behavioral index developed by Williams *et al.* (1972). New developments adapting scales tied closely to ward treatment methods can be expected. Marital interaction assessment using codes similar to those mentioned above for interview assessments would appear useful. Assessing the behavior of the partner on the same codes would add a valuable dimension to the assessment. Social skills assessments in artificial role-play situations are useful for choosing targets for interventions, and this methodology can be directly adopted in this context. Further work on developing role-playing problems specific to depression and characterizing typical depressive deficits would be valuable. In general, behavioral assessment methodologies developed for work in different problem areas could be usefully adapted to assessment of depression.

References

Abramson, L. Y., Seligman, M. E. P., & Teasdale, J. D. (1978). Learned helplessness in humans: Critique and reformulation. *Journal of Abnormal Psychology, 87*, 49-74.

Aiken, E. A., & Parker, W. H. (1965). Conditioning and generalization of positive self-evaluation in a partially structured diagnostic interview. *Psychological Reports, 17*, 459-464.

Barlow, J., Rokke, P., Carter, A., & Rehm, L. P. (1986). *An analysis of the content of current scales for assessing depression*. Manuscript in preparation.

Beck, A. T., Rush, A. G., Shaw, B. F., & Emery, G. (1979) *Cognitive therapy of depression*. New York: Guilford Press.

Beck, A. T., Ward, C. H., Mendelsohn, M., Mock, J., & Erbaugh, J. (1961). An inventory for measuring depression. *Archives of General Psychiatry, 4*, 561-571.

Bellack, A. S., Hersen, M., & Himmelhoch, J. M. (1981). Social-skills training, pharmacotherapy, and psychotherapy for unipolar depression. *American Journal of Psychiatry, 138*, 1562-1566.

Bellack, A. S., Hersen, M., & Himmelhoch, J. M. (1983). A comparison of social-skills training, pharmacotherapy and psychotherapy for depression. *Behaviour Research and Therapy, 21*, 101-108.

Brown, G. W., & Harris, T. (1978). *Social origins of depression: A study of psychiatric disorder in women*. New York: Macmillan.

Burdock, E. I., & Hardesty, A. S. (1968) *Ward Behavior Inventory (manual)*. New York: Springer.

Cone, J. D. (1977). The relevance of reliability and validity for behavioral assessment. *Behavior Therapy, 8*, 411-426.

Cone, J. D. (1978). The Behavioral Assessment Grid (BAG): A conceptual framework and a taxonomy. *Behavior Therapy, 9*, 882-888.

Coyne, J. C. (1976). Depression and the response of others. *Journal of Abnormal Psychology, 85*, 186-193.

Coyne, J. C., Kahn, J., & Gotlib, I. H. (in press). Depression. In T. Jacob (Ed.), *Family interaction and psychopathology*. New York: Plenum Press.

Derogatis, L. R. (1977). *SCL-90 administration, scoring and procedures manual — I*, Baltimore: Johns Hopkins University Press.

Farrell, A. D., & Mariotto, M. J. (1982). A multimethod validation of two psychiatric rating scales. *Journal of Consulting and Clinical Psychology, 50*, 273-280.

Ferster, C. B. (1973). A functional analysis of depression. *American Psychologist, 28*, 857-870.

Fisch, H. U., Frey, S., & Hirsbrunner, H. P. (1983). Analyzing non-verbal behavior in depression. *Journal of Abnormal Psychology, 92*, 307-318.

Frey, S., Jorns, U., & Daw, W. (1980). A systematic description and analysis of nonverbal interaction between doctors and patients in a psychiatric interview. In S. A. Corson (Ed.), *Ethology and nonverbal communication in mental health* (pp. 241-250). New York: Pergamon Press.

Hamilton, M. (1960). A rating scale for depression. *Journal of Neurology, Neurosurgery and Psychiatry, 23*. 56-61.

Hammen, C.L., & Glass, D. R., Jr. (1975). Depression, activity, and evaluation of reinforcement. *Journal of Abnormal Psychology, 84*, 718-721.

Hathaway, S. R., & McKinley, J. C. (1942). A multiphasic personality schedule (Minnesota): III. The measurement of symptomatic depression. *Journal of Psychology, 14*, 73-84.

Hautzinger, M., Linden, M., & Hoffman, N. (1982). Distressed couples with and without a depressed partner: An analysis of their verbal interaction. *Journal of Behavior Therapy and Experimental Psychiatry, 13*, 307-314.

Hersen, M., Bellack, A. S., Himmelhoch, J. M., & Thase, M. E. (1984). Effects of social skill training, amitriptyline, and psychotherapy in unipolar depressed women. *Behavior Therapy, 15*, 21-40.

Hersen, M., Eisler, R. M., Alford, G. S., & Agras, W. S. (1973). Effects of token economy on neurotic depression: An experimental analysis. *Behavior Therapy, 4*, 392-397.

Hinchliffe, M., Hooper, D., & Roberts, F. J. (1978). *The melancholy marriage*. New York: Wiley.

Hinchliffe, M., Lancashire, M., & Roberts, F. J. (1970). Eye contact and depression: A preliminary report. *British Journal of Psychiatry, 117*, 571-572.

Hinchliffe, M., Lancashire, M., & Roberts, F. J. (1971). Depression: Defense mechanisms in speech. *British Journal of Psychiatry, 118*, 417-472.

Honigfeld, G., Gillis, R. D., & Klett, J. C. (1966). NOSIE-30: A treatment-sensitive ward behavior scale. *Psychological Reports,19*, 180-182.

Ince, L. P. (1972). The self-concept variable in behavior therapy. *Psychotherapy: Theory, Research and Practice, 9*, 223-225.

Jacobson, N. S., & Anderson, E. A. (1982). Interpersonal skill and depression in college students: An analysis of the timing of self-disclosures. *Behavior Therapy, 13*, 271-282.

Kornblith, S. J. (1977). *The nature of social skills and self-evaluation in depression*. Unpublished master's thesis, University of Pittsburgh.

Kornblith, S. J., Rehm, L. P., O'Hara, M. W., & Lamparski, D. M. (1983). The contribution of self-reinforcement training and behavioral assignments to the efficacy of self-control therapy for depression. *Cognitive Therapy and Research, 7*, 499-527.

Kupfer, D. J., Detre, T. P., Foster, G., Tucker, G. J., & Delgado, J. (1972). The application of Delgado's telemetric mobility recorder for human studies. *Behavioral Biology, 7*, 585-590.

Kupfer, D. J., & Foster, F. G. (1972). Interval between onset of sleep and rapid eye movement sleep as an indicator of depression. *Lancet, 2*, 684-686.

Lamparski, D. M., Rehm, L. P., O'Hara, M. W., Kornblith, S. J., & Fitzgibbon, K. (1979, December). *Measuring overt behavioral differences in unipolar depressed, bipolar depressed and normal subjects: A multivariate analysis*. Paper presented at the meeting of the Association for Advancement of Behavior Therapy, San Francisco.

Lang, P. J. (1968). Fear reduction and fear behavior: Problems in treating a construct. In J. M. Shlien (Ed.), *Research in psychotherapy* (Vol. 3, pp. 90-102). Washington, DC: American Psychological Association.

Lazarus, A. A. (1974). Multimodal behavioral treatment of depression. *Behavior Therapy, 5*, 549-554.

Levitt, E. E., & Lubin, B. (1975). *Depression: Concepts, controversies and some new facts*. New York: Springer.

Lewinsohn, P. M. (1975). Engagement in pleasant activities and depression level. *Journal of Abnormal Psychology, 84*, 729-731.

Lewinsohn, P. M. (1976). Activity schedules in treatment of depression. In J. D. Krumboltz & C. E. Thoresen (Eds.), *Counseling methods* (pp. 74-82). New York: Holt, Rinehart & Winston.

Lewinsohn, P. M., & Amenson, C. S. (1978). Some relations between pleasant and unpleasant mood-related events and depression. *Journal of Abnormal Psychology, 87*, 644-654.

Lewinsohn, P. M., & Atwood, G. E. (1969). Depression: A clinical research approach. *Psychotherapy: Theory, Research and Practice, 6*, 166-171.

Lewinsohn, P. M., Biglan, A., & Zeiss, A. M. (1976). Behavioral treatment of depression. In P. O. Davidson (Ed.), *The behavioral management of anxiety, depression and pain* (pp. 91-146). New York: Brunner/Mazel.

Lewinsohn, P. M., & Graf, M. (1973). Pleasant activities and depression. *Journal of Consulting and Clinical Psychology, 41* (2), 261-268.

Lewinsohn, P. M., Larson, D. W., & Munoz, R. F. (1982). The measurement of expectancies and other cognitions in depressed individuals. *Cognitive Therapy and Research, 6*, 437-446.

Lewinsohn, P. M., & Libet, J. (1972). Pleasant events, activity schedules, and depression. *Journal of Abnormal Psychology, 79*, 291-295.

Lewinsohn, P. M., Mischel, W., Chaplin, W., & Barton, R. (1980). Social competence and depression: The role of illusory self-perceptions. *Journal of Abnormal Psychology, 89*, 203-213.

Lewinsohn, P. M., & Shaffer, M. (1971). The use of home observations as an integral part of the treatment of depression: Preliminary report and case studies. *Journal of Consulting and Clinical Psychology, 37*, 87-94.

Lewinsohn, P. M., & Talkington, J. (1979). Studies on the measurement of upleasant events and relations with depression. *Applied Psychological Measurement, 3*, 83-101.

Lewinsohn, P. M., Weinstein, M. S., & Alper, T. (1970). A behavioral approach to the group treatment of depressed persons: Methodological contributions. *Journal of Clinical Psychology, 26*, 525-532.

Lewinsohn, P. M., Youngren, M. A., & Grosscup, S. J. (1979). Reinforcement and depression. In R. A. Depue (Ed.), *The psychobiology of the depressive disorders: Implications for the effects of stress* (pp. 291-315). New York: Academic Press.

Libet, J. M., & Lewinsohn, P. M. (1973). Concept of social skill with special reference to the behavior of depressed persons. *Journal of Consulting and Clinical Psychology, 40*, 304-312.

Libet, J. M., Lewinsohn, P. M., & Javorek, F. (1973). *The construct of social skill: An empirical study of several measures on temporal stability, internal structure, validity, and structural generalizability*. Unpublished manuscript, University of Oregon.

Linden, M., Hautzinger, M., & Hoffman, N. (1983). Discriminant analysis of depressive interactions. *Behavior Modification, 7*, 403-422.

Lorr, M. (1961). *Manuals for the Psychotic Reaction Profile*. Los Angeles: Western Psychological Services.

Lorr, M., & Vestre, N. (1968). *Psychotic Inpatient Profile manual*. Los Angeles: Western Psychological Services.

Lyerly, S. B. (1975). *Handbook of psychiatric rating scales* (DHHS Publication No. 0-569-738). Washington, DC: U.S. Government Printing Office.

MacPhillamy, D. J., & Lewinsohn, P. M. (1974). Depression as a function of levels of desired and obtained pleasure. *Journal of Abnormal Psychology, 83*, 651-657.

Mariotto, M. J., & Paul, G. L. (1974). A multimethod validation of the Inpatient Multidimensional Psychiatric Scale with chronically institutionalized patients. *Journal of Consulting and Clinical Psychology, 42*, 497-508.

McLean, P. D., & Hakstian, A. R. (1979). Clinical depression: Comparative efficacy of outpatient treatments. *Journal of Consulting and Clinical Psychology, 47*, 818-836.

McLean, P. D., Ogston, K., & Grauer, L. (1973). A behavioral approach to the treatment of depression. *Journal of Behavior Therapy and Experimental Psychiatry, 4*, 323-330.

Merikangas, K. R., Ranelli, C. J., & Kupfer, D. J. (1979). Marital interaction in hospitalized depressed patients. *Journal of Nervous and Mental Disease, 167*, 689-695.

O'Hara, M. W., & Rehm, L. P. (1979). Self-monitoring, activity levels and mood in the development and maintenance of depression. *Journal of Abnormal Psychology, 88*, 450-453.

Paul, G. L., & Lentz, R. J. (1977). *Psychosocial treatment of chronic mental patients: Milieu versus social-learning programs*. Cambridge, MA: Harvard University Press.

Radloff, L. (1975). Sex differences in depression: The effects of occupation and marital status. *Sex Roles, 1*, 249-265.

Ranelli, C. J., & Miller, R. E. (1977, April). *Nonverbal communication in clinical depression*. Paper presented at the meeting of the Eastern Psychological Association, Boston.

Raskin, A., Schulterbrandt, J., Reating, N., & Rice, C. E. (1967). Factors of psychopathology in interview, ward behavior, and self-report ratings of hosptialized depressives. *Journal of Consulting Psychology, 31*, 270-278.

Rehm, L. P. (1977). A self-control model of depression. *Behavior Therapy, 8*, 787-804.

Rehm, L. P. (1978). Mood, pleasant events and unpleasant events: Two pilot studies. *Journal of Consulting and Clinical Psychology, 31*, 270-278.

Rehm, L. P. (1980, November). Behavioral assessment of depression in a series of therapy outcome studies. In H. Arkowitz (Chair), *The Assessment of Depression.* Symposium presented at the meeting of the Association for Advancement of Behavior Therapy, New York.

Rehm, L. P. (1981). A self-control therapy program for treatment of depression. In J. F. Clarkin & H. Glazer (Eds.), *Depression: Behavioral and directive treatment strategies* (pp. 68-110). New York; Garland Press.

Rehm, L. P., Fuchs, C. Z. Roth, D. M., Kornblith, S. J., & Romano, J. M. (1979). A comparison of self-control and assertion skills treatments of depression. *Behavior Therapy, 10*, 429-442.

Rehm, L. P., Kaslow, N. J., & Rabin, A. S. (1987). Cognitive and behavioral targets in a self-control therapy program for depression. *Journal of Consulting and Clinical Psychology, 55*, 60-67.

Rehm, L. P., Kornblith, S. J., O'Hara, M. W., Lamparski, D. M. Romano, J. M., & Volkin, J. (1981). An evaluation of major components in a self-control behavior therapy program for depression. *Behavior Modification, 5*, 459-490.

Reisinger, J. J. (1972). The treatment of "anxiety-depression" via positive reinforcement and response cost. *Journal of Applied Behavior Analysis, 5*, 125-130.

Robinson, J. C., & Lewinsohn, P. M. (1973). Behavior modification of speech characteristics in a chronically depressed man. *Behavior Therapy, 4*, 150-152.

Rush, A. J., Khatami, M., & Beck, A. T. (1975). Cognitive and behavior therapy in chronic depression. *Behavior Therapy, 6*, 398-404.

Sacco, W. P., & Hokanson, J. E. (1978). Expectations of success and anagram performance of depressives in a public and private setting. *Journal of Abnormal Psychology, 87*, 122-130.

Schwartz, G. E., Fair, P. L., Salt, P., Mandel, M. R., & Klerman, G. L. (1976). Facial muscle patterning to affective imagery in depressed and nondepressed subjects. *Science, 192*, 489-491.

Seligman, M. E. P. (1981). A learned helplessness point of view. In L. P. Rehm (Ed.), *Behavior therapy for depression: Present status and future directions* (pp. 123-142). New York: Academic Press.

Shaw, B. F. (1977). Camparison of cognitive therapy and behavior therapy in the treatment of depression. *Journal of Consulting and Clinical Psychology, 45*, 543-551.

Spitzer, R. L., Gibbon, M., & Endicott, J. (1973). *Global Assessment Scale.* New York: New York State Department of Mental Hygiene.

Szabadi, E., Bradshaw, C. M., & Besson, J. A. O. (1976). Elongation of pause-time in speech: A simple, objective measure of motor retardation in depression. *British Journal of Psychiatry, 129*, 592-597.

Taylor, F. G., & Marshall, W. L. (1977). Experimental analysis of a cognitive-behavioral therapy for depression. *Cognitive Therapy and Research, 1*, 59-72.

Teasdale, J. D., Fogarty, S. J., & Williams, J. M. G. (1980). Speech rate as a measure of shortterm variation in depression. *British Journal of Social and Clinical Psychology 19*, 271-278.

Waxer, P. (1974). Nonverbal cues for depression. *Journal of Abnormal Psychology, 83*, 319-322.

Waxer, P. (1976). Nonverbal cues for depth of depression: Set versus no set. *Journal of Consulting and Clinical Psychology, 44*, 493.

Weiss, B. L., Kupfer, D. J., Foster, F. G., & Delgado, J. (1974). Psychomotor activity, sleep, and biogenic amine metabolites in depression. *Biological Psychiatry, 9*, 45-53.

Weissman, M. M., & Paykel, E. S. (1974). *The depressed woman: A study of social relationships.* Chicago: University of Chicago Press.

Williams, J. G., Barlow, D. H., & Agras, W. S. (1972). Behavioral measurement of severe depression. *Archives of General Psychiatry, 27*, 330-333.

Williams, J. G., Barlow, D. H., & Agras, W, S. (1975). Diurnal variation in depression-Is is there? *Journal of Nervous and Mental Disease, 161*, 59-62.

Wilson, G. T. (1978). Cognitive behavior therapy: Paradigm shift or passing phase? In J. P. Foreyt & D. P. Rathjen (Eds.), *Cognitive behavior therapy: Research and application* (pp. 7-32). New York: Plenum.

Wolpe, J. (1971). Neurotic depression: An experimental analog, clinical syndromes, and treatment. *American Journal of Psychotherapy, 25*, 362-368.

Youngren, M. A., & Lewinsohn, P. M. (1980). The functional relation between depression and problematic interpersonal behavior. *Journal of Abnormal Psychology, 89*, 333-342.

Zeiss, A. M., Lewinsohn, P. M., & Munoz, R. F. (1979). Nonspecific improvement effects in depression using interpersonal skills training, pleasant activity schedules, or cognitive training. *Journal of Consulting and Clinical Psychology*, 47, 427-439.

Zung, W. W. K. (1965). A self-rating depression scale. *Archives of General Psychiatry, 12*, 63-70.

CHAPTER 8

Psychological Measurement of Depression

Overview and Conclusions

PETER M. LEWINSOHN
PAUL ROHDE
University of Oregon

INTRODUCTION

In this chapter, we review the current status of the measurement of psychological variables known, or strongly hypothesized, to be uniquely related to depression. We begin by identifying some general issues in the psychological assessment of depression; we then shift to the assessment of specific areas, asking how well these variables are being measured with currently available techniques. On the basis of this evaluation, we try to identify directions for future research.

Assessment has a number of different functions (e.g., Cronbach & Gleser, 1965). In general, it is possible to distinguish between two purposes: (1) For assistance in clinical decision making about such issues as diagnosis, assignment of patients to treatments, pinpointing of target behaviors for intervention, and assessment of change; and (2) for use in research aimed at the clarification of etiological or theoretical issues. Although these are not mutually exclusive functions, the criteria with which to evaluate assessment devices differ, depending upon which purpose is intended. For example, in clinical assessment, issues such as cost-effectiveness, ease of administration, the base rate of the phenomenon, and the sensitivity and specificity of the assessment device will influence its clinical utility. In research these issues are less relevant, the main question being whether the variables are being measured appropriately. Although our main focus here is on the measurement of psychological variables in research, many of the instruments that we evaluate are also potentially useful in the clinical management of patients.

BASIC ISSUES

Domain of Variables to Be Included

Our point of departure is the domain of psychological variables associated with depression. Ideally, such variables should have emerged from studies in which depressives differ not only from normal controls, but also from nondepressed psychiatric patients. This distinction is an important one, since measures that differentiate between depressives and normal controls may include variables on which patients with problems other than depression also are different. Although knowledge about the characteristics that depressives share with other psychiatric patients is important, the distinguishing characteristics that are uniquely related to depression can potentially shed more light on the phenomenology of depression. With relatively few exceptions, most measurement instruments have been validated by showing that they are correlated with depression, and it is often not clear whether the tests and the underlying variables differentiate depressives from persons suffering from other disorders.

An additional caveat is that the domain of psychological variables of potential importance to depression should not be restricted to those that covary with being depressed. For example, variables that are predictive of the future occurrence of depression (i.e., risk factors) may clarify the chain of events leading to depression and may thus permit the early detection of persons who are at risk for depression.

In general terms, variables that have been shown to be associated with depression can be classified into the following categories: affect; cognitions; social and other coping skills; and the subjective quality of experiences. After discussing general assessment issues, we consider each of these four categories in turn.

Levels of Observation

The distinction between data based on self-report and data that are derived from other sources is important for a number of reasons. For example, Katz *et al.* (1984) describe a "multivantaged" approach to measurement in which the existence of a specific and clinically important construct (e.g., psychomotor retardation) is postulated. The construct is assumed to manifest itself at different levels of observation (i.e., at the levels of self-report, overt behavior, psychophysiology, etc.). By obtaining data at all of these levels and combining the data into a single index, Katz *et al.* (1984) suggest that a more reliable and a more valid measure of the construct will have been obtained. Another reason for the importance of the distinction between levels of observation is that on *a priori* grounds data are often assumed to be more veridical at one level than at another. For example, "objective" data about cognitions and about social skills are probably less influenced by response biases and other sources of distortion. Thus, data from one level of observation may be used to provide evidence for the validity of data obtained at another level.

Dimensionality of Variables to Be Included

Another general issue concerns the classification of the variables that have been shown to be associated with depression. Our subdivisions — affect; cognition; social and other coping skills; and the subjective quality of experience — are obviously not the only categories that could have been advanced. Nevertheless, categorizations such as ours and that proposed by Rehm, in Chapter 7 of this volume have heuristic value and reflect current usage.

Research on the development of assessment devices has typically been motivated by theoretical considerations. Thus, investigators with a cognitive orientation to the etiology of depression have focused on the measurement of cognitive variables, whereas investigators with a social learning orientation have emphasized the assessment of social and other instrumental skills. Unfortunately, there have been very few multivariate or "multivantaged" studies of the type advocated by Katz *et al.* (1984). Consequently, we know very little about the degree of association between variables from different domains or the degree of convergence between variables within each of the categories.

To illustrate the dimensionality issue, one could begin with the hypothesis that all of the variables that have been shown to be associated with depression are manifestations of a single underlying and therefore more basic construct (e.g., self-esteem), and that all of the specific manifestations (e.g., social skills deficits, cognitive biases, etc.) are manifestations of lowered self-esteem. If this hypothesis were correct, then the critical variable to measure, of course, would be self-esteem. The dimensionality issue in the measurement of psychological variables of importance to depression is analogous to the question of whether intelligence is a single trait or whether there are several different intelligences. For the unitary theorist, the part of variance that is attributable to a general factor called "*g*" is what matters. A good test of intelligence should be as highly loaded on "*g*" as possible. The multifactorialist, on the other hand, needs tests to represent each of the dimensions assumed to be important for performance in situations requiring intelligent behavior. The resolution of the dimensionality issue has theoretical implications and is important for the development and evaluation of assessment devices. At this point in time, we know very little about the dimensionality of the variables that are of importance to depression.

Psychometric Considerations

Another general issue concerns the psychometric properties of the various instruments that have been developed (e.g., Hoch & Cattell, 1959; Jackson,

1970; Meehl, 1964). In general terms, instrument development should begin with a careful definition of the trait or construct to be measured, which should include a clear delineation of the behaviors and the situations in which the trait is likely to be expressed. This first step should be followed by the careful selection of items to sample the entire content domain. Initial forms of the instrument should then be administered to large samples of respondents. Through the application of multistage procedures, the final items should then be selected. The data so generated may then be used for scale construction, with efforts made to reduce the effects of response style and method variance as much as possible. Finally, in establishing the validity of an instrument, one should be concerned not only with concurrent and predictive validity, but also with convergent and discriminant validity (Campbell & Fiske, 1959) and with criterion or construct validity. Criterion validity is especially important for measures of cognitions, since the latter are intended to measure internal events that are usually not directly observable.

Evidence in support of the validity of most of the measures to be discussed has relied heavily on the existence of a correlation of the measure with depression. This is, of course, an important first step, but it does not obviate the need to establish criterion validity. Furthermore, the magnitude of the correlation with depression needs to be interpreted carefully. If it is very high (i.e., at the upper limit of what is posible on the basis of the reliability of the instrument), then one may wonder whether the test is just another measure of depression rather than of some other psychological construct. On the other hand, if the correlation of the measure with depression is 0, then even if the measure has high criterion validity, it may be irrelevant to depression.

Unfortunately, the effort that has gone into the psychometric development of many of the instruments to be discussed is very limited, and very few deserve high marks on the criteria above.

ASSESSMENT OF AFFECT: DYSPHORIA

An important finding is that dysphoria is probably the only invariant symptom of depression. "Dysphoria" may be defined as an unpleasant mood state experienced as a feeling of sadness, hopelessness, and helplessness that is subjectively different from anxiety. The unique importance of dysphoria for the operational definition of depression is recognized by the *Diagnostic and Statistical Manual of Mental Disorders*, third edition (DSM-III), which comes close to making persistent dysphoria a necessary condition for the diagnosis of depression.

Items relevant to dysphoria are part of most self-report depression inventories and are represented by questions intended to probe for feelings of sadness and lethargy. Factor analyses of these scales typically identify a strong first factor on which these kinds of items have high loadings. This factor has typically been labeled as a "depressed mood" factor (e.g., Roth & Lubin, 1979).

There are a number of different ways of measuring depressed mood, such as with the Beck Depression Inventory (BDI; Beck, Ward, Mendelsohn, Mock, & Erbaugh, 1961), the Self-Rating Depression Scale (Zung, 1965, 1973), and the Center for Epidemiologic Studies Depression Scale (Radloff, 1977). An even simpler method of assessing depressed affect is to have patients rate their mood on a line that is used to define a continuum ranging from "worst mood" to "best mood." Lewinsohn, Munoz, Youngren, and Zeiss (1978) used such a procedure, the Visual Analogue Scale, for the daily monitoring of mood. Little and McPhail (1973) compared Visual Analogue ratings with BDI scores obtained over a period of 16 months for eight female outpatients. While these authors found a ceiling effect for the Visual Analogue ratings, they have also emphasized its ease of administration and sensitivity to mood changes. Other advantages of the Visual Analogue Scale in clinical settings are described by Folstein and Luria (1973).

Another useful measure for the measurement of depressed affect is the Depression Adjective Check List (DACL) developed by Lubin (1967, 1977). The DACL has seven alternate forms, consisting of either 32 or 34 nonoverlapping adjectives. The existence of alternate forms and ease of administration make the DACL especially useful as a repeated measure. Lubin (1977) has reported on the extensive psychometric development of this scale, including normative data for different age groups. The DACL has been translated into Spanish, Portuguese, French, Hebrew, and Chinese.

Another method for assessing depressed mood or dysphoria is via ratings of facial expression. Initially given impetus by Schlosberg's (1941) reports that judgments of emotions from facial expression could reliably be made on several dimensions including sadness, Tomkins (1962, 1963) provided a theoretical rationale for studying the face as a means for learning about emotion. To the extent that there is universality in the facial expression of different emotions, ratings of facial expression provide a method for assessing affect that is relatively free of particular cultural values.

More reliable but also more cumbersome methods for assessing facial expression have been developed such as Ekman and Friesen's (1982b) Emotional Facial Action Coding System (EMFACS), which is a simplification of their earlier facial measurement technique (FACS; Ekman & Friesen, 1978). Ekman and Friesen (1982a) used FACS with samples of interviews with patients with major and minor depressive, manic, and schizophrenic disorders. Composite scores were then generated corresponding to the emotions measured by FACS. A greater number of composites held to comprise "sadness" discriminated the major depressives from the other groups. EMFACS was developed for increased practical utility and seems promising, although the validity of this coding system is still being established.

In a study by Youngren and Lewinsohn (1980), facial expression was rated on two dimensions ("unpleasant-pleasant" and "sleep-arousal") for depressed subjects, nondepressed psychiatric controls, and normal controls who were observed in a group interaction situation. Interrater reliability was intermediate — .69 for the pleasantness and .59 for the arousal ratings. Significant differences between the means of the three groups on these two measures of facial expression were obtained, but planned contrasts showed that both pathological groups differed from the normal controls but not from each other.

Facial electromyogram (EMG) studies have shown that depressed individuals manifest higher EMG activity on certain facial muscles than do nondepressed individuals. Schwartz, Fair, Salt, Mandel, and Klerman (1976) recorded EMG activity from several facial muscle sites in 12 depressed and 12 nondepressed subjects who were instructed to "re-experience the feelings" associated with happy or sad imagery items. The depressed subjects were observed to show greater corrugator muscle site activity than the controls. Problematic in this study was the fact that the diagnosis of depression was based solely on a self-report measure and no nondepressed psychiatric control group was used. Oliveau and Wilmuth (1979) used affective imagery and more stringent diagnostic criteria in a partial replication of the Schwartz *et al.* (1976) study and failed to discriminate depressives from nondepressed controls. However, using "resting" EMG of selected facial sites, Carney, Hong, Kulkarni, and Kapila (1982) found higher EMG levels in depressed than in nondepressed individuals. Teasdale and Bancroft (1977) found that within depressed patients, ratings of mood correlated with corrugator region EMG activity.

While these studies have generated promising findings, a limitation is that they have focused on one measure of overt behavior and psychophysiological expression (i.e., facial expression) in isolation from other psychophysiological indices of emotion. As has frequently been suggested (e.g., Cacioppo, Marshall-Goodell, & Dorfman, 1983), studying the total pattern of psychophysiological responsivity has many advantages, and the simultaneous inclusion of several of these measures should provide a fruitful area for future research on the assessment of dysphoria. Such studies may be expected to clarify the psychophysiology of emotions (and of dysphoria). They also provide a method to evaluate the criterion validity of self-report measures of dysphoria. Psychophysiological measures of emotion also have the advantage of being relatively free of particular cultural values, and therefore should be useful in cross-cultural studies of depression.

ASSESSMENT OF COGNITIVE FUNCTIONS

The construction of assessment measures for the study of cognitive functions in depression is a relatively recent development. Kendall and Kogerski (1979) were among the first to emphasize the importance of developing cognitive instruments in order to assess change in cognitive therapy. After all, cognitive therapy is specifically designed to alter cognitions, and it is therefore important to construct reliable measures of the target behavior. Kendall and Kogerski's admonition has elicited a hearty response, and many of these measures are described by Rush in Chapter 9 of this volume.

In addition to questions about their psychometric properties, a number of other issues can be raised about these instruments. One issue concerns their dimensionality. Since they have been developed to test hypotheses about specific theoretical formulations, only one of the cognitive measures has typically been given to the same subjects. Thus the degree of intercorrelation between the cognitive measures and their factorial structure remains to be addressed. There have been some exceptions. For example, Blaney, Behar, and Head (1980) gave the Cognitive Bias Questionnaire (Hammen & Krantz, 1976; Krantz & Hammen, 1979) and the Attributional Style Questionnaire (Peterson *et al.*, 1982) to the same subjects and found that the correlation between these scales tended to be modest. Lewinsohn, Larson, and Munoz (1982) computed the intercorrelations between the Cognitive Events Schedule (Munoz & Lewinsohn, 1976a), the Personal Beliefs Inventory (Munoz & Lewinsohn, 1976b), and the Subjective Probability Questionnaire (Munoz & Lewinsohn, 1976c) and subjected the data to factor analysis, which suggested a rather weak underlying dimension. The results of a factor analysis of items empirically found to be most discriminating between depressed and nondepressed subjects indicated considerable specificity in the types of cognitions associated with depression. The dimensionality issue is unresolved, and future research should address the issue of whether all of the cognitive measures reflect a unitary cognitive change that occurs when people are depressed, or whether there are indeed several different kinds of changes, as implied by the various cognitive theorists. Placing themselves with the unitary theorists, Kuiper (e.g., Kuiper & MacDonald, 1982) and Davis (Davis & Unruh, 1981) hypothesize a depressogenic "self-schema" to account for many of the specific cognitive changes that have been found to characterize depressives.

Another important issue concerns the criterion validity of the cognitive instruments. By definition, cognitions refer to internal events, and consequently it is not easy to demonstrate their criterion validity. Nevertheless, Heiby (1983b) and Peterson and Seligman (1983) have conducted studies that provide evidence for the criterion validity of their respective instruments.

Cognitive instruments can roughly be divided into those that measure self-esteem, irrational beliefs, expectancies, attributions of causality, self-reinforcement, and cognitive distortions. For a more detailed review, the reader is referred to Merluzzi, Glass, and Genest (1981) and to Chapter 9 of this volume.

Measures of Self-Esteem

Lowered self-esteem is a major manifestation of depression, and it is therefore surprising that relatively little systematic work has been done on the assessment of lowered self-esteem in depression. A host of simple self-esteem measures are available, including Jackson's (1976) recent Personality Inventory. For a more detailed discussion of this literature, the reader is referred to Wylie (1979).

Measures of Irrational Beliefs

"Irrational beliefs" can be defined as a set of generalized life rules or philosophical beliefs that are hypothesized to play an important role in the development of emotional disorders (Ellis, 1962). These beliefs are assumed to represent relatively stable cognitive structures.

The first test devised to measure these beliefs was Jones's (1968) Irrational Beliefs Test. Munoz and Lewinsohn (1976b) and Nelson (1977) independently developed the Personal Beliefs Inventory (PBI) along the same lines. These tests consist of statements for the beliefs (e.g., "To be successful is very important in life"), and subjects indicate their degree of agreement on a 5-point scale. Munoz and Lewinsohn (1976b) and Nelson (1977) found their scales to discriminate significantly between depressed and nondepressed groups. Test-retest reliability for the PBI ranged from .60 to .79 over a 1-month period. Most and least discriminating items were identified. Their content and their factorial structure is discussed elsewhere (Lewinsohn *et al.*, 1982).

As discussed by Rush in Chapter 9 of this volume, another commonly used measure aimed at the ideosyncratic beliefs and assumptions held by depressives is the Dysfunctional Attitudes Scale (DAS; A. N. Weissman & Beck, 1978). The DAS was found to significantly differentiate depressed from nondepressed groups, but since no nondepressed psychiatric control group was included, the uniqueness of the cognitive changes identified by the DAS for depression has not been established.

Hollon and Kendall's (1980) Automatic Thoughts Questionnaire (ATQ), while conceptually related to the Irrational Beliefs Test, includes many items that represent common depression symptoms (e.g., "I hate myself," "I am so weak," "My life is a mess"). Not surprisingly, the scale is highly correlated with depression (Dobson & Breiter, 1983), but its discriminant validity with respect to anxiety may be problematic. Thus, Hollon and Kendall (1980) found the ATQ to be highly correlated ($r = .79$) with anxiety. An issue deserving further study is the more specific delineation of the specific beliefs that are uniquely associated with depression, as against those that may also (and perhaps even especially) be important for anxiety and other emotional reactions (Goldfried & Sobocinski, 1975).

Measures of Expectancies

Negative expectancies play an important role in Beck's (1967) theory, and the Hopelessness Scale (Beck, Weissman, Lester, & Trexler, 1974), a 20-item true-false measure, was developed to assess expectancies. This scale was found to have a high degree of internal consistency, showed good correlation with clinical ratings of hopelessness, and was sensitive to changes in the patients' depression level.

Also derived from Beck's theory is Munoz and Lewinsohn's (1976c) Subjective Probability Questionnaire (SPQ). This test consists of 80 items representing three dichotomous and crossed dimensions: "positive" versus "negative," "self" versus "world," and "present" versus "future." Subjects rate the probability (from 0% to 100%) that the statement is or will be true. Scores on this test significantly differentiated depressed from psychiatric and normal control groups, and 29 items (27 of which refer to "self" rather than "world") were found to be most discriminating between these groups. Over a 1-month period, test-retest reliability was moderate (r = .61-.83). Consistent with theoretical expectations, depressives attached higher probabilities to the occurrence of negative events and lower probabilities to the occurrence of positive events. Interestingly, these findings applied only to items pertaining to "self" and not to "world" items.

A recent measure of expectancy is the Expected BDI (Steinmetz, Lewinsohn, & Antonuccio, 1983), which involves having patients complete the 21-item BDI according to how they expect to feel at the end of treatment. The Expected BDI was found to be a good predictor of posttreatment depression in a multiple-regression analysis (Steinmetz *et al.*, 1983). What is especially interesting about this measure is that its correlation with the BDI was found to be relatively low (r = .40). Thus, people who are equally depressed seem to differ in how optimistic they are about getting better, and this expectation apparently is predictive of treatment response.

Measures of Attributions of Causality

Seligman's reformulated attributional theory of depression hypothesizes that individuals who make internal, stable, and global attributions for negative events become depressed (Abramson, Seligman, & Teasdale, 1978) The oldest measure of attribution is the Internal-External (I-E) Locus of Control Scale (Rotter, 1966). While group norms are available for young adult populations and adolescents, similar norms for the elderly are not available. This scale has not been found to be particularly correlated with depression. By far the most commonly used measure of attributions is the Attributional Style Questionnaire, developed by Peterson *et al.* (1982), which is discussed in greater detail in Chapter 9 of this book. A Children's Attributional Style Questionnaire (Peterson & Seligman, 1983), which consists of 48 forced-choice items in which the child chooses between one of two possible explanations for each event, has also been developed.

Another attributional measure that has had considerable psychometric development is the Multidimensional, Multiattributional Causality Scale (MMCS; Lefcourt, von Baeyer, Ware, & Cox, 1979). The items for this test were generated to fit a four-factor design: "internal" versus "external," "ability" versus "effort," "success" versus "failure," and "achievement" versus "affiliation." The factors have been shown to have adequate internal consistency, and test-retest correlations over 1-week to 4-month periods have ranged from .50 to .70. The correlation between the achievement and affiliation factors was low, suggesting that these factors are not measuring the same construct. Normative data are provided for an adult population. One possible problem is suggested by the significant correlation between the achievement factor of the MMCS and the Marlowe-Crowne Social Desirability Scale (Lefcourt, 1979). The correlation of attributional scales with social desirability has also been a problem for other locus of control scales (Rotter, 1966).

Measures of Self-Reinforcement

Several measures have been designed to assess self-reinforcement. Munoz and Lewinsohn (1976a), in developing the Cognitive Events Schedule (CES), hypothesized that depressed subjects would report fewer and less pleasant positive thoughts, and more frequent and more disturbing negative thoughts. The CES consists of 160 items (e.g., "I'm pretty smart," "What's the use?"), which the subject rates for frequency of occurrence (3-point scale) and for impact (5-point scale) during the past month. The items were selected to generate eight rationally derived scales along three dimensions ("positive-negative," "self-world," and "present-future"). Over a 1-month period, the test-retest reliability was fair for the frequency ratings (mean $r = .58$) and for the impact ratings (mean $r = .54$). Depressed subjects had an elevated number of negative thoughts and significantly fewer positive thoughts than the control group scoring high on the Minnesota Multiphasic Personality Inventory (MMPI) or the normal control group. Depressives reported higher negative impact for negative events and lower positive impact for positive events. A subset of items was identified that discriminated most strongly between the depressed and the control groups. As was found for the SPQ, the most discriminating items heavily involved "self" rather than "world" items.

Recently, a new instrument to measure self-reinforcement was developed by Heiby (1983a) — the Frequency of Self-Reinforcement Attitudes Questionnaire (FSRAQ). This scale consists of 30 items regarding self-reinforcement (e.g., "I silently praise myself even when others do not praise me"). Norms based on an undergraduate sample are available. Test-retest reliability over an 8-week period was .92. Split-half reliability was found to be .87. Criterion validity was demonstrated by correlating test scores with average amount of self-praise on an analogies task ($r = .69$, $p < .0001$). The FSRAQ is a carefully developed test that deserves to be studied further.

Measures of Cognitive Distortions

Assessment of cognitive distortions was stimulated by Beck's (1967; Beck, Rush, Shaw, & Emery, 1979) theorizing about the nature of specific cognitive distortions associated with depression (e.g., magnification, personalization). These distortions are described in greater detail in Chapter 9 of this volume. Assessment of these types of cognitive distortions has been incorporated into the Interpretation Inventory (II; Warren, Stake, & McKee, 1982). This scale consists of 21 items describing an event and a cognitive response to that event (e.g., "A friend walks by and does not appear to see you. Do you think that your friend is just avoiding you?"). The subject then rates the item on a 5-point scale from "never think that way" to "always think that way." Cognitive distortions as measured by the II were found to be correlated with a depression measure in a college population. Just how specific these distortions are to depression cannot be determined from this study, since no psychiatric control group was included. The II has good internal consistency, but it needs to be evaluated with populations other than college students.

Studies using more traditional tests (e.g., the Thematic Apperception Test and the Rorschach) to assess the motivational influences on thinking in depression are rare, but Klinger and his associates (Klinger, 1983; Klinger, Barta, & Maxeiner, 1981) have developed two instruments — the Interview Questionnaire (Klinger, 1983) and the Concerns Dimension Questionnaire (Klinger *et al.*, 1981) — to evaluate and study frequently occurring thoughts. These measures are relatively time-consuming (the Interview takes approximately 2 hours), but they may represent an interesting new methodology for studying cognitive processes in depression. Another new methodological development for the study of cognitive processes is represented by the work of Davis (1979), Kuiper (1978), Lloyd and Lishman (1975), and Teasdale and his associates (e.g., Teasdale & Fogarty, 1979). Using relatively simple reaction time and recall measures, these investigators have been studying the effects of cognitive schemas on information processing. This methodology should prove fruitful in the future study of the cognitive biases and distortions associated with depression. Also potentially relevant to the study of cognition are developments in the study of the psychophysiological correlates of cognitions, as summarized in the writings of Cacioppo and Sandman (1981). These methodologies may prove quite useful for the further delineation of the specific cognitive patterns associated with depression, as well as for work aimed at establishing the criterion validity of cognitive (self-report) instruments.

It appears that while considerable progress has been made to develop instruments to measure cognitions deemed important in depression, there remain both specific and more general problems deserving further study. Specifically, the discriminant validity of the cognitive instruments in relation to other psychopathological conditions, especially anxiety, needs to be addressed. At this point in time, the hypothesis that many of the cognitions currently thought to be uniquely related to depression are also problematic for other psychiatric populations would be hard to refute with empirical data.

ASSESSMENT OF SOCIAL AND OTHER COPING SKILLS

Even though there is no question that social skills deficits have been shown to be associated with depression (e.g., M. M. Weissman & Paykel, 1974), two major issues remain unresolved. First, are these deficits unique to depression, or do they characterize other psychiatric patients as well? Second, are the social skills deficits that have been found to characterize depressives situation-specific, or are they indicative of a more general interpersonal deficiency?

Before specific problems in the assessment of social skills deficits can be discussed, the more general issue of defining social skills and competence must be addressed briefly. The most common method has been to define social competence in terms of the person's adjustment in important life roles and to measure it with the types of social adjustment scales reviewed by John and Weissman in Chapter 12 of this volume. With such measures, depressed individuals have consistently been shown to be less socially competent.

The other end of the continuum is represented by behavioral approaches, which focus on specific behaviors of depressed individuals and the environmental consequences of such behaviors. Lewinsohn, Libet, and Javorek (1973) have defined "social skill" as the ability to emit behaviors that are positively reinforced by others or that terminate negative consequences from others. On the basis of data generated from observations of interpersonal interactions, these investigations attempted to operationalize this definition in terms of (1) being active, (2) being quick to respond, (3) being fairly insensitive to aversive responses from others, (4) not missing a chance to react, (5) distributing one's behavior evenly among others, and (6) emitting behaviors that reinforce the behavior of others. With the above-mentioned criteria, depressed subjects were found to be less socially skillful.

A similar approach to the definition of social skills is represented by the work of Romano and Bellack (1980), who attempted to empirically identify the distinguishing characteristics of socially skillful individuals. Subjects role-played assertive scenes and were rated for overall skillfulness to pinpoint specific behaviors that distinguished more skilled subjects.

While the two types of approaches to the definition of social skills may be seen as representing opposite poles of a continuum, there are other approaches and points of view (McFall, 1982), and their implications for assessment have been discussed by Cairns (1979) and Argyle (1969).

Methods that have been used to assess social skills may roughly be divided into those that make use of global ratings of adjustment, those that measure specific aspects of a depressed person's behavior in interaction with others, and those that focus on the impact that depressed people have on others.

Studies making use of methods attempting to identify the specific social skills problems of depressed individuals are exemplified by the studies by Lewinsohn *et al.* (1973), Rehm (1976), and Jacobson and Anderson (1982). The methods involved are very labor-intensive, and, without attempting a careful review of this literature, the results may be said to have been disappointing. In general, the findings have not gone beyond showing that depressives are less active, smile less, maintain less eye contact, report more discomfort in social interaction, and rate themselves as less socially skillful.

Ilfeld (1977), Biglan, Hops, Sherman, Friedman, and Arthur (1983), and Arkowitz, Holliday, and Hutter (1982) have looked at the interactions of depressed people and their spouses. In general, depressed couples have higher levels of tension and hostility, and lower levels of positive nonverbal behavior (Hinchliffe, Hooper, & Roberts, 1978).

In terms of impact on others, the depressed are seen as less competent (Youngren & Lewinsohn, 1980). They also generate negative affect in others (Coyne, 1976; Hammen & Peters, 1978). Other studies that indicate that in meeting new people the depressed have a negative impact on others are those by Howes and Hokanson (1979) and Strack and Coyne (1983). Coyne (1976) suggests that depressives self-disclose too much and that this is perceived by others as inappropriate.

When assessing social skills, it is especially important to distinguish self-report data from data generated by observers or raters. While self-report measures of social competence are important in their own right, they are undoubtedly strongly influenced by the general negative response set that characterizes depressed individuals. Measures based on objective data are more likely to represent "real" skill deficits, which can then become the targets for treatment intervention.

Self-Report Measures

The Interpersonal Events Schedule (IES; Youngren, Zeiss, & Lewinsohn, 1977) consists of 160 items involving interpersonal activities or cognitions regarding these activities. Subjects rate both the frequency and impact of each item for the past month. The IES incorporates eight rationally derived subscales: Social Activity, Assertion, Cognition, Conflict, Give Positive, Receive Positive, Give Negative, and Receive Negative. Youngren and Lewinsohn (1980) report that the IES significantly discriminated depressed subjects from both psychiatric and normal control groups, with depressed subjects reporting (1) lower activity levels, (2) being less comfortable in activities, (3) giving and receiving less positive reinforcement for their interactions, and (4) being less comfortable in assertive behavior. As depressed subjects improved, their IES scores became indistinguishable from those of normals (Zeiss & Lewinsohn, 1984). A set of the most discriminating IES items has been generated, based on one-way analyses of covariance controlling for age and sex.

The Social Interaction Self-Statement Test (Glass, Merluzzi, Bierer, & Larsen, 1982) consists of 30 self-statements (15 positive, 15 negative). A factor analysis identified four factors that accounted for 91.5% of the variance and that were labeled "self-depreciation," "positive anticipation," "fear of negative evaluation," and "coping." The concurrent validity of this instrument was evaluated by the inclusion of other measures of social anxiety and skill.

Problems with assertion have long been hypothesized to be important for depression (Lazarus, 1968; Wolpe, 1971), and assertion tests have frequently been used with depressed individuals. The results have been consistent with theoretical expectations in showing that the depressed report themselves as less assertive. Most measures of assertion are based on self-report — for example, the Wolpe-Lazarus Assertiveness Scale (Wolpe & Lazarus, 1966) and the Conflict Resolution Inventory (McFall & Lillesand, 1971). Relying on self-report measures may be problematic, since self-described nonassertive subjects were found to be behaviorally indistinguishable from subjects self-described as assertive (Alden & Cappe, 1981).

Measures of General Problem-Solving Skills

A potentially useful test of general problem-solving ability is the Self-Control Scale, developed by Rosenbaum (1980) as a measure of "learned resourcefulness." The scale is composed of 36 items, which are divided into four subscales: Cognitions, Problem-Solving, Delay of Gratification, and Self-Efficacy. Test-retest reliability over a 4-week period indicated that the Self-Control Scale is fairly stable over time (r = .86). Coefficient alpha for 6 samples of subjects ranged from .78 to .86, suggesting a high internal consistency.

Another measure of general problem-solving skills is the Means-End Problem-Solving Procedure, developed by Platt and Spivack (1975), in which subjects try to resolve a series of interpersonal conflict situations. Platt and Spivack (1975) found that depressed subjects generated significantly fewer relevant solutions to the situations than nondepressed controls. Recent reviews of the literature dealing with the assessment of general problem-solving skills can be found in Butler and Meichenbaum (1981) and D'Zurilla and Nezu (1982).

Behavioral Measures

A number of different behavioral coding systems have been developed to assess the interpersonal skills deficits of depressed individuals. The systems code both verbal and nonverbal behavior.

An elaborate attempt to code the verbal behavior of depressed individuals in interpersonal interactions was described by Lewinsohn (1976). In this system, behavior interactions are seen as having a source and an object. Actions are followed by reactions that can be coded as either positive (e.g., expressions of affection, approval, interest) or negative (e.g., expressions of criticism, disapproval, lack of interest). Interjudge agreement for the major scoring categories has been quite high (Libet & Lewinsohn, 1973). This system has been used in coding the behavior of depressed individuals in their own homes (Libet & Lewinsohn, 1973) and in group therapy (Lewinsohn, Weinstein, & Alper, 1970).

A more recently developed comprehensive coding system for observing the behavior of depressed individuals in their homes is the Living in Familial Environments (LIFE) recording system (Arthur, Hops, & Biglan, 1982). This system records the context (e.g., playing, working), content (e.g., physical and psychological complaint, self-disclosure, worry), and affect (e.g., happy, caring, irritable) contained in familial interaction. The LIFE system has been shown to have good interrater reliability and to discriminate between depressed and nondepressed mothers (Hops, Biglan, Sheman, Arthur, & Friedman, 1983).

Jacobson and Anderson (1982) developed a coding system for assessing dyadic interaction that focuses on the frequency and timing of self-disclosive statements. These authors emphasize the importance of focusing on sequences of behavior and their conditional probabilities, rather than merely the frequency with which different behaviors occur. Other behavioral coding systems include the Ward Behavioral Checklist (Williams, Barlow, & Agras, 1982); the systems developed by Reisinger (1972) and Liberman and Roberts (1974); and the Behavioral Assertiveness Test (Eisler, Miller, & Hersen, 1973). The latter was designed to provide simulated *in vivo* situations requiring assertive responses. The subject's responses are taped and rated on a number of verbal and nonverbal dimensions, such as duration of reply, latency of response, loudness of speech, compliance content, content requesting new behavior, affect, and overall assertiveness. This test did not discriminate between depressed and nondepressed subjects (Sanchez, 1976).

By way of summarizing a rather large number of studies aimed at the delineation of the behavioral social skills deficits of depressed individuals, one is impressed with the wide range of behaviors that have been studied and with the range of measures and coding systems that have been developed. The types of situations that have been the focus of attention have included the familial behavior of depressed individuals, dyadic interaction, group interaction, and marital interaction (e.g., Arkowitz *et al.*, 1982). The results are not easy to summarize, and part of the problem is that there are ambiguities and often serious disagreements about the definition and operationalization of "social skills" that have not been sufficiently addressed.

The construct validity and criterion validity of many of the measures have also not been sufficiently demonstrated. In general, it seems that depressed individuals are less socially skilled in situations that involve close and intimate relationships and in those that require them to interact with more than one person. Aspects of social interaction that may be suggested for further research are these:

1. General communication (sending and receiving) skills. These skills have typically been studied in the context of therapist skills (Strupp & Hadley, 1979; Truax & Carkhuff, 1967). While these skills are probably important for effective therapy, they may also be hypothesized to be important for all successful human interaction.
2. Conflict resolution skills.
3. Parenting skills.

ASSESSMENT OF SUBJECTIVE QUALITY OF EXPERIENCES

In this section, we discuss the assessment of the subjective quality of experiences, or what has also sometimes been called the quality of life.

Enjoyment of Pleasant Events

One of the more commonly used measures for assessing the degree of enjoyment of pleasant events is the Pleasant Events Schedule (PES), developed by MacPhillamy and Lewinsohn (1971, 1982). The item generation process was intended to sample a large number of pleasant activities for the age range from adolescence to old age. Extensive work was done to establish the psychometric properties of the PES (MacPhillamy & Lewinsohn, 1976, 1982). Concurrent validity was studied by comparing the subjects' ratings with those of peers and trained observers. Predictive validity was evaluated against subsequent self-monitoring and choice behavior. From a study of the relationship between engaging in pleasant activities and daily mood (Lewinsohn & Graf, 1973), 49 mood-related activities were identified. Cluster and factor analyses indicated that these items fell into four categories: positive social interactions, sex, activities that are incompatible with feeling sad (e.g., being relaxed, laughing), and activities that make one feel more competent (e.g., completing a task). Modifications of the PES have been developed by Bootzin (1982), Fuchs and Rehm (1975), and Amenson and Lewinsohn (1981).

Cautela and Kastenbaum (1967) have developed a somewhat similar measure, the Reinforcement Survey Schedule (RSS). The RSS is designed to identify stimuli with relatively high reinforcement value. The scale consists of 54 items, most with many subdivisions, and it takes approximately 20 to 30 minutes to complete. Kleinknecht, McCormick, and Thorndike (1971) reported the test-retest reliability coefficients for the PSS over 1-, 3-, and 5-week periods to be .73, .66, and .71, respectively. Cautela, Steffan, and Wish (1970) found that imagining scenes of stimuli rated high on reinforcement value increased the probability of over- or under-estimating circle size, while imagining stimuli with neutral reinforcement value had no such effect. Mermis (1971) found a significant relationship between time spent looking at slides of items from the RSS and the rated reinforcement value of those items. Modifications of the RSS have been developed for use with children (Philips, 1971) and for psychiatric inpatients (Cautela, 1972).

Both the PES and the RSS were developed within the framework of reinforcement theory, which assumes that depression and reinforcement are related phenomena. A theoretically somewhat different but nevertheless related concept is anhedonia. "Anhedonia" has been defined as the lowered ability to experience pleasure. Chapman, Chapman, and Raulin (1976) devised two true-false scales, a 40-item Physical Anhedonia Scale (e.g., "The beauty of sunsets is greatly overrated") and a 48-item Social Anhedonia Scale (e.g., "Getting together with old friends is one of my greatest pleasures"). The internal consistency of these scales was found to be high (between .70 and .80), and the correlation between the two scales was .60 for males and .51 for females, suggesting that the scales are to a considerable extent measuring the same underlying construct. Chapman *et al.* developed the anhedonia scales for clinical use with schizophrenics (who score more anhedonic) and as potential predictors of future schizophrenia. It would be of interest to know to what extent the pattern of reduced pleasure in schizophrenia resembles that seen in depression.

From the above-mentioned studies, it is clear that the degree of enjoyment experienced by people in their daily activities can be measured quite reliably and apparently also quite validly with the PES and with other similar instruments. Because these are all self-report measures, the influence of response bias factors cannot be completely eliminated. However, it is unlikely that response bias factors are entirely responsible for the differences that have been reported. Arguments relevant to this issue have been presented elsewhere (Lewinsohn & Amenson, 1978; MacPhillamy & Lewinsohn, 1982).

Stressful and Aversive Events

Stressful life events and aversive experiences have long been recognized as contributing factors in the development of depression (e.g., Paykel *et al.*, 1961). The oldest and most popular of the life events or stress measures are the Schedule of Recent Experience and the closely related Social Readjustment Rating Scale (Holmes & Rahe, 1967; Rahe, Meyer, Smith, Kjaer, & Holmes, 1969). More recent scales include Sarason, Johnson, and Siegel's (1978) Life Experiences Survey; Kanner, Coyne, Schaefer, and Lazarus's (1981) Hassles Scale; Dohrenwend, Krasnoff, Askenasy, and Dohrenwend's (1978) Psychiatric Epidemiology Research Interview life events scale; and a scale developed by Paykel, Prusoff, and Uhlenhuth (1971).

A limitation of currently available life events inventories concerns the number and the kinds of events assessed. Selection of specific events for inclusion in these lists has typically been arbitrary, with an emphasis on very stressful and very infrequently occurring events. The events of the Schedule of Recent Experience also emphasize events of young adulthood (e.g., start or end of formal schooling, marriage, changing to a new school, assuming a mortgage), and, as a result, young adults typically report twice as many events as people over 60 years of age (Dekker & Webb, 1974). Assuming that there are numerous minor and more frequently occurring stressful life events, Kanner *et al.* (1981) developed the Hassles Scale specifically to measure these. This instrument consists of 117 items and includes events such as "losing things," "auto maintenance," and "unexpected company."

Normative data have also not been systematically obtained for most currently available scales. Score distributions are typically markedly skewed to the right, and it is common to obtain standard deviations that are as large as the mean on the Schedule of Recent Experience (Wershow & Reinhart, 1974). Test-retest reliabilities for the Schedule of Recent Experience have been reported as ranging from .26 to .90 (Rahe *et al.*, 1974), and Sarason, de Monchaux, and Hunt (1975) suggest that the reliability of this particular instrument is lower than required by good research standards. The test-retest reliabilities for instruments that include a larger number of ongoing and/or more frequently recurring events, such as the Life Experiences Survey (Sarason *et al.*, 1978) and the Hassles Scale (Kanner *et al.*, 1981), have been found to be more satisfactory.

The Unpleasant Events Schedule (UES; Lewinsohn & Talkington, 1979) was designed to be a self-report inventory assessing the frequency of occurrence and the subjective impact of aversive events in people's lives. The UES has gone through several revisions, and normative data are available on a large sample of adults heterogeneous with regard to age, sex, and demographic characteristics (Lewinsohn, Mermelstein, Alexander, & MacPhillamy, 1983).

The UES and the PES were designed to cover most of the total life span. Both Teri and Lewinsohn (1982) and Gallagher and Thompson (1982) have modified the PES and UES for use with the elderly. These scales are shorter and therefore easier to use.

Summary

By way of summarizing the state of the art in regard to the assessment of the quality of life experiences, it appears that a range of instruments have been developed and that investigators have been responsive to some of the criticism made by Dohrenwend and Dohrenwend (1974). The fact that all instruments in this area rely so heavily on self-report is a shortcoming that can be remedied by using behavioral and psychophysiological measures and by making more use of a multivantaged approach as advocated by Katz *et al.* (1984).

DISCUSSION AND RECOMMENDATIONS

It is clear that an almost overwhelming number of assessment devices have been developed to measure the psychological variables that are important in regard to depression. All of this work has been done with unipolar depressives, and one obvious recommendation is that attempts to replicate findings with bipolar depressives be made in order to determine how applicable these results are to bipolar depression.

The psychometric properties of the assessment devices vary, but several criticisms can be leveled against most of them. For one thing, the degree to which the variables are uniquely associated with depression is often not clear, and many of the assessment devices may lack discriminant validity. More work needs to be done to try to determine to what extent the variables that have been shown to be associated with depression are also associated with other psychopathological states, especially anxiety. Because measures of anxiety and of depression are always highly intercorrelated, the extent to which the psychological correlates of depression and of anxiety differ is especially important. As has been stressed throughout this chapter, this issue can be addressed by including clearly defined nondepressed psychiatric control groups in studies.

The criterion validity of many of the instruments has also not been adequately demonstrated. This is especially true of the cognitive and social skills measures. The assessment of depressogenic cognitions has relied very heavily on self-report procedures, and consequently is vulnerable to questions about the degree to which people are able and willing to report their cognitive processes. Recently, sophisticated experimental procedures to assess the extent to which motivational and affective states influence information processing have been developed (Bower & Gilligan, 1979; Kuiper, 1978; Rogers, Kuiper, & Kirker, 1977; Teasdale & Fogarty, 1979). In these studies, it has been shown that the depressed state produces systematic changes in the way information about the self is processed, so that negative information about the self is processed more efficiently. This is the opposite of what is found in the nondepressed state, in which positive information about the self is processed more efficiently. These experimental procedures promise to be useful not only for aiding in the further clarification of the cognitive mechanisms that are associated with depression, but also for evaluating the criterion validity of the self-report measures. New techniques such as those developed by Klinger (1983; Klinger *et al.*, 1981) for the identification of the specific content of the thoughts experienced by depressed individuals may also help clarify the nature of the underlying cognitive changes and distortions seen in depression, as well as help establish the criterion validity of currently available cognitive instruments. Investigators may want to use these newer experimental techniques in conjunction with the self-report measures that have already been developed.

Corresponding to the differences that exist between theorists as to which specific cognitive processes are critical for the occurrence of depression, a wide variety of cognitive instruments has been developed. It would be of considerable interest to investigate the degree to which all of these instruments measure similar or different cognitive processes.

Measures of affect, which have also been largely self-reports, can probably be refined by using them in conjunction with psychophysiological and other less subjective methods, such as those that have been described by Cacioppo and Petty (1981), Ekman (1982), and Fridlund and Izard (1983). These methods are also less sensitive to cultural factors and therefore may be very useful with populations that differ in important respects from those that were used to develop currently the available self-report measures.

In the social skills area, self-report measures have consistently been found to produce large differences between depressed and nondepressed individuals. However, attempts to cross-validate such findings with behavioral observations typically have found much smaller effects. Furthermore, the degree of association between the self-report data and the observational data is often quite small. Since the procedures for collecting behavioral data are often quite cumbersome, require trained observers, and so on, it is understandable that investigators have shown a strong preference for self-report measures. The discrepancy between the findings from self-reports and behavioral observations raises basic questions about the specific nature of the social skills deficits associated with depression. Clearly, more research is needed to clarify the criterion validity of all social skills measures. Other directions for future research might follow Jacobson's (1981) recommendation that social skills assessment focus more sharply on the interpersonal behavior of depressed individuals with specific others (e.g., spouses, children) in specific contexts (e.g., conflict resolution). Another suggestion might be to focus on specific communication skills, such as being able to send messages that are clearly understood by others and being able to understand messages from others. The distinction between the possession of these specific social skills and their actual use in daily intercourse may also be important. Clearly, more research is needed to clarify the nature of the social skills deficits associated with depression and to develop assessment devices that go beyond the fact that depressed individuals evaluate themselves negatively on everything, including their social skills.

To shift to a more general level, it is apparent that investigators would be well advised to approach assessment from a multitrait-multimethod vantage point in order to deal with some of the above-mentioned problems. Studies should also include more than one measure for variables within and across domains, not only to address issues of convergent and discriminant validity, but also to ascertain to what extent deficits associated with depression in one domain are associated with deficits in other domains.

Another general issue that can be raised is the fact that most available assessment devices are "static"; that is, they measure a person on a variable at a given point in time, with the assumption that the person's score on the measure describes that person's standing on the variable (i.e., as if it were a trait). For many of the variables important for depression, it may be useful to look at behavioral sequences and at changes over time. For example, Jacobson and Anderson (1982) found no difference in the overall frequency of self-disclosures between depressed and nondepressed subjects, but did find a significant difference in the types of statements that preceded these disclosures.

Most of the assessment devices reviewed in this chapter were developed to test specific hypotheses derived from current psychological theories, and relatively little has been done to adapt these instruments for use in clinical practice. Many of them are quite lengthy, and the absence of norms limits their clinical utility. This is especially critical because many of the instruments were developed for use with younger and often highly educated persons. The psychometric development of the instruments with the goal of making them clinically useful would probably permit considerable shortening of many of them, because they undoubtedly incorporate a great deal of redundancy. The potential clinical utility of many of the assessment procedures described in this chapter is felt to be quite substantial, since many of them address variables that are of great importance for depression.

References

Abramson, L. Y., Seligman, M. E. P., & Teasdale, J. D. (1978). Learned helplessness in humans: Critique, and reformulation. *Journal of Abnormal Psychology, 87*, 49-74.

Alden, L., & Cappe, R. (1981). Nonassertiveness: Skill deficit or selective self-evaluation? *Behavior Therapy, 12*, 107-114.

Amenson, C. S., & Lewinsohn, P. M. (1981). An investigation into the observed sex difference in prevalence of unipolar depression. *Journal of Abnormal Psychology, 90*, 1-13.

Argyle, M. (1969). *Social interaction*. Chicago: Aldine.

Arkowitz, H., Holliday, S., & Hutter, M. (1982). *Depressed women and their husbands: A study of marital interaction and adjustment*. In *Depression and intimate relations*. Symposium conducted at the annual meeting of the Association for Advancement of Behavior Therapy, Los Angeles.

Arthur, J. A., Hops, H., & Biglan, A. (1982). *LIFE (Living in Familial Environments) coding system*. Unpublished manuscript, Oregon Research Institute.

Beck, A. T. (1967). *Depression: Clinical, experimental, and theoretical aspects*. New York: Harper & Row.

Beck, A. T., Rush, A., J., Shaw, R. F., & Emery, G. (1979). *Cognitive theraphy of depression*. New York: Guilford press.

Beck, A. T., Ward, C. H., Mendelson, M., Mock, J., & Erbaugh, J. (1961). An inventory for measuring depression. *Archives of General Psychiatry, 4*, 561-571.

Beck, A. T., Weissman, A., Lester, D., Trexler, L. (1974). The measurement of pessimism: The Hopelessness Scale. *Journal of Consulting and Clinical Psychology, 42*, 861-865.

Biglan, A., Hops, H., Sherman, L., Friedman, L. S., & Arthur, J. (1983). *A direct observation study of spousal interaction in maternal depression*. Unpublished manuscript, Oregon Research Institute.

Blaney, P. H., Behar, V., & Head, R. (1980). Two measures of depressive cognitions: Their association with depression and with each other. *Journal of Abnormal Psychology, 89*, 678-682.

Bootzin, R. R. (1982). A skill deficit approach to loneliness. In K. R. Blankenstein & J. Polivy (Eds.), *Self-control and self-modification of emotional behavior* (pp. 101-115). New York: Plenum Press.

Bower, G. H., & Gilligan, S. G. (1979). Remembering information related to one's self. *Journal of Research in Personality, 13*, 420-432.

Butler, L., & Meichenbaum, D. (1981). The assessment of interpersonal problem solving skills. In P. C. Kendall & S. D. Hollon (Eds.), *Assessment strategies for cognitive-behavioral interventions* (pp. 197-226). New York: Academic Press.

Cacioppo, J. T., Marshall-Goodell, B., & Dorfman, D. D. (1983). Skeletal muscular patterning: Topographical analysis of the integrated electromyogram. *Psychophysiology, 20*, 269-283.

Cacioppo, J. T., & Petty, R. E. (1981). Electromyograms or measures of extent and affectivity of information-processing. *American Psychologist, 36*, 441-456.

Cacioppo, J. T., & Sandman, C. A. (1981). Psychophysiological functioning, cognitive responding, and attitudes. In R. E. Petty, T. M. Ostrom, & T. C. Brock (Eds.), *Cognitive responses in persuasion* (pp. 81-103). Hillsdale, NJ: Erlbaum.

Cairns, R. B. (Ed.). (1979). *The analysis of social interactions: methods, issues and illustrations.* Hillsdale, NJ: Erlbaum.

Campbell, D. T., & Fiske, D. W. (1959). Convergent and discriminant validation by the multitrait-multimethod matrix. *Psychological Bulletin, 56*, 81-105.

Carney, R. M., Hong, B. A., Kulkarni, S., & Kapila, A. (1982). A comparison of EMG and SCL in normal and depressed subjects. *Pavlovian Journal of Biological Science, 16*, 212-216.

Cautela, J. R. (1972). Reinforcement Survey Schedule: Evaluation and current application. *Psychological Reports, 30*, 683-690.

Cautela, J. R., & Kastenbaum, R. (1967). A reinforcement survey schedule for use in therapy, training, and research. *Psychological Reports, 20*, 115-130.

Cautela, J. R., Steffan, J., & Wish, P. (1970). *Covert reinforcement: An experimental test.* Paper presented at the annual meeting of the American Psychological Association, Miami, F1.

Chapman, L. J., Chapman, J. P., & Raulin, M. L. (1976). Scales for physical and social anhedonia. *Journal of Abnormal Psychology, 85*, 374-382.

Coyne, J. C. (1976). Depression and the response of others. *Journal of Abnormal Psychology, 85*, 186-193.

Cronbach, L. J., & Gleser, G. C. (1965). *Psychological tests and personnel decisions.* Urbana: University of Illinois Press.

Davis, H. (1979). Self-reference and the encoding of personal information in depression. *Cognitive Therapy and Research, 3*, 97-110.

Davis, H., & Unruh, W. R. (1981). The development of the self-schema in adult depression. *Journal of Abnormal Psychology, 90*, 125-133.

Dekker, D. J., & Webb, J. T. (1974). Relationships of the Social Readjustment Rating Scale to psychiatric patient status, anxiety and social desirability. *Journal of Psychosomatic Research, 18*, 125-130.

Dobson, D. S., & Breiter, H. T. (1983). Cognitive assessment of depression: Reliability and validity of three measures. *Journal of Abnormal Psychology, 92*, 107-109.

Dohrenwend, B. S., & Dohrenwend, B. D. (1974). *Stressful life events: Their nature and effects.* New York: Wiley.

Dohrenwend, B. S., Krasnoff, L., Askenasy, A. R., & Dohrenwend, B. P. (1978). Exemplification of a method for scaling life events: The PERI life events scale. *Journal of Health and Social Behavior, 19*, 205-229.

D'Zurilla, T. J., & Nezu, A. (1982). Social problem solving in adults. In P. C. Kendall (Ed.), *Advances in cognitive-behavioral research and therapy* (Vol. 1, pp. 201-274). New York: Academic Press.

Eisler, R., Miller, P., & Hersen, M. (1973). Components of assertive behavior. *Journal of Clinical Psychology, 3*, 295-299.

Ekman, P. (1982). *Emotion in the human face* (2nd ed.). Elmsford, NY: Pergamon Press.

Ekman, P., & Friesen, W. V. (1978). *The Facial Action Coding System*. Palo Alto, CA: Consulting Psychologists Press.

Ekman, P., & Friesen, W. V. (1982a). *Facial expressions and psychopathology*. Unpublished manuscript.

Ekman, P., & Friesen, W. V. (1982b). Felt, false, and miserable smiles. *Journal of Nonverbal Behavior, 6*, 238-252.

Ellis, R. J. (1962). *Reason and emotion in psychotherapy*. New York: Lyle Stuart.

Folstein, M. F., & Luria, R. (1973). Reliability, validity and clinical application of the Visual Analogue Mood Scale. *Psychological Medicine, 3*, 479-486.

Fridlund, A. J., & Izard, C. E. (1983). Electromyographic studies of facial expressions of emotions and patterns of emotions. In J. T. Cacioppo & R. E. Petty (Ed.), *Social psychophysiology: A sourcebook* (pp. 243-286). New York: Guilford Press.

Fuchs, C., & Rehm, L. P. (1975). *The treatment of depresson through the modification of self-control behaviors*. Paper presented at the annual meeting of the Association for Advancement of Behavior Therapy, San Francisco.

Gallagher, D., & Thompson, L. W. (1982). *Stressful events, coping, and relapse rates in depressed elderly*. Paper presented at the annual meeting of the Amnerican Psychological Association, Washington, DC.

Glass, C. R., Merluzzi, T. V., Biever, J. L., & Larsen, K. H. (1982). Cognitive assessment of social anxiety: Development and validation of a self-statement questionnaire. *Cognitive Therapy and Research, 6*, 37-55.

Goldfried, M. R., Sobocinski, D. (1975). Effect of irrational beliefs on emotional arousal. *Journal of Consulting and Clinical Psychology, 43*, 504-510.

Hammen, C. L., & Peters, S. D. (1978). Interpersonal consequences of depression: Responses to men and women enacting a depressed role. *Journal of Abnormal Psychology, 87*, 322-332.

Hammen, C. L., & Krantz, S. (1976). Effect of success and failure on depressive cognitions. *Journal of Abnormal Psychology, 85*, 577-586.

Heiby, E. M. (1983a). Assessment of frequency of self-reinforcement. *Journal of Personality and Social Psychology, 44* (6), 1304-1307.

Heiby, E. M. (1983b). Depression as a function of the interaction of self- and environmentally-controlled reinforcement. *Behavior Therapy, 14*, 430-433.

Hinchliffe, M. K., Hooper, D., & Roberts, F. J. (1978). *The melancholy marriage: Depression in marriage and psychosocial approaches to therapy*. New York: Wiley.

Hoch, P. H., & Cattell, J. P. (1959). The diagnosis of pseudoneurotic schizophrenia. *Psychiatric Quarterly, 33*, 17-43.

Hollon, S. D., & Kendall, P. C. (1980). Cognitive self-statements in depression: Development of an Automatic Thoughts Questionnaire. *Cognitive Therapy and Research, 4*, 383-395.

Holmes, T. H., & Rahe, R. H. (1967). The Social Readjustment Rating Scale. *Journal of Psychosomatic Research, 11*, 213-218.

Hops, A., Biglan, A., Sherman, L., Arthur, J., & Friedman, L. (1983, August). *A direct observation study of family processes in maternal depression*. Paper presented at the annual meeting of the American Psychological Association, Anaheim, CA.

Howes, M. J., & Hokanson, J. E. (1979). Conversational and social responses to depressive interpersonal behavior. *Journal of Abnormal Psychology, 88*, 625-634.

Ilfeld, F. W. (1977). Current social stressors and symptoms of depression. *American Journal of Psychiatry, 134*, 161-166.

Jacobson, N. S. (1981). Assessment of overt behavior. In L. P. Rehm (Ed.), *Behavior therapy for depression* (pp. 279-300). New York: Academic Press.

Jacobson, N. S., & Anderson, E. A. (1982). Interpersonal skill and depression in college students: An analysis of the timing of self-disclosures. *Behavior Therapy, 13*, 271-282.

Jackson, D. N. (1970). A sequential system for personality scale development. In C. D. Spielberger (Ed.), *Current topics in clinical and community psychology* (Vol. 2, pp. 61-96). New York: Academic Press.

Jackson, D. N. (1976). *Jackson Personality Inventory Manual.* Port Huron, MI: Research Psychologists Press.

Jones, R. G. (1968). *A factored measure of Ellis' Irrational Belief System.* Wichita, KS: Test Systems.

Kanner, A. D., Coyne, J. C., Schaefer, C., & Lazarus, R. S. (1981). Comparison of two modes of stress measurement. Daily hassles and uplifts versus major life events. *Journal of Behavioral Medicine, 4*, 1-39.

Katz, M. M., Koslow, S. H., Berman, N., Secunda, S. K., Maas, J. R., Casper, R., Kocsis, J., & Stokes, P. (1984). A multivantaged approach to the measurement of behavioral and affect states for clinical and psychobiological research. *Psychological Reports, 55*, 619-671.

Kendall, P. C., & Korgeski, G. P. (1979). Assessment and cognitive-behavioral interventions. *Cognitive Therapy and Research, 3*, 1-21.

Kleinknecht, R. A., McCormick, C. E., & Thorndike, R. M. (1971). *Stability of reinforcers as measured by the Reinforcement Survey Schedule.* Paper presented at the annual meeting of the Association for Advancement of Behavior Therapy, Washington, D.C.

Klinger, E. (1983). *The Interview Questionnaire technique: Reliability and validity of a mixed idiographic-nomothetic measure of motivation.* Paper presented at the Eighth International Congress on Personality Assessment, Copenhagen.

Klinger, E., Barta, S. G., & Maxeiner, M. E. (1981). Current concerns: Assessing therapeutically relevant motivation. In P. C. Kendall & S. D. Hollon (Eds.), *Assessment strategies for cognitive-behavioral interventions* (pp. 161-196). New York: Academic Press.

Krantz, S., & Hammen, C. (1979). Assessment of cognitive bias in depression. *Journal of Abnormal Psychology, 88*, 611-619.

Kuiper, N. A. (1978). Depression and causal attributions for success and failure. *Journal of Personality and Social Psychology, 36*, 236-296.

Kuiper, N. A., & MacDonald, M. R. (1982) Self and other perception in mild depressives. *Social Cognition, 1*, 223-239.

Lazarus, A. A. (1968). Learning theory and the treatment of depression. *Behaviour Research and Therapy, 6*, 83-89.

Lefcourt, H. M. (1979). Locus of control for specific goals. In L. C. Perlmuter & R. A. Monty (Eds.), *Choice and perceived contol* (pp. 209-220.) Hillsdale, NJ: Erlbaum.

Lefcourt, H. M., von Baeyer, C. L., Ware, E. E., & Cox, D. J. (1979). The Multidimensional-Multiattributional Causality Scale: The development of a goal specific locus of control scale. *Canadian Journal of Behavioral Science, 11*, 286-304.

Lewinsohn, P. M. (1976). Manual of instructions for the behavior ratings used for the observation of interpersonal behavior. In E. J. Mash & L. G. Terdal (Eds.), *Behavior-therapy assessment* (pp. 335-345). New York: Springer.

Lewinsohn, P. M., & Amenson, C. (1978). Some relationships, between pleasant and unpleasant mood related activities and depression. *Journal of Abnormal Psychology, 87*, 644-654.

Lewinsohn, P. M., & Graf, M. (1973). Pleasant activities and depression. *Journal of Consulting and Clinical Psychology, 41*, 261-268.

Lewinsohn, P. M., Larson, D. W., & Munoz, R. F. (1982). The Measurement of expectancies and other cognitions in depressed individuals. *Cognitive Therapy and Research, 6*, 437-446.

Lewinsohn, P. M., Libet, J. M., & Javorek, R. (1973). *The construct of social skill: An empirical study of several behavioral measures on temporal stability, internal structure, validity, and situational generalizability.* Unpublished mimeograph, University of Oregon.

Lewinsohn, P. M., Mermelstein, R. M., Alexander, C., & MacPhillamy, D. J. (1983). *The Unpleasant Events Schedule: A scale for the measurement of aversive events*. Unpublished mimeograph, University of Oregon:

Lewinsohn, P. M., Munoz, R. R., Youngren, M. A., & Zeiss, A. M. (1978). *Control your depression*. Englewood Cliffs, NJ: Prentice-Hall.

Lewinsohn, P. M., & Talkington, J. (1979). Studies on the measurement of unpleasant events and relations with depression. *Applied Psychological Measurement, 3*, 83-101.

Lewinsohn, P. M., Weinstein, M., & Alper, T. (1970). A behavioral approach to the group treatment of depressed persons: A methodological contribution. *Journal of Clinical Psychology, 26*, 525-532.

Liberman, R. P., & Roberts, J. (1974). Contingency management of neurotic depression and marital disharmony. In H. J. Eysenck (Ed.), *Case histories in behavioral therapy*. London: Routledge & Kegan Paul.

Libet, J. M., & Lewinsohn, P. M. (1973). The concept of social skill with special reference to the behavior of depressed persons. *Journal of Consulting and Clinical Psychology, 40*, 304-312.

Little, J. C., & McPhail, N. I. (1973). Measures of depressive mood at monthly intervals. *British Journal of Psychiatry, 122*, 447-452.

Lloyd, G. G., & Lishman, W. A. (1975). Effect of depression on the speed of recall of pleasant and unpleasant experiences. *Psychological Medicine, 5*, 173-180.

Lubin, B. (1967). *Depression Adjective Check Lists: Manual*. San Diego: Educational and Industrial Testing Service.

Lubin, B. (1977). *Bibliography for the Depression Adjective Check Lists: 1966-1977*. San Diego: Educational and Industrial Testing Service.

MacPhillamy, D. J., & Lewinsohn, P. M. (1971). *A scale for the measurement of positive reinforcement*. Unpublished mimeograph, Ulniversity of Oregon.

MacPhillamy, D. J., & Lewinshon, P. L. (1976). *Manual for the Pleasant Events Schedule*. Unpublished mimeograph, University of Oregon.

MacPhillamy, D. J., & Lewinsohn, P. M. (1982). The Pleasant Events Schedule: Studies on reliability, validity, and scale intercorrelation. *Journal of Consulting and Clinical Psychology, 50*, 363-380.

McFall, R. M. (1982). A review and reformulation of the concept of social skills. *Behavior Assessment, 4*, 1-33.

McFall, R. M., & Lillesand, D. B. (1971). Behavior rehearsal with modeling and coaching in assertion training. *Journal of Abnormal Psychology, 77*, 313-323.

Meehl, P. E. (1964). *Manual for use with checklist of schizotypic signs*. Unpublished manuscript, University of Minnesota.

Merluzzi, T. V., Glass, C. R., & Genest, G. (Eds). (1981). *Cognitive assessment*. New York: Guilford Press.

Mermis, B. J. (1971). *Self-report of reinforcers and looking time*. Unpublished doctoral dissertation, University of Tennessee.

Munoz, R. F., & Lewinsohn, P. M. (1976a). *The Cognitive Events Schedule*. Unpublished mimeograph, University of Oregon.

Munoz, R. F., & Lewinsohn, P. M. (1976b). *The Personal Beliefs Inventory*. Unpublished mimeograph, University of Oregon.

Munoz, R. F., & Lewinsohn, P. M. (1976c). *The Subjective Probability Questionnaire*. Unpublished mimeograph, University of Oregon.

Nelson, R. E. (1977). Irrational beliefs in depression. *Journal of Consulting and Clinical Psychology, 45*, 1190-1191.

Oliveau, D., & Willmuth, R. (1979). Facial muscle electromyography in depressed and nondepressed hospitalized subjects. A partial replication. *American Journal of Psychiatry, 136*, 548-550.

Paykel, E. S., Meyers, J. K., Dienelt, M. N., Klerman, G. L., Lindenthal, J. J., & Pepper, M. P. (1961). Life events and depression: A controlled study. *Archives of General Psychiatry, 21*, 753-760.

Paykel, E. S., Prusoff, B. A., & Uhlenhuth, E. H. (1971). Scaling of life events. *Archives of General Psychiatry, 25*, 340-347.

Peterson, C., & Seligman, M. E. P. (1983). *Casual explanations as a risk factor for depression: Theory and evidence*. Unpublished mimeograph, University of Pennsylvania.

Peterson, C., Semmel, A., von Baeyer, C., Abramson, L. Y., Metalsky, G. I., & Seligman, M. E. P. (1982). The Attributional Style Questionnaire. *Cognitive Therapy and Research, 6*, 287-300.

Philips, I. (1971). *Children's Reinforcement Survey Schedule*. Unpublished manuscript, Temple University Medical School.

Platt, J., & Spivack, G. (1975). *The MEPS procedure manual*. Unpublished manuscript, Community Mental Health/Mental Retardation Center, Hahnemann Medican College and Hospital, Philadelphia.

Radloff, L. S. (1977). The CES-D Scale: A self-report depression scale for research in the general population. *Applied Psychological Measurement, 1*, 385-401.

Rahe, R. H., Meyer, M., Smith, M., Kjaer, G., & Holmes, T. H. (1969). Social stress and illness onset. *Journal of Psychosomatic Research, 8*, 35-44.

Rehm, L. P. (1976). Assessment of depression. In M. Hersen & A. S. Bellack (Eds.), *Behavioral assessment* (pp. 233-260). Oxford: Pergamon Press.

Reisinger, J. J. (1972). The treatment of "anxiety-depression" via positive reinforcement and response cost. *Journal of Applied Behavior Analysis, 5*, 125-130.

Rogers, T. B., Kuiper, N. A., & Kirker, W. S. (1977). Self-reference and the encoding of personal information. *Journal of Personality and Social Psychology, 35*, 677-688.

Romano, J. M., & Bellack, A. S. (1980). Social validation of a component model of assertive behavior. *Journal of Consulting and Clinical Psychology, 48*, 478-490.

Rosenbaum, M. (1980). A schedule for assessing self-control behaviors: Preliminary findings. *Behavior Therapy, 11*, 109-121.

Roth, A. V., & Lubin, B. (1979). *Factors underlying the Depression Adjective Check Lists*. Unpublished mimeograph.

Rotter, J. B. (1966). Generalized expectancies for internal versus external control of reinforcement. *Psychological Monographs, 80*, 1-28.

Sanchez, V. C. A. (1976). *A comparison of depressed, psychiatric control and normal control subjects on two measures of assertiveness*. Unpublished master's thesis, University of Oregon.

Sarason, I. G., de Monchaux, C., & Hunt, T. (1975). Methodological issues in the assessment of life stress. In L. Levi (Ed.), *Emotions: Their parameters and measurements*. New York: Raven Press.

Sarason, I. G., Johnson, J. H., & Siegel, J. M. (1978). Assessing the impact of life changes: Development of the Life Experiences Survey. *Journal of Consulting and Clinical Psychology, 46*, 932-946.

Schlosberg, H. (1941). A scale for the judgement of facial expression. *Journal of Experimental Psychology, 29*, 497-510.

Schwartz, G. E., Fair, P. L., Salt, P., Mandel, M. R., & Klerman, G. L. (1976). Facial muscle patterning to affective imagery in depressed and nondepressed subjects. *Science, 192*, 489-491.

Steinmetz, J. L., Lewinsohn, P. M., & Antonuccio, D. O. (1983). Prediction of individual outcome in a group intervention for depression. *Journal of Consulting and Clinical Psychology, 86*, 235-241.

Strack, S., & Coyne, J. C. (1983). Social confirmation of dysphoria: Shared and private reactions to depression. *Journal of Personality and Social Psychology, 44*, 798-806.

Strupp, H. H., & Hadley, S. W. (1979). Specific vs. nonspecific factors in psychotherapy. *Archives of General Psychiatry, 36*, 1125-1136.

Teasdale, J. D., & Bancroft, J. (1977). Manipulation of thought content or a determinant of mood and corrugator activity in depressed patients. *Journal of Abnormal Psychology, 86*, 235-241.

Teasdale, J. D., & Fogarty, S. J. (1979). Differential effects of induced mood on retrieval of pleasant events from episodic menory. *Journal of Abnormal Psychology, 88*, 248-257.

Teri, L., & Lewinsohn, P. M. (1982). Modification of the pleasant and unpleasant events schedules for use with the elderly. *Journal of Consulting and Clinical Psychology, 50*, 444-445.

Tomkins, S. S. (1962). *Affect, imagery, consciousness: Vol. 1. The positive affects*. New York: Springer.

Tomkins, S. S. (1963). *Affect, imagery, consciousness: Vol. 2. The negative affects*. New York: Springer.

Truax, C. B., & Carkhuff, R. R. (1967). *Toward effective counseling and psychotherapy*. Chicago: Aldine.

Warren, N. J., Stake, J. E., & McKee, D. C. (1982). Cognitive distortions, coping behavior, and depression in college students. *College Health, 30*, 279-283.

Weissman, A. N., & Beck, A. T. (1978). *Development and validation of the Dysfunctional Attitude Scale*. Paper presented at the annual meeting of the Association for Advancement of Behavior Therapy, Chicago.

Weissman, M. M., & Paykel, E. S. (1974). *The depressed woman: A study of social relationships*. Chicago: University of Chicago Press.

Wershow, H. J., & Reinhart, G. (1974). Life change and hospitalization; A heretical view. *Journal of Psychosomatic Research, 18*, 393-401.

Williams, J. G., Barlow, D., & Agras, W. (1972). Behavioral measurement of severe depression. *Archives of General Psychiatry, 27*, 330-337.

Wolpe, J. (1971). Neurotic depression: Experimental analog, clinical syndromes, and treatment. *American Journal of Psychotherapy, 25*, 362-368.

Wolpe, J., & Lazarus, A. A. (1966). *Behavior therapy techniques*. Oxford: Pergamon Press.

Wylie, R. C. (1979). *The self-concept: Theory and research on selected topics* (Vol. 2). Lincoln: University of Nebraska Press.

Youngren, M. A., & Lewinsohn, P. M. (1980). The functional relationship between depression and problematic interpersonal behavior. *Journal of Abnormal Psychology, 89*, 334-341.

Youngren, M. A., Zeiss, A., & Lewinsohn, P. M. (1977). *Interpersonal Events Schedule*. Unpublished mimeograph, University of Oregon.

Zeiss, T., & Lewinsohn, P. M. (1984). *Changes in vulnerability for future episodes of depression as a function of duration of since previous episode*. Unpublished mimeograph, University of Oregon.

Zung, W. K. (1965). A self-rating depression scale. *Archives of General Psychiatry, 12*, 63-70.

Zung, W. K. (1973). From art to science: The diagnosis and treatment of depression. *Archives of General psychiatry, 29*, 328-337.

CHAPTER 9

Measurement of the Cognitive Aspects of Depression

A. JOHN RUSH
University of Texas Health Science Center at Dallas

INTRODUCTION

Cognition

The term "cognition" has a variety of meanings, ranging from the capacity to process, comprehend, or recall specific types of information (measured by mental status examination or neuropsychologic testing) to particular symptoms noted in various syndromes such as major depression (e.g., suicidal ideation, trouble concentrating or making decisions, self-criticism, or guilt). Neisser (1967) defined "cognition" as "all the processes by which the sensory input is transformed, reduced, elaborated, stored, recovered, and used" (p. 4). Thus, cognitive processes include sensation, perception, imagery, attention, recall, memory, problem solving, and thinking.

While cognitive symptoms of depression are derived, defined, and operationalized on an empirical or clinical basis, other cognitive aspects of depression refer to psychological *constructs* suggested by different psychological theories of depression. These constructs include notions such as attributional style (Abramson, Seligman, & Teasdale, 1978), dysfunctional attitudes or schemata (Beck, 1976), or anger turned on the self (Freud, 1917/1957). Such constructs are hypothesized to underlie or form the basis for cognitive, behavioral, affective, and other clinically apparent symptoms of depression. These constructs are based on or derived from inferences about the nature of depression and particular symptoms.

Thorough recent reviews of information processing or neuropsychological deficits found in some depressions are available elsewhere (W. R. Miller, 1975; Weingartner & Silberman, 1984). Therefore, this chapter focuses on those cognitive aspects of depression that are based on empirical clinical findings, as well as those derived from theoretical psychological models of depression. An excellent and thorough review of this area has recently been made available (Hammen & Krantz, 1985). This chapter highlights the methodological and interpretive problems and reviews some of the commonly used measures of the cognitive aspects of depression.

Depression

Just as the term "cognition" has multiple meanings, so does the term "depression." Most studies of the cognitive aspects of depression have focused on symptomatic patients with unipolar major depression. Studies of bipolar depressed or manic-phase patients are rare, perhaps because of both the difficulties inherent in obtaining compliance from manics and the dearth of psychological theories of mania. Perhaps another cause for this information vacuum is the unspoken abrogation of mania to the biologists, implying that psychological methods and measures will contribute little to our understanding of this disorder. This position, I believe, is both premature and ill-founded. A brief look at the symptoms of mania, and even more particularly hypomania, will reveal a plethora of cognitive malfunctions (e.g., pressured thinking, involvement in activities with an apparent disregard for the dangerous or painful consequences, inflated sense of self-esteem, grandiosity, sharpened wit, sense of creativity, etc.). Furthermore, clinicians often observe that certain life events may precede (and by implication, facilitate) the onset of manic or hypomanic episodes, although empirical studies of these observations are lacking. In addition, a clarification of the psychology of mania or hypomania might well result in improved methods to obtain compliance with pharmacotherapy or other prescriptions for improved psychosocial functioning. Thus, while much clinical data argue for the need to clarify the psychology of mania/hypomania, little effort has been expended in this direction.

A further deficit in the current literature is the total absence of studies of the cognitive aspects of dysthymic disorder. This deficiency is even more puzzling, as at least some dysthymics may be suitable candidates for psychosocial interventions. However, this clinical notion is neither supported nor discounted by empirical psychotherapy outcome studies.

Some Methodological Problems

In addition to the above-noted limitations in the populations studied, several methodological difficulties are apparent in this field (Hammen & Krantz, 1985; Hollon & Bemis, 1981). Perhaps the most long-standing and pivotal difficulty is that of measurement itself. Most measures of cognition depend on patient self-reports, which may take the form of paper-and-pencil tests or ratings of emotional or cognitive responses to predefined stimuli (e.g., insoluble anagrams, written vignettes, videotaped stimuli, or role-played interpersonal situations). This heavy reliance on self-report has a built-in problem

— namely, that depressed patients have a biased recall of actual events (DeMonbruen & Craighead, 1977; Kuiper, 1978; Lloyd & Lishman, 1975).

If one wishes to measure this bias, one strategy is to objectively measure the event itself, as well as the subject's view of the event. This strategy, which is common in experimental psychology, has the advantage of high reliability and replicability, while restricting generalizability to laboratory situations. Furthermore, if self-reports are conducted within a particular context that is known to the subject (e.g., measurement of cognitions as part of a psychotherapeutic program aimed at changing cognitions), the subject's self-report responses may be more or less influenced by the demand characteristics of the situation, even without the subject's awareness.

How to validate self-reports of private mental events remains a central question for this field. Concurrent use of multiple measures of cognitions can increase one's certainty in one respect — namely, that the subject is being consistent. Yet this strategy does not directly address the question of whether the subject, for example, actually solves interpersonal problems in the manner he or she reports on a written test. Similarly, if subjects do not endorse dysfunctional attitudes on self-reports, do they actually not act on such attitudes on a day-to-day basis? That is, how are we to know whether the self-reports are valid?

A second methodological problem that confounds this field is that the most transparent or easily observed aspects of cognitions are most easily measured. For example, suicidal ideation can be measured by simple self-monitoring procedures that count the frequency or duration of such thoughts, or the actual thought content. The Suicidal Ideation Scale (Beck, Schuyler, & Herman, 1974; see below) captures reliably many aspects of suicidal ideation. Much greater difficulty is encountered when one attempts to assess "deeper structures" or "constructs" that are not in the subject's immediate awareness (e.g., schemata, attributional style). These constructs must bc inferred from patterns of emotional or behavioral resposes, problem-solving behaviors, interpersonal relationships, and so on.

A third methodological problem centers around the fluctuating nature of depressive symptomatology. If the cognitions to be measured are highly state-dependent, then establishing test-retest reliability becomes a two-horned dilemma. If the two test occasions are close together in time, then responses to the first test are more easily recalled and may therefore affect results with the second test. If the two tests are separated by more time to counter this concern, then symptomatic status will be more likely to fluctuate and therefore to reduce test-retest reliability. One possible solution to this dilemma is to develop two or more variations of the same test that can be used as interchangeable instruments. For example, there are two forms of the Dysfunctional Attitude Scale (Weissman, 1979; see below).

A fourth methodological difficulty encountered in the measurement of cognitive aspects of depression derives from the likelihood that culture affects cognitive content. Maudsley was the first to emphasize the influence of society and culture on both the symptoms and the mental content of depressives. Senegalese, Indonesians, non-Westernized Arabs, native American Indians, and others may not evidence guilt or self-blame, and may even have a lower frequency of suicidal ideation (Marsella, 1980), although a variety of methodological problems still inhere in most studies upon which the contention above is based. Virtually all studies of the perceptions of the self, world (experience), and future, for example, have been conducted on Westernized patients. Therefore, one must be cautious in generalizing findings about the cognitive aspects of depression to patients form non-Western cultures.

Given these four methodological difficulties, we are also likely to encounter several interpretive errors (Hammen & Krantz, 1985; Hollon & Bemis, 1981). One cannot assume that a particular cognitive abnormality found in, say, depression, is specific to this disorder. Other psychopathological conditions must be studied to determine whether specificity is noted. This stipulation is particularly critical with regard to depression. Many psychopathological conditions are not classified descriptively as affective disorders, yet some depressive symptoms may accompany these disorders (e.g., anorexia nervosa, agoraphobia, panic disorder, bulimia, etc.) (American Psychiatric Association, 1980). Thus, constrast groups must be obtained without such variably associated affective symptomatology.

Conversely, one cannot assume without empirical evaluation that since a particular cognitive abnormality is associated with unipolar depression, for example, it is also present in bipolar depression, dysthymia, or grief. A third error is to infer etiology from the finding that certain cognitive or, for that matter, biological abnormalities are found in depression. Such abnormalities may be simple accompaniments of the state (e.g., suicidal or self-critical thinking) or consequences of the state once it has developed (e.g., excess alcohol ingestion to self-medicate the depression once it is present). Even abnormalities that precede a particular clinical episode may be longer-term consequences (residues) of prior episodes of illness.

Similarly, whether or not the cognitive abnormality disappears with clinical remission bears only indirectly on whether the abnormality is of etiological importance. Those abnormalities that are specific to depression and precede, are present during, and are present following a clinical episode are more likely to be vulnerability factiors (i.e., to play an important role in the pathopsychology or pathophysiology of depression) than are those abnormalities that are highly state-dependent. Unfortunately, there are few longitudinal studies of patients before, during, and following an episode of depression. Such data are essential to determine whether etiological importance can be inferred.

Finally, the advent of cognitive therapies to treat some depressions provides yet another opportunity for illogical interpretation. If cognitive therapy is associated with symptom reduction, one cannot infer either (1) that cognitive theory has been validated or (2) that cognitions are of etiological importance.

Conversely, if medication is effective in reducing symptoms and correcting certain cognitive abnormalities, one cannot conclude (1) that cognitive theory is invalid or (2) that cognitions have no etiological or pathopsychological relevance.

Given all of these pitfalls and problems, why even try to measure cognitions? I would propose, much as for biological measurements, that such measures may improve our ability to perform one or more of the following tasks: diagnosis, treatment selection, treatment monitoring, clarification of the pathopsychology of these disorders, testing of etiological theories of depression, prognostication, or the identification of those vulnerable to developing a depression. In addition, one might use such measures to clarify the relationship, if any, between biological and psychological aspects of depression. To date, however, only minimal assistance in each of these tasks has been gained from cognitive measurements of depression.

It should be noted that a particular cognitive measure may meaningfully address one or more of the above-listed tasks, but may be irrelevant to other tasks. For instance, a particular measure may help in treatment selection, but may be unrelated to descriptive differential diagnosis. A similar commentary applies to biological measures that may subserve one but not others of the tasks above.

For the following review, I have divided strategies for measuring cognitions into those that aim at assessing the more prominent aspects of depression and those that attempt to measure particular theoretically derived constructs. This subdivision is not the only one possible. For example, Shaw and Dobson (1981) have argued the importance of distinguishing cognitive content (e.g., images, assumptions, ideation, automatic thoughts) from cognitive processes (e.g., transfer of infomation from short-term to long-term memory).

This chapter reviews some of the attempts to assess selected cognitive aspects of depression. It is not intended to be encyclopedic. Rather, commonly used or better developed instruments are reviewed, with an emphasis on both the problems and promises that remain. At this time, there is no consensus about which aspects of cognition are most critical to our understanding of depression, or about which measures are optimal.

COGNITIVE MEASURES RELEVANT TO BECK'S THEORY OF DEPRESSION

Before discussing particular cognitive measures, we must briefly review the major cognitive psychological theories of depression, as these theories form the basis for the development of many cognitive measures. The empirical data that support or fail to support each theory are presented in various reviews (Beck & Rush, 1978; Seligman, Klein, & Miller, 1976).

Table 9-1 summarizes those psychological theories of depression that con-

TABLE 9-1 Psychological Theories of Depression Containing Important Cognitive Elements

Author	Hypotheses
Bandura (1971)	1. Depressives show a decrease in self-reinforcing activities (overt and covert).
Costello (1972)	1. Loss of reinforcer effectiveness leads to a generalized disruption in chains of behavior.
Abramson, Seligman, & Teasdale (1978); Seligman (1974, 1975)	1. Learned helplessness ensues from previous experience of noncontingent positive or negative reinforcement schedules. 2. Negative events are attributed to self (vs. other), stable (vs. unstable), and global (vs. specific) characteristics. 3. When (1) and (2) are combined, depression follows.
Rehm (1977)	1. Depressives engage in selective monitoring of negative events. 2. Depressives engage in selective monitoring of immediate (vs. delayed) consequences of behavior. 3. Depressives have stringent self-evaluative criteria. 4. Depressives make inaccurate attributions of responsibility. 5. Depressives engage in insufficient self-reward and excessive self-punishment.
Beck (1967, 1976)	1. Negative views of self, world, and future participate in symptom maintenance. 2. Schemata (silent assumptions) form basis for (1) and account for vulnerability.

tain important cognitive elements. This chapter focuses primarily on the two dominant cognitive theories, Beck's and Seligman's, because they have led to the development of many of the cognitive measures.

Introduction to Beck's Theory

Table 9-2 summarizes Beck's cognitive theory of depression (Beck, 1964, 1976; Rush, 1983). Depression is viewed in terms of the activation of three major thinking patterns (the cognitive triad) through which depressed persons regard themselves, their experiences, and their future in an unrealistically negative manner.

TABLE 9-2 Cognitive Theory of Depression

1. Cognitive triad
   A. The cognitive triad is an unrealistically negative view of self, future, and world.
   B. The triad explains symptoms of depressive syndrome.
   C. It is evident in cognitions.
   D. It is based on schemata.
   E. The triad is reinforced by interpretations of current events.
   F. It varies with severity of depression.
2. Schemata
   A. Schemata consist of unspoken, inflexible general rules or silent assumptions (beliefs, concepts).
   B. They develop as enduring concepts from past (early) experiences.
   C. Schemata serve as a basis for screening, discriminating, weighing, and coding stmuli.
   D. They serve as a basis for categorizing and evaluating experiences, making judgments, and distorting reality situations.
   E. Which schemata are activated in a situation determines the content of cognitions formed in the situation and the affective responses to it.
   F. Schemata increase vulnerability to depression.
3. Logical errors
   A. Logical errors in thinking result from hyperactive schemata because of misinterpretations of events that reinforce the cognitive triad.
   B. These errors include arbitrary inference, magnification or minimization, dichotomous thinking, overgeneralizations, personalization, selective abstraction, and rigid thinking.

According to Beck's cognitive formulation, depressed patients have a systematic negative bias in their beliefs and self-evaluations. They see themselves as deficient, inadequate, and unworthy, and they tend to attribute their unpleasant experiences to physical, mental, or moral deficits in themselves. They believe that they are undesirable and worthless because of these defects. They believe they lack the attributes that they consider essential for attaining contentment and happiness.

Depressed persons also interpret their experiences in a distorted manner. They see the world as making exorbitant demands on them or as presenting insurmountable obstacles to achieving their life goals. They systematically misinterpret situations in negative ways, even though more plausible interpretations are available. They consistently construe interactions with their environment as representing defeat or deprivation.

Also, depressed persons see the future in a negative way. They anticipate that their current difficulties will continue indefinitely. They expect to fail when undertaking tasks. They cannot see the future as more promising than their current reality.

The cognitive triad contributes to, maintains, or exacerbates the signs and symptoms of the depressive syndrome. For example, if patients incorrectly *think* that they are being rejected, they will react with the same affect that occurs with *actual* rejection. If they are pessimistic about the future and anticipate negative outcomes, they will feel low in energy, will be apathetic, and will be reluctant to initiate various tasks. Suicidal wishes are more likely if the patients desire to escape from what *appear* to be unbearable situations or insoluble problems. Seeing themselves as inept, they overestimate the difficulty of normal tasks in life. Indecision follows from their belief that any decisions they make will be wrong.

These negative views of self, world, and future are apparent in how such patients consciously think (their automatic thoughts). These views are also mutually reinforcing, such that even objectively pleasant or desired events are misconstrued in a negative way. The views are based on enduring concepts or "schemata," which are inflexible, unspoken general rules, beliefs, or silent assumptions developed from early experience. An example of such a schema might be "In order to be loved or worthwhile, I must be successful in my work." These schemata form the basis for screening, weighing, categorizing, and evaluating experiences, and for making judgments about situations. Judgments based on hypervalent schemata are distorted.

Specific situations activate certain schemata. For example, correction from a superior at work might activate the schemata above. The activated schema determines how the person evaluates the specific situation (the correction from the boss is construed as "I am totally worthless"). This evaluation (automatic thought) leads to feelings of guilt and sadness. According to theory, schemata increase a person's vulnerability to depression and account for the relapsing, recurrent nature of many depressions. The schemata are present both during clinical episodes and between the episodes. They are hypervalent (i.e., are more active, are more apparent, and exert more influence) during the episode, however.

Finally, cognitive theory posits the existence of a number of structural errors in the thinking of depressed persons. These structural errors, or errors of logic, are evident in the depressed persons' misinterpretations of events. They include arbitrary inference, selective abstraction, over generalization, magnification or minimization, personalization, and dichotomous thinking.

"Arbitrary inference" refers to drawing a conclusion in the absence of evidence to support the conclusion. "Selective abstraction" consists of focusing on a detail taken out of context, while ignoring other salient features of the situation, and conceptualizing the whole experience based on this detail. For example, a secretary who makes a typographical error in one letter, while typing another 30 letters without error, may illogically conclude "I can't type" if he or she focuses only on the letter typed in error. "Overgeneralization" refers to the pattern of drawing a conclusion on the basis of a single incident. "Magnification" and "minimization" are different ways of assigning unusual weight or importance to certain aspects of a situation and drawing an illogical conclusion from the situation. "Personalization" refers to a patient's tendency to relate external events (usually negative events) to himself or herself without a basis for making such a connection. "Dichotomous thinking" refers to the tendency to think in terms of black and white or bipolar opposites. An example would consist of thinking that one is either a great success or a total failure. These logical or structural errors are present in association with depressed persons' misconceptualizations of events, themselves, and their future, and are a consequence of hyperactive schemata.

A number of measures to assess negative thinking have undergone validation procedures. In general, the content of depressives' perceptions (e.g., of themselves, of experience, and of the future) has received a large amount of study (Beck & Rush, 1978). This emphasis undoubtedly derives from the common clinical observation in Western cultures that depressives view themselves in a negative or self-critical fashion. This observation has been so well agreed upon that the *Diagnostic and Statistical Manual of Mental Disorders*, third edition (DMS-III; American Psychiatric Association, 1980), lists self-criticism/guilt as a criterion symptom for the diagnosis of the syndrome of major depression.

The Automatic Thoughts Questionnaire

The Automatic Thoughts Questionnaire (ATQ; Hollon & Kendall, 1980) was derived empirically to identify common depressive automatic thoughts. Students were asked to recall a depressing situation, and then to list their thoughts in that situation. After redundant and incomprehensible items were eliminated, the remaining 100 items were given to another student group along with the Beck Depression Inventory (BDI) to identify those items that discriminated between depressed and nondepressed students. The 30 most discriminating items were used in the final scale. Table 9-3 provides exemplar ATQ items.

Internal reliability for the ATQ has been found to be high. The split-half reliability coefficient was .97, and coefficient alpha (Cronbach, 1951) was .96 (both p's $< .001$). These findings were replicated with student subjects (Dobson & Breiter, 1983) and with mental health center and medical outpatients (Harrell & Ryon, 1983). Test-restest reliability has not been reported.

Construct validity is suggested by the fact that ATQ scores differed between depressed and nondepressed students (Hollon & Kendall, 1980). Harrell and Ryon (1983) also found that depressed outpatients had significantly higher ATQ scores than nondepressed psychiatric and medical patient controls. ATQ scores and depressive symptom severity ratings were correlated among students (r's $= .62$ for females and .64 for males, both p's $< .001$) (Dobson & Breiter, 1983). The correlation between depression severity and ATQ scores was higher than correlations with two other cognitive measures, including the Dysfunctional Attitude Scale (Weissman, 1979; see below).

Four ATQ factors have been reported: (1) personal maladjustment and desire for change (e.g., "What's wrong with me?"); (2) negative self-concept

TABLE 9-3 Exemplar Items from the ATQ

How frequently (1-5) did this thought occur to you in the last week?

1. I feel like I'm up against the world.
2. I'm no good.
3. I've let people down.
4. I'm a loser.

Note. Reprinted by permission of S. D. Hollon.

and expectations (e.g., "My future is bleak"); (3) low self-esteem (e.g., "I'm worthless"); and (4) giving up and helplessness (e.g., "I can't finish anything") (Hollon & Kendall, 1980). These factors are similar to the cognitive distortions described by Beck (1976).

The ATQ is a brief and easily administered measure of automatic thoughts. While it appears promising, Coyne and Gotlieb (1983) have questioned whether subjects can reliably estimate how often automatic negative thoughts occur to them in a week, given Beck's (Beck, Rush, Shaw, & Emery, 1979) belief that specific training in "catching" automatic thoughts may be required. Furthermore, since items were derived from recalled situations in a nonclinical population, the degree to which these specific thoughts (items) are a valid representation of a depressed patient's actual thinking can be questioned. On the other hand, some construct validity can be inferred from a recent report (Eaves & Rush, 1984) in which depressed patients had high ATQ scores when symptomatic and had normal scores when clinically remitted — as would be predicted by Beck's theory.

Cognitive Bias Questionnaire

The Cognitive Bias Questionnaire (CBQ; Hammen & Krantz, 1976; Krantz & Hammen, 1979) is a self-report that assesses depressive negative thinking and evaluates negative bias, independent of dysphoric tone. Six problematic situations that are commonly encountered by college students (Hammen & Krantz, 1976) or by psychiatric inpatients (Krantz & Hammen, 1979) are presented in vignette form. Three vignettes have an interpersonal focus, and three have an achievement focus. Four multiple-choice questions about the protagonist's thoughts and feelings follow each story (except one, which has three questions). The multiple-choice questions were designed to assess two crossed dimensions — "distorted" "nondistorted," and "depressed" "nondepressed." The distorted-nondistorted dimension depends on whether or not inferences are made that go beyond the available information. The depressed-nondepressed dimension depends on the presence or absence of dysphoria (not syndromal depression). Each depressed/distorted option includes one or more of Beck's logical errors (e.g., arbitrary inference, overgeneralization, etc.). Table 9-4 provides an exemplar vignette from the CBQ.

TABLE 9-4 Exemplar Vignette from the CBQ

Shelly, a college sophomore living in the dorms, is one of the few women remaining on her floor Friday evening. The other residents are out for the evening or away for the weekend. Imagine as vividly as possible what Shelly might think and feel about being alone on a Friday night.

a. Doesn't bother me because I figure I'll have a date next weekend for sure [nondepressed/nondistorted].
b. Upsets me and makes me feel lonely [depressed/nondistorted].
c. Upsets me and makes me start to imagine endless days and nights by myself [depressed/distorted].
d. Doesn't bother me because one Friday night alone isn't that important; probably everybody has spent one night alone [nondepressed/nondistorted].

Note. Reprinted by permission of C. Hammen.

Coefficients of internal consistency were only moderate in two student samples (α's = .62 and .69). Test-retest correlations over 4-8 weeks were satisfactory in these two samples (*r*'s = .48 and .60, both *p*'s $<$ .001). Test-retest reliability in depressed patients remains to be determined. Hammen and Krantz (1985) suggest that the modest alpha coefficients may reflect the heterogeneity in the construct of cognitive distortions.

Krantz and Hammen (1979) reported on the validity of the CBQ in clinically depressed outpatients, depressed and nondepressed psychiatric inpatients, and four independent student samples. In depressed outpatients, Krantz and Hammen (1979) reported significant correlations between depressed/distorted CBQ and BDI scores. Furthermore, CBQ scores were sensitive to treatment for depression. Finally, depressed subjects gave significantly more depressed/distorted responses than nondepressed subjects.

These findings have been replicated by other investigators. Norman, Miller, and Klee (1983) found that the depressed/distorted CBQ scores differentiated two depressed groups (depression was the primary diagnosis in one and the secondary diagnosis in the other) from a nondepressed, schizophrenic inpatient sample. Blaney, Behar, and Head (1980) reported that depressed/distorted CBQ scores were significantly correlated with depressive symptom severity in two different student samples (*r*'s = .26 and .44, both *p*'s $<$ .001). Frost and MacInnis (1983) found significant correlations between BDI scores (obtained 3-10 weeks before and 2 days after the CBQ) and the depressed/distorted score (*r*'s = .43 and .51, both *p*'s $<$ .005) in depressed college women. Significant correlations between several observed behavioral indices of depression (*r*'s ranged from .34 to .50, *p*'s $<$ .05) and distortion scores were also found. However, after the variance shared with depression was controlled for, hostility was correlated with the depressed/distorted CBQ score ($r = .29$, $p < .05$); this raises a question about the specificity of this cognitive abnormality to depression.

The correlational studies are consistent with findings from experimental manipulations of mood states. With a modified version of the CBQ, Goodwin and Williams (1982) found that induction of a sad mood significantly increased distortion scores, although the effect different somewhat by the type of mood induction (self-referent or somatic). Riskind and Rholes (1983) also found that the induction of a sad mood led to significant elevations in CBQ scores with a self-devaluative mood induction procedure but not with a somatic induction procedure.

Several cautions regarding the CBQ have been suggested by Hammen and Krantz (1985). The concept of cognitive bias is an extremely complex one. The authors themselves have voiced concern that CBQ items may represent considerable heterogeneity of interpretations, attributions, predictions, and so on (Krantz & Hammen,1979). Allthough the instrument appears sensitive to variations in depressed mood, depressed/distorted responses are typically less than the possible 6 out of 23 even in depressed persons. That is, there may be some insensitivity in the instrument. Finally, a potential practical limitation is that the measure is tied to specific socioenviornmental contexts and populations. The two existing versions were designed for and validated in student and psychiatric populations. Thus, its use may be limited to these groups, and other forms may be required for adolescent and geriatric populations, for example. This problem is common to some other measures as well. By attempting to present personally poignant and relevant vignettes, problem situations, or other stimuli, the investigator must narrow the focus of the instrument. In so doing, the instrument may not be useful in different populations. The development of several forms may ensue, but how can one be certain that they are equally sensitive (i.e. are the scores actually interchangeable)?

Dysfunctional Attitude Scale

The Dysfunctional Attitude Scale (DAS; Weissman, 1979) is available in two 40-item self-reports. This instrument is based upon Beck's silent assumptions or schemata found in depression and other psychiatric conditions. The subjects indicate the degree to which they agree or disagree with each item on a 7-point scale (from "agree very much" to "neutral" to "disagree very much"). The items include perfectionistic standards, concern about approval from others, requirements for being happy or feeling adequate, and so on. Table 9-5 provides exemplar items from the DAS.

Good internal consistency and stability over time have been demonstrated. Coefficient alpha ranged from .89 to .92, and the test-retest correlation was .84 over an 8-week period (Weissman, 1979). These findings were replicated (Hamilton & Abramson, 1983; O'Hara, Rehm & Campbell, 1982), although Hamilton and Abramson (1983) reported a slightly lower test-retest correlation (.71).

Construct validity of the DAS can be inferred from both clinical and

TABLE 9-5 Exemplar Items from the DAS

1. It is difficult to be happy unless one is good-looking, intelligent, rich, and creative.
2. People will probably think less of me if I make a mistake.
3. If a person asks for help, it's a sign of weakness.
4. If someone disagrees with me, it probably indicates he does not like me.
5. Being isolated from others is bound to lead to unhappiness.

Note. Reprinted by permission of A. N. Weissman.

nonclinical studies. The DAS was correlated .36 and .47 (p's $< .001$) with two measures of depressive symptoms in a student population (Weissman, 1979). Depressed inpatients had higher DAS scores than nondepressed psychiatric patients or nondepressed community volunteers (Hamilton & Abramson, 1983). With treatment, DAS scores dropped significantly, so that these between-group differences disappeared. O'Hara *et al.* (1982) reported a correlation between DAS and BDI scorres during the second trimester of pregnancy ($r = .28$, $p < .001$). However, the DAS score did not add significantly to the prediction of postpartum depression obtained with the second-trimester BDI score. Dobson and Breiter (1983) found similar correlations between DAS and BDI scores among students (r's $= .30$ for females and .36 for males, both p's $< .001$). The DAS correlates .52 with the CBQ (Weissman, 1979).

The DAS is sensitive to clinical improvement obtained with cognitive therapy, as well as pharmacotherapy (Eaves & Rush, 1984; Silverman, Silverman, & Eardley, 1984; Simons, Garfield, & Murphy, 1984; Simons, Murphy, Levine, & Wetzel, 1986). A recent study (Eaves & Rush, 1984) found that the DAS score was greater than normal control levels in both endogenous and nonendogenous symptomatic unipolar major depression, as did a slightly earlier study (Giles & Rush, 1982). With symptom remission lasting 3-4 weeks, the DAS scores remained elevated compared to those of controls, although they were lower than during the symptomatic state in both depressed groups (Eaves & Rush, 1984). In a follow-up study 6 months later, both BDI and Hamilton Rating Scale for Depression scores were predicted by DAS scores with recent remission (Rush, Eaves, & Weissenburger, 1986). This finding is consistent with a recent report by Simons *et al.* (1986) that DAS scores during remission predicted symptom severity 6 months later in formerly depressed outpatients.

While the DAS has good psychometric properties and its test-retest reliability is high, the DAS score is affected by the state of depression (Eaves & Rush, 1984; Hamilton & Abramson, 1983; Silverman *et al.*, 1984; Simons *et al.*, 1986; Weissman, 1979). Thus, the DAS does not measure an enduring trait found in depression. In fact, whether patients with other conditions also have elevated DAS scores is unclear. On the other hand, Beck's theory predicts an increase in dysfunctional attitudes during the depression. One problem with the DAS is that it is supposed to measure *silent* assumptions (those out of the patient's awareness). Yet the self-report states the assumptions plainly. Whether a response to the DAS is a *valid* measure of the actual assumptions of the patient is thus uncertain.

Irrational Beliefs Test

The Irrational Beliefs Test (IBT; Jones, 1969) is designed to measure irrational beliefs that Ellis has linked to a variety of psychiatric disorders, including (but not limited to) depression. Ellis's irrational beliefs overlap considerably with Beck's notions of silent assumptions. Both Beck and Ellis indicate that these beliefs are present in various psychopathological conditions (Beck, 1976; Ellis, 1962).

The IBT is a 100-item self-report. Respondents rate the degree of agreement with each item on a 5-point scale. The IBT has 10 subscales: High Self-Expectations, Demand for Approval, Blame Proneness, Frustration Reactivity (becoming overly upset with undesired outcomes), Emotional Irresponsibility (belief that unhappiness is caused by factors outside one's control), Anxious Overconcern (excessive worry about potential difficulties in the future), Avoidance, Dependency, Helplessness, and Perfectionism. These subscales were created by means of a factor analysis performed on student's responses to items that were originally generated on intuitive grounds and validated by consensus of independent judges. With minor differences, this factor structure has been replicated (Lohr & Bonge, 1980).

Good internal consistency is suggested by item-total correlations for the subscales that range from .66 to .80 (mean = .74) Test-retest reliabilities for total scores range from .92 over 24 hours (Jones, 1969) to .79 over 8 weeks (Lohr & Bonge, 1980), with Trexler and Karst (1972) reporting .88 over an undefined time period.

The original validations were conducted with general psychiatric inpatients. Recent studies suggest that elevated IBT scores are associated with depressive symptomatology among students. Nelson (1977) found that the IBT and BDI scores correlated .53 in students. LaPointe and Crandell (1980) found significant differences between depressed and nondepressed, nonneurotic (defined by the Neuroticism subscale of the Maudsley Personality Inventory) students on all IBT subscales. The depressed group had a higher total IBT score than students with high Neuroticism scores but *low* depression scores. Thus, the IBT may tap beliefs that are particularly characteristic of depression (Hammen & Krantz, 1985).

Hammen and Krantz (in press) caution that interpretations of the IBT may be confounded by its inverse correlations with intelligence and education level, as well as by the significant sex differences reported by Jones (1969) and partially replicated by Nelson (1977).

In sum, the IBT has good psychometric properties. The IBT *may* assess beliefs that are somewhat specific to depression. However, whether the IBT measures enduring, trait-like beliefs requires longitudinal studies of symptomatic and later remitted subjects that are yet to be conducted. Furthermore, as most work to date has been with students, the research and clinical value of the IBT in clinically depressed patients remains to be established.

COGNITIVE MEASURES RELEVANT TO SELIGMAN'S REFORMULATED LEARNED HELPLESSNESS THEORY OF DEPRESSION

Introduction to Seligman's Theory

Seligman's reformulated learned helplessness theory of depression indicates that depressive symptoms result from the causal attributions made by people when confronted with undesired, uncontrollable outcomes (Abramson *et al.*, 1978; I. W. Miller & Norman, 1979; Seligman, Abramson, Semmel, & von Baeyer, 1979). This theory suggests that depressive symptoms follow from the individual's belief that the causes of undesired events are located inside the self (internal locus of causality); that they will persist over time (stable); and that these causes will have widespread effects (global). For example, when a business executive believes that recent financial reverses were caused by his or her own mistakes (internal), which result from enduring personality characteristics (stable) and which will affect other business dealings (global), depression is likely. On the other hand, depression is less likely if the financial reversals are viewed as results of a poor economic climate (external), which occurs sporadically (unstable) and will not affect other aspects of the executive's life (specific) (see Figure 9-1).

While attributions made in particular situations were originally thought to be stable, Metalsky and Abramson (1981) recently argued that attributions are based *both* on individual, stable, generalized beliefs *and* on the information inherent in the particular situation. The relative contribution of individual and situational factors may vary, depending on the situation.

Hammen and Krantz (1985) have identified two general approaches to the assessment of causal attributions. These two approaches differ in the level of abstraction asked of the respondents. With first-order attribution measures, respondents rate the degree to which each of several causes, described in a specific and concrete manner, influence a particular outcome. For example, the subjects might rate the influence of low ability in producing failure outcomes in an experimental task (e.g., card sorting, anagram solving). These responses are used to infer the locus of causality, stability, or globality based on *a priori* assumptions about the dimensional properties of the specific causes. For instance, those who attribute experimental task failure largely to poor ability are thought to make internal, stable attributions.

Second-order measures, on the other hand, ask subjects to evaluate par-

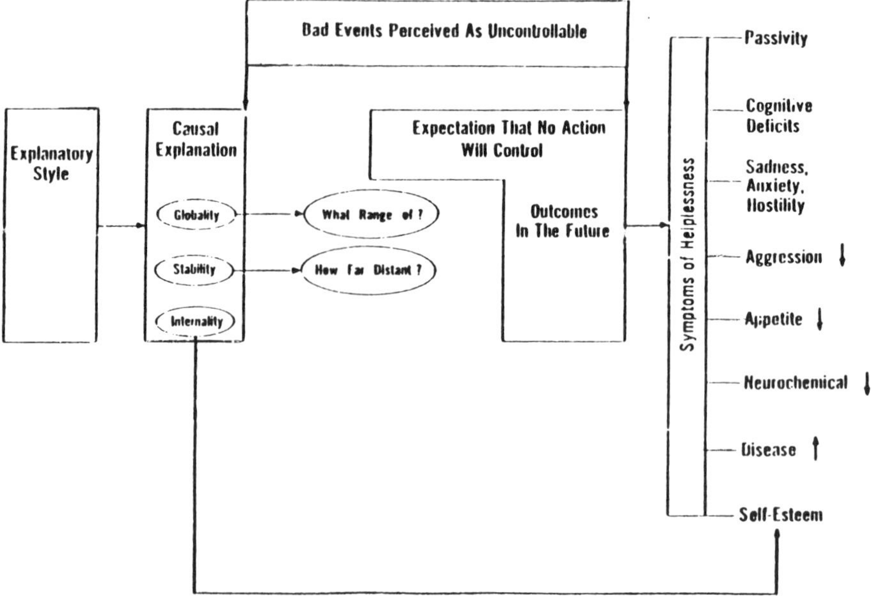

FIGURE 9-1 Seligman's model of learned helplessness. (From "Causal Explanations as a Risk Factor for Depression: Theory and Evidence" by C. Peterson & M. E. P. Seligman, 1984, *Psychological Review, 91*, 347-374. Reprinted by permission.)

ticular aspects or dimensions of the causes rather than the particular causes themselves. Laypeople appear not to construe the attributes of specific causes in the same way as do scientists. Indeed, Krantz and Rude (in press) found poor agreement between nonscientists and scientists on the dimensional properties of specific causes, and it was also found that the correlations between attributions obtained from first- and second-order methods were not impressive (Hammen & Krantz, 1985).

Attributional Style Questionnaire

The Attributional Style Questionnaire (ASQ; Peterson *et al.*, 1982) is the best-developed, best-standardized procedure for assessing attributions. This self-report provides scores for the explanation of undesired and desired events along three dimensions: "internal-external," "stable-unstable," and "global-specific." Twelve vignettes are presented, half of which describe undesired events (e.g., "You go out on a date and it goes badly") and half describe desired events (e.g., "You meet a friend who compliments you on your appearance"). After each vignette, the subject writes down "the one major cause" of the event. Next, this cause is rated by the respondent along the three attributional dimensions using a 7-point Likert-type scale. The internal-external dimension is rated, for example, from "totally due to the other person or circumstance" to "totally due to me" (see Table 9-6).

The ASQ was designed to avoid giving preselected choices in hopes of providing a more valid sample of actual thinking (Falbo & Beck, 1979). On the other hand, it avoids the problems that many open-ended questionnaires of attributional style have-namely, that they are time-consuming to score and may have low reliability (Elig & Frieze, 1979). The ASQ is easily scored. However, as with other vignette-based questionnaires, it presents only selected situations that may not tap areas of specific concern to the individual (e.g., poor physical health, death of a child, etc.) Various different age-related ASQs that provide more appropriate vignettes for particular groups may be needed (e.g., for adolescents, the elderly, etc.).

The internal consistency and test-retest reliability of the ASQ have been assessed. Peterson *et al.* (1982) reported that the composite good-outcome and composite bad-outcome scores show moderate internal consistency (α's = .75 and .72 for desired and undesired outcomes, respectively). The alphas for the internal, stable, and global dimensions individually, however, were less impressive (from .44 to .58 for good outcomes; from .46 to .69 for bad outcomes). Others found similar internal-consistency figures (Golin, Sweeny, & Schaeffer, 1981; Manly, McMahon, Bradley, & Davidson, 1982). The alpha coefficients for good and bad affiliative achievement situations were even lower — from .21 to .53 (Peterson *et al.*, 1982). As no differences between affiliation and achievement situations were found, these two types of situations may be combined to circumvent the problem of low reliability. However, the affiliative or achievement situations should not be used alone, as the internal consistency of these situations is poor.

TABLE 9-6 Exemplar Items from the ASQ

1. You can't get all the work done others expect of you.
2. You go out on a date and it goes badly.
3. You have been looking for a job unsuccessfully for some time.

Write down the *one* major cause.

Totally due to the other person or circumstance	1	2	3	4	5	6	7	Totally due to me [internal-external]
Will never happen again	1	2	3	4	5	6	7	Will always be present [stable-unstable]
Influences just this particular situation	1	2	3	4	5	6	7	Influences all situations in my life [global-specific]
Not at all important	1	2	3	4	5	6	7	Extremely important

Note. Reprinted by permission of C. Peterson.

Peterson *et al.* (1982) reported reasonable test-retest correlations over a 5-week period (r's = .70 for good and .64 for bad composite scores). The coefficients for the three dimensions within each of the good and bad outcomes ranged from .58 to .69 (mean = .62). These findings were replicated over a 4-week period (Golin *et al.*, 1981) (r = .67 for both desired and undesired composite scores).

A variety of studies (Cutrona, 1983; Golin *et al.*, 1981; Manly *et al.*, 1982; I. W. Miller, Klee, & Norman, 1982; Mukherji, Abramson, & Martin, 1982; O'Hara, Rehm, & Campbell, 1982; Peterson *et al.*, 1982; Raps, Peterson, Reinhard, Abramson, & Seligman, 1982; Seligman *et al.*, 1979) have revealed that attributions for undesired outcomes are somewhat more strongly related to depressive symptoms than are attributions for desired outcomes. However, there is a wide range in the reported degree to which ASQ scores related to depressed mood. The greatest association (r = .48) was reported by Seligman *et al.* (1979), whereas other correlations ranged from .03 to .35 (mean = .20). If, however, attributional style is more trait-like, then one would expect only a modest relationship between ASQ scores and depressive symptoms.

The ASQ has a problem of a restricted range of vignettes — a problem that also confronts the CBQ (Hammen & Krantz, 1976), the Cognitive Response Test (Watkins & Rush, 1983), and other measures. Whether vignette-based questionnaires are differentially sensitive for males versus females, for homosexuals versus heterosexuals, or for persons of various racial, socioeconomic, or religious backgrounds remains to be seen. It is likely, however, that the personal and emotional relevance of a particular vignette will vary substantially, depending on the age, sex, occupation, and prior life experience of the subject. For example, the response of a 40-year-old Army veteran to a notice of call to active duty may be one of self-righteous anger or even laughter over a presumed computer error, while a 19-year-old college freshman may respond with fear or sadness. Furthermore, the responses to such situations are likely to be highly influenced by the culture (e.g., such a notice in Iran may elicit a dramatically different cognitive-emotional response than a similar notice in the USSR or the US), and are also likely to be relatively time-dependent (e.g., the nature of the draft system varies over time in both dictatorships and democracies). To make matters worse, culturally bound, time-dependent events may have the greatest emotional charge, and therefore may be the most personally relevant of all potential events. Thus, the dilemma of emotional relevance (a clinical variable) versus generalizability and replicability (reseach variables) is encountered. Perhaps a decision-tree-based, computerized presentation with potentially interchangeable items (depending on the relevant demographic, cultural, political, etc., variables) might solve this problem.

In order to extend the range of subjects whose attributional style can be assessed, a children's version of the ASQ (the CASQ) has been created. A forced-choice format is used to simplify test taking. Whether this format reduces validity is unclear, although it does appear to increase reliability (Peterson & Seligman, 1984). The hypothetical good or bad events are followed by two possible explanations, which vary one of the explanatory dimensions while holding the other constant. From the pair, the child chooses the cause that better describes why the event occurred. Sixteen questions pertain to each of the three dimensions (half refer to good events and half to bad events). Thus, the 48 questions consist of 8 items for each of the factorial combinations of internal-external, stable-unstable, global-specific, and desirability (good, bad).

The CASQ is scored by assigning 1 to each internal, stable, or global response, and 0 to each external, unstable, or specific response. Scales are formed by summing these scores across the appropriate questions for each of the three dimensions, separately for good and for bad events. Scores for each scale range form 0 to 8. Exemplar CASQ items ae shown in Table 9-7.

Hammen and Krantz (1985) in their excellent recent review of cognitive measures, suggest several concerns about the ASQ. They cite the rather weak association between ASQ and depressive symptom scores, the poor alpha coefficients for each of the three attributional dimensions (though the alpha coefficients for the composite scores are adequate), and findings that subjects do not show the same attributional pattern on the ASQ as they do in attributions for stressful life events or for laboratory tasks (I. W. Miller *et al.*, 1982).

If the ASQ measures an enduring trait-like attribution style, its correlation

TABLE 9-7 Exemplar Items from the Children's ASQ

	Dimensions	
Item [valence]	Varied	Constant
1. A good friend tells you that he hates you [bad].		
a. My friend was in a bad mood.	External	Stable
b. I wasn't nice to my friend that day.	Internal	Global
2. You get all the toys you want for your birthday [good].		
a. People always guess what toys you want for your birthday.	Stable	Internal
b. This birthday people guessed right as to what toys I wanted.	Unstable	Global

Note. Reprinted by permission of C. Peterson.

with measures of depressive symptoms should be low. That is, it should *not* be strongly influenced by whether or not the subject is depressed. A recent study (Eaves & Rush, 1984) found very little change in ASQ composite scores for depressed patients studied when symptomatic and later when clinically remitted. Furthermore, correlations between ASQ and BDI scores were low. Whether attributional style as assessed by ASQ is validated by other attempts to measure attribution has yet to be resolved. Several studies (Metalsky, Abramson, Seligman, Semmel, & Peterson, 1982; Peterson, Luborsky, & Seligman, 1983) are available to indicate predictive validity, however (for a review, see Peterson & Seligman, 1984). Given the reasonable success of this first attempt to measure attributional style, further research in this direction is called for.

COGNITIVE MEASURES RELEVANT TO REHM'S SELF-CONTROL MODEL OF DEPRESSION

Rehm (1977) has proposed that depressive symptoms follow from deficient self-control behaviors. This self-control model of depression derives largely from Kanfer's (1971) self-control model of psychopathology. This model hypothesizes that individuals use three sequential processes (self-monitoring, self-evaluation, and self-reinforcement) to acquire and maintain behaviors that are needed to meet their goals. The depressed person is thought to exhibit deficits in each of these phases. Depressed individuals selectively attend to negative events and to immediate as opposed to delayed outcomes (self-monitoring deficit). As self-monitored behaviors are compared to internal criteria that are too rigid or perfectionistic, self-evaluation is impaired. These overly high standards discourage efforts at goals that are realistic, and they set the stage for the perception of failure if the person attempts these goals. Finally, the discrepancy between observed behavior and internal performance standards lead to self-punishment, which discourages future goal-directed behaviors. This lack of goal-directed behavior may lead to the psychomotor retardation, inhibition, and low response rates typically found in depression.

The measurement of self-control processes is less well developed, compared to the measures described thus far. Two measures, the Self-Control Questionnaire (SCQ; Rehm, Kornblith, *et al.*, 1981) and the Self-Control Schedule (SCS; Rosenbaum, 1980) are available.

Self-Control Questionnaire

The SCQ (Rehm, Kornblith, *et al.*, 1981) contains 41 items that assess attitudes and beliefs about self-control behavior. Exemplar SCQ items are shown in Table 9-8. In preliminary reports, both internal consistency and test-retest reliability of the SCQ have been satisfactory. Alpha coefficients of

TABLE 9-8 Exemplar Items from the SCQ

Rate each item from *very characteristic* to *very uncharacteristic* of me:

1. When I do something right, I take time to enjoy the feeling.
2. I depend heavily on other people's opinions to evaluate objectively what I do.
3. Planning each step of what I have to do helps me get things done well.

Note. Reprinted by permission of L. P. Rehm.

.82 (O'Hara *et al.*, 1982) and .88 (Rude, 1983) are good, and O'Hara *et al.* (1982) found a good test-retest correlation over a 5-week period ($r = .86$).

The construct validity of the SCQ is less clear. O'Hara *et al.* (1982) found that SCQ obtained from women during the second trimester of pregnancy correlated modestly ($r = .31$ $p < .001$) with BDI scores obtained, on average, 12 weeks after delivery. On the other hand, Rude (1983) found no correlation between the SCQ and two measures of depressive symptoms in depressed outpatients (r's = .05 with the BDI and .11 with the Minnesota Multiphasic Personality Inventory [MMPI] Depression [*D*] subscale). SCQ scores change during self-control interventions for depression (Rehm, Kornblith, *et al.*, 1981), though the prediction of post-treatment depression was not enhanced by pretreatment SCQ scores (Rehm, Kaslow, Rabin, & Willard, 1981). Further studies of the construct validity of the SCQ are needed.

In addition, the SCQ measures "attitudes and beliefs" about self-control, not *actual* self-control behaviors and cognitions. As the self-control processes, not attitudes about self-control, are presumed to be critical to depression, and as the relation between these two constructs is not established, a more direct measure of self-control process may be needed (Hammen & Krantz, 1985).

Self-Control Schedule

The SCS (Rosenbaum, 1980) is a 36-item self-report that assesses cognitive strategies to (1) combat unpleasant emotional and physical states; (2) solve everyday problems; (3) delay gratification; and (4) evaluate oneself or one's situation (Hammen & Krantz, 1985). Like the IBT (Jones, 1969), the SCS is not particularly designed for depression, although the cognitive processes evaluated may be especially relevant to depression. It has had limited use in depression research, although it is the only available measure that attempts to measure self-control *behaviors* rather than attitudes about self-control (Hammen & Krantz, 1985). Table 9-9 shows exemplar SCS items.

In the development of the SCS, two experienced psychologists judged 60 items that described self-control behaviors or self-efficacy perceptions. The self-control behavior items were judged on whether the situation described was likely to be experienced by a wide range of people and by whether the

TABLE 9-9 Exemplar Items from the SCS

1. When I do a boring job, I think about the less boring parts of the job and the reward that I will receive when I am finished.
2. When I am feeling depressed, I try to think about pleasent events.
3. I cannot avoid thinking about mistakes I have made in the past.
4. When I am faced with a difficult problem, I try to approach its solution in a systematic way.
5. When I plan to work, I remove all the things that are not relevant to my work.

Note. Reprinted by permission of M. Rosenbaum.

item reflected an effective use of a self-control strategy. Both judges agreed on 44 items, which were given to a sample of students. The final 36 items were chosen to elicit a wide range of responses.

Rosenbaum (1980) conducted psychometric studies on four samples of Israeli students, one sample of U.S. students, and one sample of Israeli men. The internal reliability (alpha coefficient) of the SCS was good (range .78-.88). Test-retest reliability over 4 weeks (Rosenbaum, 1980) was good ($r = .86$).

Little information on the validity of the SCS in depression is available. Rehm, Kaslow, *et al.* (1981) found that SCS scores were not among the more important predictors of the outcomes of self-control interventions. Rude (1983) failed to find an association between depressive symptoms and the SCS (r's $= -.08$ for the BDI and $-.28$ for 30-item MMPI *D* (Depression) scale, both n.s.), although a restricted score range was found in this clinically depressed sample. On the other hand, the SCS was correlated .54 ($p < .01$) with the SCQ.

Recently, Simons, Lustman, and Murphy (1985) found that pretreatment SCS scores predicted symptomatic outcome following cognitive therapy and pharmacotherapy in depressed outpatients. High pretreatment SCS scores were associated with a better outcome for cognitive therapy. The converse tended to be true for drug-treated patients (i.e., lower pretreatment SCS scores were associated with a better drug response). These findings provide some evidence of predictive validity for the measure, although further studies are needed.

OTHER MEASURES OF DEPRESSIVE COGNITIONS

Several additional self-report questionnaires to assess cognitive processes in depression have been developed. Weintraub, Segal, and Beck (1974) developed a story completion test to measure negative cognitions. Scores on this test correlated with depressed mood in male college students. Lefebvre (1981) developed a Cognitive Error Questionnaire, patterned after Hammen and Krantz's CBQ. This measure consists of 24 short vignettes, each of which is followed by a dysphoric cognition representing selected cognitive errors, which subjects rate based on whether they would think that way. Raters could not distinguish between various types of logical errors as specified by Beck *et al.* (1979), though higher distortion scores were found in depressed inpatients than in normals. Lefebvre reported reliability data that indicate adequate psychometric properties.

Lewinsohn and colleagues have deveoped a Subjective Probability Questionnaire, a Personal Beliefs Inventory, and a Cognitive Events Schedule, the psychometric data for which have been reported (Munoz, 1977). Lewinsohn, Steinmetz, Larson, and Franklin (1981) found that scores on these measures and those of other cognitions were associated with current depressed mood, but they appeared to be neither antecedents nor consequences of symptomatic depression in a longitudinal study. While higher scores on these measures were associated with the persistence of depressive symptoms, they appeared not to measure a stable trait independent of current mood. Thus, as cognitive theory would predict, negative cognitions about the self, world, or future covary with the severity of depressive symptoms.

All of the instruments described above employ fixed-choice formats in which the content of items is set *a priori.* Such a format, however, may not tap actual thoughts (i.e., are they valid?). An open-ended format may circumvent this problem of transparency. One attempt to measure instantaneous "automatic thoughts" in response to various interpersonal situations is the Cognitive Response Test (CRT; Watkins & Rush, 1983). The final form contains 36 items, the responses to which are grouped into four categories: "rational," "irrational/depressed," irrational/nondepressed," and "nonscorable." Table 9-10 shows exemplar CRT items.

Irrational/depressed scores differentiated depressed from nondepressed subjects and correlated with BDI ratings ($r = .58$). Judges had reasonable interrater agreement (.72-.88) on scoring the responses with a standardized scoring manual. While the CRT avoids the transparency problems present in fixed-choice formats, it is more time-consuming to score. Whether it is a more valid reflection of actual moment-to-moment thinking remains yet to be established.

TABLE 9-10 Exemplar Items from the CRT

1. Lately my work has become more and more demanding.
   I think ____

2. When I consider being married, my first thought is ____________________

3. A fellow employee who has been with the company less time than I has been promoted. My immediate thought is ______________________________

Crandell and Chambless (1981) developed the Crandall Cognitions Inventory (CCI) to assess the frequency of negative cognitions in a population of clinically depressed individuals with comparison groups of depressed and nondepressed psychiatric patients and normal controls. The scale was reduced from an initial 100 items to 34 items that maximally differentiated these groups. The 34-item version also was employed in a cross-validation study. Internal cosistency was high (α = .95). When demographic variables were partialed out, the CCI correlated with the BDI (r = .69) and with the DAS (r = .52). As expected, a better correlation was found with the state-dependent measure (the BDI).

A factor analysis revealed four factors: "thoughts of detachment," "inferiority," "helplessness," and "hoplessness" (see Table 9-11 for exemplar items). Inferiority (negative view of self) and hopelessness (negative view of future) reflect two components of Beck's (1976) cognitive triad. The CCI is a promising instrument, although further evidence of discriminant validity is needed (e.g., can it differentiate cognitions of anxious versus depressed patients?).

The Hopelessness Scale (HS; Beck, Weissman, Lester, & Trexler, 1974) was designed to measure an individual's negative expectancy about events in the future — a component of Beck's (1976) cognitive triad. The HS contains 20 true-false items that assess expectations about overcoming unpleasant life situations or attaining things of value. The HS differs from other measures (e.g., the CCI) in that it is designed to measure one general construct. It should reflect the individual's current, relatively labile views about reaching desired goals. Consequently, it should be highly state-dependent, as should automatic thoughts in contrast to underlying schemas.

The HS correlates with the BDI (r = .68) (Minkoff, Bergman, Beck, & Beck, 1973) and with clinical ratings of hopelessness. In addition, the HS was administered along with the BDI and the Suicidal Intent Scale (SIS; Beck, Schuyler, & Herman, 1974) to suicide attempters within 48 hours following hospital admission. The SIS is a clinician-completed scale that assesses the

TABLE 9-11 Exemplar Items from the CCI

Item	Almost never	Seldom	Sometimes	Frequently	Almost always
1. I'm just a nobody.					
2. I've made such a mess of my life.					
3. My life is so confused, I'll never straighten it out.					
4. I wish people would just leave me alone.					

Note. Reprinted by permission of C. J. Crandell.

level of the subject's "desire" to end his or her life, based on objective circumstances (e.g., extent of preparation) and subjective factors (e.g., the subject's notion of the potential lethality of the method chosen). When attempters were divided according to high versus low BDI scores and high versus low HS scores, with the SIS as the dependent variable, an analysis of variance produced a significant interaction effect such that high HS scores were associated with high SIS scores, whether BDI scores were high or low (Beck, Kovacs, & Weissman, 1975). These findings indicate that hopelessness is a critical cognitive factor mediating the relationship between depression and suicidality; they also provide construct validity data for the HS (for a review, see Beck & Epstein, 1982).

We (Rush, Beck, Kovacs, Weissenburger, & Hollon, 1982) found that the HS was a sensitive measure of treatment outcome with depressed patients treated with cognitive therapy or antidepressant medication. Cognitive therapy produced a more rapid decrease in hopelessness.

The Self-Concept Test (SCT; A. T. Beck, personal communication, 1985) was developed to measure individuals' views of themselves, another component of Beck's cognitive triad (Beck, 1976). SCT should be state-dependent to the degree it reflects current negative automatic thoughts, but it also is likely to tap underlying schemata about the self and thus to reflect a moderate degree of stability (perhaps more so than the HS). The 25-item scale differs from other self-concept/self-esteem questionnaires in that respondents compare themselves on 25 characteristics to others they know, rather than some unspecified standard. Thus, each rating is based on a reference point that has clear personal meaning.

In an initial sample of 198 outpatients at the University of Pennsylvania, internal consistency was adequate ($\alpha = .80$), as was a 1-week test-retest correlation ($r = .88$). A principal-component factor analysis with varimax rotation yielded five significant factors: "assessing intellectual abilities" "achievement," "negative interpersonal traits," "personal attractiveness," and "positive social qualities." These factors were replicated in a nonclinical sample ($n = 146$).

Some validation for the SCT was provided by correlations with measures of theoretically related constructs. In the initial clinical sample ($n = 198$), the SCT correlated with the BDI ($r = -.47$, $p < .001$), the MMPI *D* ($r = -.46$, $p < .001$), the MMPI *Pt* (Psychasthenia) scale ($r = -.52$, $p < .001$), the MMPI *Si* (Social Introversion) scale ($r = -.55$, $p < .001$), the Hamilton Rating Scale for Anxiety ($r = -.19$, $p < .001$), and the Hamilton Rating Scale for Depression ($r = -.37$, $p < .001$).

In a sample of 146 nonclinical subjects and 70 outpatients, the SCT correlated ($r = .55$, $p < .001$) with the Rosenberg Self-Esteem Scale (Rosenberg, 1979). The SCT scores of the 146 nonclinical subjects were significantly higher than those of the 70 patient subjects, mainly due to the achievement and sociability items. In the combined sample of 216, males scored slightly higher than females ($r = -.19$, $p < .01$). Overall, the SCT appears very promising as a measure of self-concept.

CONCLUSIONS

A variety of measures are available to assess selected aspects of thinking processes and thought content in depressed patients. Major problems that face this field, however, are establishing (1) specificity and (2) validity. Do other psychiatric syndromes differ from depression in these measures? Are responses to paper-and-pencil tests reflective of actual thought processes? More studies of predictive validity might approach the latter question. Further developments of new measures are needed before a consensus can be reached as to an optimal cognitive test battery for depression.

Acknowledgments

I wish to express my appreciation to Mr. David Savage for his secretarial assistance and to Kenneth Z. Altshuler, M. D., for his administrative support.

References

Abramson, L. Y., Seligman, M. E. P., & Teasdale, J. D. (1978). Learned helplessness in humans: Critique and reformulation. *Journal of Abnormal Psychology, 87*, 49-74.

American Psychiatric Association. (1981). *Diagnostic and statistical manual of mental disorders* (3rd ed.). Washington, D.C.: Author.

Bandura, A. (1971). Vicarious and self-reinforcement processes. In R. Glaser (Ed.), *The nature of reinforcement* (pp. 228-278). New York: Academic Press.

Beck, A. T. (1964). Thinking and depression: 2. Theory and therapy. *Archives of General Psychiatry, 10*, 561-571.

Beck, A. T. (1967). *Depression: Clinical, experimental and theoretical aspects*. New York: Harper & Row.

Beck, A. T. (1976). *Cognitive therapy and the emotional disorders*. New York: International Universities Press.

Beck, A. T., & Epstein, N. (1982). *Cognitions, attitudes and personality dimensions in depression*. Paper presented at the annual meeting of the Society for Psychotherapy Research, Smugglers Notch, VT.

Beck, A. T., Kovacs, M., & Weissman, A. (1975). Hopelessness and suicidal behavior: An overview. *Journal of the American Medical Association, 234*, 1146-1149.

Beck, A. T., & Rush, A. J. (1978). Cognitive approaches to depression and suicide. In G. Serban (Ed.), *Cognitive defects in development of mental illness* (pp. 235-257). New York: Brunner/ Mazel.

Beck, A. T., Rush, A. J., Shaw, B. F., & Emery, G. (1979). *Cognitive therapy of depression*. New York: Guilford Press.

Beck, A. T., Schuyler, D., & Herman, I. (1974). Development of suicidal intent scales. In A. T. Beck, H. L. P. Resnik, & D. J. Lettieri (Eds.), *The prediction of suicide* (pp. 45-56). Bowie, MD: Charles Press.

Beck, A. T., Weissman, A., Lester, D., & Trexler, L. (1974). The measurement of pessimism: The Hopelessness Scale. *Journal of Consulting and Clinical Psychology, 42*, 861-865.

Blaney, P. H., Behar, V., & Head, R. (1980). Two measures of depressive cognitions: Their association with depression and with each other. *Journal of Abnormal Psychology, 89*, 678-682.

Costello, C. G. (1972). Depression: Loss of reinforcement or loss reinforcer effectiveness? *Behavior Therapy, 3*, 240-247.

Coyne, J. C., & Gotlieb, I. H. (1983). The role of cognition in depression: A critical appraisal. *Psychological Bulletin, 94*, 472-505.

Crandell, C. J., & Chambless, D. L. (1981). *The validation of an inventory for measuring depressive thoughts: The Crandell Cognitions Inventory*. Paper presented at the annual meeting of the Association for Advancement of Behavior Therapy, Toronto.

Cronbach, L. J. (1951). Coefficient alpha and the internal structure of tests. *Psychometrika, 16*. 297-334.

Cutrona, C. (1983). Causal attributions and perinatal depression. *Journal of Abnormal Psychology, 92*, 161-172.

DeMonbreun, B. G., & Craighead, W. E. (1977). Selective recall of positive and neutral feedback. *Cognitive Therapy and Research, 1*, 311-329.

Dobson, K. S., & Breiter, H. J. (1983). Cognitive assessment of depression: Reliability and validity of three measures. *Journal of Abnormal Psychology, 92*. 107-109.

Eaves, G., & Rush, A. J. (1984). Cognitive patterns in symptomatic and remitted unipolar major depression. *Journal of Abnormal Psychology, 93*. 31-40.

Elig, T. W., & Frieze, I. H. (1979). Measuring causal attributions for success and failure. *Journal of Personality and Social Psychology, 37*, 631-634.

Ellis, A. (1962). *Reason and emotion in psychotherapy*. New York: Lyle Stuart.

Falbo, T., & Beck, R. C. (1979). Naive psychology and the attributional model of achievement. *Journal of Personality, 47*, 185-195.

Freud, S. (1957). Mourning and melancholia. In J. Strachey (Ed. and Trans.), *Standard edition of the complete psychological works of Sigmund Freud* (Vol. 14, pp. 243-260). London: Hogarth Press. (Original work published 1917).

Frost, R. O., & MacInnis, D. J. (1983). The Cognitive Bias Questionnaire: Further evidence. *Journal of Personality Assessment, 47*, 173-177.

Giles, D. E., & Rush, A. J. (1982). Relationship of dysfunctional attitudes and dexamethasone response in endogenous and nonendogenous depression. *Biological Psychiatry, 17*, 1303-1314.

Golin, S., Sweeney, P. D., & Schaeffer, D. E. (1981). The causality of causal attributions in depression: A cross-lagged panel correlation analysis. *Journal of Abnormal Psychology, 90*, 14-22.

Goodwin, A. M., & Williams, J. M. G. (1982). Mood induction research: Its implication for clinical depression. *Behaviour Research and Therapy, 20*, 373-382.

Hamilton, E. W. & Abramson, L. Y. (1983). Cognitive patterns and major depressive disorders: A longitudinal study in a hospital setting. *Journal of Abnormal Psychology, 92*, 173-184.

Hammen, C., & Krantz, S. E. (1976). Effects of success and failure on depressive cognitions. *Journal of Abnormal Psychology, 85*, 577-586.

Hammen, C., & Krantz, S. E. (1985). Measures of psychological prophecies in depression. In E. E. Beckham & W. R. Leber (Eds.), *Handbook of depression: Treatment, assessment and research* (pp. 408-444). Homewood, IL: Dorsey Press.

Harrell, T. H., & Ryon, N. B. (1983). Cognitive-behavioral assessment of depression: Clinical validation of the Automatic Thoughts Questionnaire. *Journal of Consulting and Clinical Psychology, 51*, 721-725.

Hollon, S. D., & Bemis, K. M. (1981). Self-report and the assessment of cognitive functions. In M. Hersen & A. S. Bellack (Eds.), *Behavioral assessment: A practical handbook* (pp. 125-174). New York: Pergamon Press.

Hollon, S. D., & Kendall, P. (1980). Cognitive self-statements in depression: Development of an Automatic Thoughts Questionnaire. *Cognitive Therapy and Research, 4*, 383-396.

Jones, R. G. (1969). A factored measure of Ellis' irrational belief system, with personality and maladjustment correlates (Doctoral dissertation, Texas Technological College, 1969). *Dissertation Abstracts International, 29*, 4379B-4380B.

Kanfer, F. H. (1971). The maintainence of behavior by self-generated stimuli and reinforcement. In A. Jacobs & L. B. Sachs (Eds.), *The psychology of private events* (pp. 39-75). New York: Academic Press.

Krantz, S. E., & Hammen, C. L. (1979). Assessment of cognitive bias in depression. *Journal of Abnormal Psychology, 88*, 611-619.

Krantz, S. E., & Rude, S. S. (in press). The selection of different causes or the assignment of different dimensional meanings? *Journal of Personality and Social Psychology*.

Kuiper, N. A. (1978). Depression and causal attibutions for success and failure. *Journal of Personality and Social Psychology, 36*, 236-246.

LaPointe, K. A., & Crandell, C. J. (1980). Relationships of irrational beliefs to self-reported depression. *Cognitive Therapy and Research, 4*, 247-250.

Lefebvre, M. F. (1981). Cognitive distortion and cognitive errors in depressed psychiatric and low back pain patients. *Journal of Consulting and Clinical Psychology, 49*. 517-525.

Lewinsohn, P. M., Steinmetz, J. L., Larson, D. W., & Franklin, J. (1981). Depression-related cognitions: Antecedent or consequence. *Journal of Abnormal Psychology, 90*, 213-219.

Lloyd, G. G., & Lishman, W. A. (1975). Effect of depression on the speed of recall of pleasant and unpleasant experiences. *Psychological Medicine, 5*, 173-180.

Lohr, J. M., & Bonge, D. (1980). Retest reliability of the Irrational Beliefs Test. *Psychological Reports, 47*, 1314.

Manly, P. C., McMahon, R. J., Bradley, C. F., & Davidson, P. O. (1982). Depressive attributional style and depression following childbirth. *Journal of Abnormal Psychology, 91*, 245-254.

Marsella, A. J. (1980). Depressive experiences and disorder across cultures. In H. Triandis & J. Draguns (Eds.), *Handbook of cross-cultural psychology* (Vol. 6, pp. 237-289). Boston: Allyn & Bacon.

Metalsky, G. I., & Abramson, L. Y. (1981). Attribution styles: Toward a framework for conceptualization and assessment. In P. C. Kendall & S. D. Hollon (Eds.), *Assessment strategies for cognitive-behavioral interventions* (pp. 13-58). New York: Academic Press.

Metalsky, G. I., Abramson, L. Y., Seligman, M. E. P., Semmel, A., & Peterson, C. (1982). Attributional styles and life events in the classroom: Vulnerability and invulnerability to depressive mood reactions. *Journal of Personality and Social Psychology, 43*, 612-617.

Miller, I. W., Klee, S. H., & Norman, W. H. (1982). Depressed and nondepressed inpatients' cognitions of hypothetical events, experimental tasks and stressful life events. *Journal of Abnormal Psychology, 91*, 78-81.

Miller, I. W., & Norman, W. H. (1979). Learned helplessness in humans: A review and attribution theory model. *Psychological Bulletin, 86*, 93-119.

Miller, W. R. (1975). Psychological deficit in depression. *Psychological Bulletin, 82*, 238-260.

Minkoff, K., Bergman, E., Beck, A. T., & Beck, R. (1973). Hopelessness, depression, and attempted suicide. *American Journal of Psychiatiry, 130*, 455-459.

Mukherji, B. R., Abramson, L. Y., & Martin, D. J. (1982). Induced depressive mood and attributional patterns. *Cognitive Therapy and Research, 6*, 15-22.

Munoz, R. F. (1977). *A cognitive approach to the assessment and treatment of depression*. Unpublished doctoral dissertation, University of Oregon.

Nelson, R. E. (1977). Irrational beliefs in depression. *Journal of Consulting and Clinical Psychology, 45*, 1190-1191.

Neisser, U. (1967). *Cognitive psychology*. New York: Appleton-Century-Crofts.

Norman, W. H., Miller, I. W., & Klee, S. H. (1983). Assessment of cognitive distortion in a clinically depressed population. *Cognitive Therapy and Research, 7*, 133-140.

O'Hara, M. W., Rehm, L. P., & Campbell, S. B. (1982). Predicting depressive symptomatology: Cognitive-behavioral models and post-partum depression. *Journal of Abnormal Psychology, 91*, 457-461.

Peterson, C., Luborsky, L., & Seligman, M. E. P. (1983). Attributions and depressive mood shifts: A case study using the symptoms-context method. *Journal of Abnormal Psychology, 92*, 96-103.

Peterson, C., & Seligman, M. E. P. (1984). Causal explanations as a risk factor for depression: Theory and evidence. *Psychological Review, 91*, 347-374.

Peterson, C., Semmel, A., von Baeyer, C., Abramson, L. Y., Metalsky, G. I., & Seligman, M. E. P. (1982). The Attributional Style Questionnaire. *Cognitive Therapy and Research, 6*, 287-300.

Raps, C. S., Peterson, C., Reinhard, K. E., Abramson, L. Y., & Seligman, M. E. P. (1982). Attributional style among depressed patients. *Journal of Abnormal Psychology, 91*, 102-108.

Rehm, L. P. (1977). Self-control model of depression. *Behavior Therapy, 8*, 787-804.

Rehm, L. P., Kaslow, N. J., Rabin, A. C., & Willard, R. (1981). *Prediction of outcome in a self-control behavior therapy program for depression*. Paper presented at the annual meeting of the American Psychological Association, Los Angeles.

Rehm, L. P., Kornblith, S. J., O'Hara, M. W., Lamparski, D. M., Romano, J. M., & Volkin, J. I. (1981). An evaluation of major components in a self-control therapy program for depression. *Behavior Modification, 5*, 459-489.

Riskind, J., & Rholes, W. S. (1983). Somatic versus self-evaluative statements in the Velten Mood Induction Procedure: Effects on negativistic interpretations and on depressed mood. *Journal of Social and Clinical Psychology, 1*, 300-311.

Rosenbaum, M. (1980). A schedule for assessing self-control behaviors: Preliminary findings. *Behavior Therapy, 11*, 109-121.

Rosenberg, M. (1979). *Conceiving the self*. New York: Basic Books.

Rude, S. S. (1983). *An investigation of differential response to two treatments of depression*. Unpublished doctoral dissertation, Stanford University.

Rush, A. J. (1983). Cognitive therapy for depression. In M. Zales (Ed.), *Affective and schizophrenic disorders: New approaches to diagnosis* (pp. 178-206). New York: Brunner/Mazel.

Rush, A. J., Beck, A. T., Kovacs, M., Weissenburger, J., & Hollon, S. D. (1982). Comparison of effects of cognitive therapy and pharmacotherapy on hopelessness and self-concept. *American Journal of Psychiatry, 139*, 862-866.

Rush, A J., Eaves, G. G. & Weissenburger, J. (1986). Do thinking patterns predict depressive symptoms? *Cognitive Therapy and Research, 10*, 225-236.

Seligman, M. E. P. (1974). Depression and learned helplessness. In R. J. Freedman & M. M Katz (Eds.), *The psychology of depression: Contemporary theory and research* (pp. 83-113). Washington, DC: Winston.

Seligman, M. E. P. (1975). *Helplessness: On depression, development and death*. San Francisco: W. H. Freeman.

Seligman, M. E. P., Abramson, L. Y., Semmel, A., & von Baeyer, C. (1979). Depressive attibutional style. *Journal of Abnormal Psychology, 88*, 242-248.

Seligman, M. E. P., Klein, D. C., & Miller, W. R. (1976). Depression. In H. Leitenberg (Ed.), *Handbook of behavior modification and behavior therapy* (pp. 168-210). Englewood Cliffs, NJ: Prentice-Hall.

Shaw, B. F., & Dobson, K. S. (1981). Cognitive assessment of depression. In T. V. Merluzzi, C. R. Glass, & M. Genest (Eds.), *Cognitive assessment* (pp. 361-387). New York: Guilford Press.

Silverman, J. S., Silverman, J. A., & Eardley, D. A. (1984). Do maladapative attitudes cause depression? *Archives of General Psychiatry, 41*, 28-30.

Simons, A. D., Garfield, S. L., & Murphy, G. E. (1984). The process of change in cognitive therapy and pharmacotherapy for depression. *Archives of General Psychiatry, 41*, 45-51.

Simons, A. D., Lustman, P. J., & Murphy, G. E. (1985). Predicting response to cognitive therapy: The role of learned resourcefulness. *Cognitive Therapy and Research, 9*, 79-90.

Simons, A. D., Murphy, G. E., & Levine, J. L., & Wetzel, R. D. (1986). Cognitive therapy and pharmacotherapy for depression. Sustained improvement over one year. *Archives of General Psychiatry, 43*, 43-48.

Trexler, L. D., & Karst, T. O. (1972). Rational emotive therapy, placebo, and no treatment effects on public speaking anxiety. *Journal of Abnormal Psychology, 79*, 60-67.

Watkins, J. T., & Rush, A. J. (1983). Cognitive Response Test. *Cognitive Therapy and Research, 7*, 425-436.

Weingartner, H., & Silberman, E. K. (1984). Cognitive changes in depression. In R. M. Post & J. C. Ballenger (Eds.)., *Neurobiology of mood disorders* (pp. 121-135). Baltimore: Williams & Wilkins.

Weintraub, M., Segal, R. M., & Beck, A. T. (1974). An investigation of cognition and affect in the depressive experiences of normal men. *Journal of Consulting and Clinical Psychology, 42*, 911.

Weissman, A. N. (1979). The Dysfunctional Attitude Scale: A validation study (Doctoral dissertation, University of Pennsylvania, 1979). *Dissertation Abstracts International, 40*, 1389B-1390B.

CHAPTER 10

The Multivantaged Approach to the Measurement of Affect and Behavior in Depression

MARTIN M. KATZ
Albert Einstein College of Medicine-Montefiore Medical Center

INTRODUCTION

The measurement of psychological attributes, many of which are subjective in nature, in psychiatrically disturbed patients is difficult, and the field is in a continuing state of development. Psychologists find it useful when considering issues of measurement to categorize psychological functions into classes, such as affect, cognition, activity level, social behavior, and perception.

The area of affect or emotion examplifies the multiform problems of measurement. It is by definition an experiential or subjective state — one that only the person can "know," even if he or she does not always have words with which to describe it. Through the use of inventories of descriptors, psychologists try to present the person with the right words, but these terms can only be approximations of what any patient is likely to feel. When self-report is used as a vehicle, there are other barriers to attaining accurate measurement of a "feeling" state. It turns out that subjects may have constraints of various types that prevent them from providing a frank picture of their internal state. For example, there are additional complications when dealing with very disturbed patients, who may in many cases be unable to indicate how they feel.

Investigators, therefore, seek other ways of assessing affect states. In most instances of clinical research, they will ask the experts to examine the patients and then, on the basis of their observations, to judge the extent to which a given state (e.g., anxiety or depression) exists. The experts in this case are psychiatrists, psychologists, and nurses who see the patients in different interview and ward settings. Psychologists will use other tools in the course of their studies that assist them in gauging the intensity of a particular affect, such as anxiety.

This use of several perspectives acknowledges that from no one of these perspectives is it possible to obtain a comprehensive and reliable estimate of the depth and extent of an affect state; validity and reliability of measurement of the state are enhanced by combining these perspectives. In addition, combining such measurements assumes that the more intensive or severe a state such as anxiety, the more likely it is that it will be manifested in more situations. It also assumes the converse — that is, to the extent that the state is only mildly present, it will be less likely to appear in all situations, and may be detectable only in one or two of those described.

In measuring psychological qualities, we also use such terms as "constructs." A construct is an abstraction; it implies that from a physical or objective standpoint the quality itself may not be measurable, but that there are aspects of it in subjects, overt behavior or in their description of their state that appear to occur together, and that help to define it. Thus, "anxiety" is something that we cannot actually see, but that we believe exists because there are a number of aspects occuring together (e.g., subjective fear, uncomfortable physical feelings, jitteriness) that help to define it. From the multiperspective approach, a patient can usually describe the fear, but it requires outsiders to observe the jitteriness and the other aspects of its physical expression.

Many of the constructs we use in psychopathology are overinclusive and thus very complex. Clinicians, for example, use such terms as "cognitive impairment" to describe serious thinking disorders. In examining aspects of this construct, we note the inclusion of such varying disturbances as difficulties in concentration and in memory, loss of insight, and confusion and poor judgment. Some of these impairments can only be discovered by examining the performance of the patient, others only by expert observation, and still others only by the patient's own report.

Thus, in all of these areas of psychological functioning, we find it necessary to rely on a multiperspective approach to attain both validity and comprehensiveness, since in regard to the latter, certain characteristics of the construct can only be measured by applying a certain type of instrument.

When we approached the tasks set out by the National Institute of Mental Health (NIMH) Collaborative Program on the Psychobiology of Depression (Katz, Secunda, Hirschfeld, & Koslow, 1979) — namely, the comprehensive study of the nature of the depressive disorders, and the testing of a wide range of psychobiological and psychosocial hypotheses — it was necessary, in order to accomplish these goals, that certain critical psychological and behavioral qualities of depressed patients be measured.

In the case of the Collaborative Program's Biological Studies (Maas *et al.*, 1980), which are focused on the role of neurochemistry in depression, four affect and behavioral constructs were critical for the testing of the central hypotheses. The affect constructs were "anxiety" and "depressed mood," and the behavioral activity constructs were "motor retardation" and "agitation."

Because we also had a number of clinical hypotheses concerning the basic phenomenology of depression and the pattern of action of tricyclic drugs, a structure was created for the measurement of behavior in these studies that would extend beyond the four constructs and be more comprehensive in scope.

The first part of this chapter describes (1) the kinds of methods applied to the study of affect, behavior, and cognition; (2) the manner in which the constructs were derived and how the facets came to comprise the system; and (3) the nature of the constructs and how they are related. The chapter then describes some of the applications to which the constructs have been put in investigating a number of issues relevant to the nature and treatment of the depressive disorders. These applications include studies of the following.

1. The relationship between neurochemistry and behavior (Redmond *et al.*, 1986).
2. The comparative clinical phenomena of unipolar and bipolar depression (Katz, Robins, Croughan, Secunda, & Swann, 1982).
3. The timing and specificity of tricyclic drug actions (Katz, Koslow, Maas, & Bowden, 1987).
4. Predicting tricyclic drug response in the clinical situation.

For the purposes of this chapter, the applications to be focused on are the analyses of the actions and the timing of the effects of tricyclic drugs, and the clinical prediction of drug response (i.e., items 3 and 4 in the list above).

DEVELOPMENT AND CHARACTERISTICS OF THE METHOD

The development of this multivantaged approach is described elsewhere in detail (Katz *et al.*, 1984). The main features of this approach are briefly described here.

The system consists of 11 state constructs and their associated factors and vantages. These constructs span the areas of the psychological functions of affect, activity level, cognition, perception, somatization, and social behavior.

In Table 10-1, the methods used in the Biological Studies of the NIMH Collaborative Program are presented. They include standard observational rating instruments for use by experienced doctors (e.g., the Hamilton Rating Scale for Depression [HRSD]; Hamilton, 1960); instruments (e.g., the Global Ward Behavior Scale [GWBS]) for ratings by nurses; self-report inventories to be completed by the patients themselves (e.g., the Symptom Checklist — 90 [SCL-90]); and psychomotor performance tests.

In the Biological Studies, the objectives include the investigation of the relationships of changes in central nervous system chemistry to behavior over time, and of the action of tricyclic drugs on these systems over the course of treatment. Thus, "change" in behavior and affect is an important issue for measurement. To enhance measurement capacity in this sphere, new methods

TABLE 10-1 Methods for Measuring State and Outcome Constructs

- I. Observational rating methods
  - A. "Live" interview (doctors)
    1. Hamilton Rating Scale for Depression (HRSD)
    2. SADS—Change scale (SADS-C)
    3. Video Interview Behavior and Symptom Scale (VIBES)
  - B. Video interview (doctors at different centers)
    1. VIBES
    2. Ching K-S Social Behavior Scale
    3. Expressive Movement Scale
    4. HRSD
  - C. Ward behavior (nurses)
    1. Affective Disorder Rating Scale (ADRS)
    2. NIMH Mood Scale
    3. Global Ward Behavior Scale (GWBS)
- II. Patient testing
  - A. Self-report scale
    1. Symptom Checklist — 90 (SCL-90)
    2. NIMH Mood Scale
  - B. Psychomotor performance
    1. Reaction time
    2. Tapping speed
    3. Dot placing
    4. Tracking

Note. Reprinted with permission of publisher from: Katz, M. M., Koslow, S. H., Berman, N., Secunda, S., Maas, J. W., Casper, R., Kocsis, J., & Stokes, P. A multi-vantaged approach to measurement of behavioral and affect states for clinical and psychobiological research. *Psychological Reports*, 1984, *55*, 619-671. Monograph Supplement 1 V55. Table 1.

that rely on standard brief video interviews were refined. Separate scales for application for the rating of the patients in these interviews were devised for doctors, nurses, and movement experts. Up to this point in the Collaborative Program, only the doctor ratings have been analyzed. Use of the other "vantages" and of the specially devised scales awaits subsequent studies of these data.

In the Biological Studies, 125 hospitalized depressives (both unipolar and bipolar) from six field centers, a sample of 80 outpatient and hospitalized "normal" controls, and smaller samples of manic and schizophrenic patients, were available for study (see Table 10-2). Administering this battery of instruments to the study population during the admission phase made a very large sample and data base available for the development of a measurement framework.

To reaffirm the objectives, the instruments were selected so that sound measures could be developed of (1) four constructs critical to the testing of the major neurochemical-behavioral hypotheses; and (2) other major com-

TABLE 10-2 Biological Studies Sample: Demographic and Clinical Characteristics

	Number of subjects			Mean age			Mean duration in weeks of current episode	
Diagnostic class[a]	Total	Male	Female	Male	Female	Age range	Male	Female
Major depressive disorder	132	70	62	47.7	46.8	20-78	33.4	32.1
Unipolar depression	85	39	46	50.7	48.2	23-78	42.0	37.0
Bipolar depression	47	31	16	43.9	42.9	20-68	22.6	18.1
Manic disorder	19	12	7	44.8	43.9	23-74	4.5	8.0
Schizophrenia	15	13	2	32.8	32.5	19-52	204.4	225.0
Normal controls	80	38	42	45.4	46.3	21-76		
Nonhospitalized controls	47	23	24	43.7	45.1	21-76		
Hospitalized controls	33	15	18	47.9	47.8	24-72		
Total	246	133	113	45.3	46.2	19-78		

Note. Reprinted with permission of publisher from: Katz, M. M., Koslow, S. H., Berman, N., Secunda, S., Maas, J. W., Casper, R., Kocsis, J., & Stokes, P. A multi-vantaged approach to measurement of behavioral and affect states for clinical and psychobiological research. *Psychological Reports*, 1984, *55*, 619-671. Monograph Supplement 1 V55. Table 2.

[a] In accord with administration of the Schedule for Affective Disorders and Schizophrenia (SADS; Endicott & Spitzer, 1978) and the Research Diagnostic Criteria (RDC; Spitzer, Endicott, & Robins, 1978).

ponents of the depressive disorders, previously identified in research, which could then be applied to studies of the phenomenology of unipolar and bipolar depression and to the analysis of the actions of tricyclic drugs.

The approach to developing measures of the state and outcome constructs involved the following:

1. The articulation of operational definitions of the major constructs.
2. The segregation of scales within the battery that were presumed to measure each of these constructs.
3. The analysis, within each construct realm, of the relationships among the various measures and of the realm's factor composition.
4. The development of a scoring system for each construct that would both (a) take advantage of several procedures used to measure it, thus providing optimal reliability; and (b) preserve its multifaceted nature (i.e., derive measures of each of the factors or vantages that comprise it).

This process resulted in the derivation of 11 state and 3 outcome constructs, each comprised of 1 to 4 factors or vantages. These are presented in Table 10-3. The "operational" definitions referred to in item 1 of the list above were then revised to fit more closely the scales used to measure them.

In Table 10-4, the internal consistencies of the factors associated with each state construct are presented. In most cases, the factors simply represent the different vantages from which the construct is measured. In other constructs (specifically, cognitive impairment), the factors represent different components of the construct (i.e., confusion and lack of insight, and impaired thinking and concentration).

Basic psychometric studies of the reliability and validity of the constructs, conducted prior to their application to the Biological Studies' hypotheses, are summarized elsewhere (Katz *et al.*, 1984). Essentially, these studies showed the constructs, when measured prior to drug treatment, to be relatively stable over the pretreatment period of 2 weeks. They showed the factors within constructs to be relatively homogeneous and to measure different facets of the same basic construct. Regarding validity, the state constructs were capable of discriminating between patient groups and normals (a relatively simple task); in a more demanding test, they were capable of distinguishing between the behavioral characteristics of two subtypes of depression, the unipolar and bipolar types (Katz *et al.*, 1982). The measures indicated differences in the behavior and affect of different age groups in both normals and depressives (Katz *et al.*, 1984).

Following their applications to issues in the Biological Studies, certain of the constructs have been shown to correlate with levels of neuroamines and their metabolities in cerebrospinal fluid, both in depressed patients and in manics (Redmond *et al.*, 1986; Swann *et al.*, 1987). There has been, in other words, a steady accumulation of evidence that the constructs are not only valid, but capable of detecting rather fine relationships between neurochemistry and the expression of behavior in affective syndromes.

TABLE 10-3 State and Outcome Constructs: Definitions and Factor Composition

Construct	Factor	Vantages
State constructs		
I. *Depressed Mood.* Describes a central mood that is expressed through feelings of sadness, downheartedness, worthlessness, loneliness, and an inability to enjoy anything. The construct, as defined, does not extend beyond the mood element of the depressive disorder.	1	Patients' reports of subjective state.
	2	Doctors' ratings based on live interview observations.
	3	Nurses' ratings based on ward behavior.
II. *Anxiety.* Describes a mood and somatic state characterized by manifestations of fear, apprehension, severe tension bordering on a state of panic; the subjects exhibit these characteristics and use such terms to describe themselves, with evidence of both psychic and autonomic components.	4	Doctors' ratings based on live interviews.
	5	Nurses' ratings based on ward behavior.
	6	Doctors' ratings based on video interviews.
	7	Patients' reports of subjective state.
III. *Retardation of Movement and Speech.* Describes a slowing down of motor movement, reactivity, and speech, reflecting a reduction of available energy or retardation of central nervous system functioning generally.	8	Doctors' ratings based on live and video interviews.
	9	Patients' psychomotor performance.
	10	Nurses' ratings based on ward behavior.
IV. *Agitation.* Describes physical and mental restlessness that is expressed by the level and type of motor activity, with associated signs of hyperactivity, nervousness, and irritability.	11	Doctors' ratings based on video interviews.
	12	Doctors' ratings based on live interviews.
	13	Nurses' ratings based on ward behavior.
V. *Hostility.* The entire range of hostile affect and behavior, from covert, "felt" anger and resentment to outward expressions of irritability, threats, and other verbally aggressive behavior.	14	Doctors' ratings based on video interviews.
	15	Patients' reports of subjective state.
	16	Nurses' ratings based on ward behavior.
VI. *Somatization.* The extent to which psychopathology is expressed through physical symptoms. A range of symptoms usually or potentially reflective of anxiety and depression, which can involve any or all of the systems of the organism.	17	Doctors' ratings based on live and video interviews, and patients' self-reports.
VII. *Distressed Expression.* The extent to which emotional distress is manifested overtly in facial expression, with such signs as tearfulness, sagging of the mouth, and eyebrows drawn.	18	Doctors' ratings based on live and video interviews.
VIII. *Interpersonal Sensitivity.* Extends from self-consciousness and minor sensitivity to criticism, to suspiciousness of the motives of others and "ideas of reference." Thus, shyness and "feelings easily hurt" would characterize patients with a moderate amount of this affect, while high scores would border on strong paranoidal tendencies.	19	Patients' reports of subjective state.
	20	Doctors' ratings from video interviews, and nurses' ratings from ward behavior.

Table 10-3 (cont'd)

Construct	Factor	Vantages
IX. *Positive Adaptation.* Reflects generally positive affect and effective social behavior. Indicates extent to which there is good feeling within the self; friendliness; and comfortable, assertive, open behavior with others.	21	Doctors' ratings from video interviews, and nurses' ratings from ward behavior (adaptive social behavior)[a]
	22	Patients' reports of subjective state (friendliness, positive self-feelings).[a]
X. *Cognitive Impairment.* Extent to which judgment, concentration, memory, and thinking generally are impaired, from minimum disturbance to the degree that there is actual confusion and psychotic impairment.	23	Doctors' ratings from live and video interviews, and nurses' ratings from ward behavior (confusion and lack of insight).[a]
	24	Doctors' ratings from live and video interviews, and patients' reports of subjective state (impaired concentration).[a]
XI. *Sleep Disorder.* The extent to which the normal sleep pattern is disturbed, as manifested by early, middle, or late insomnia, early awakening, difficulty falling a asleep, and apparent troubled sleep.	25	Doctors' ratings from live interviews, and patients' reports of subjective state.
Outcome constructs		
XII. *Global Improvement.* The extent to which patients improve overall during course of treatment (or over time), as judged by doctors and nurses, and from their own reports on the extent of symptom distress at the end of the treatment period.	26	Doctors' ratings based on live interviews, patients' self-reports, and nurses' ratings based on ward behavior.
XIII. *Depressed State.* This is a general measure of the severity of the depressive syndrome. It takes into account all of the major characteristics of the depressive disorder (i.e., subjective state, activity level, appearance, and somatic symptoms) and assesses the extent to which the "depressed state" is present.	27	Doctors' ratings based on live and video interviews.
	28	Patients' reports of subjective state.
	29	Nurses' ratings based on ward behavior.
XIV. *General Psychopathology.* This is a general measure of the severity of psychopathology. It essentially summarizes the extent to which elements of severe disturbance other than those specifically associated with the depressed state are present, but emphasizes those elements associated with cognitive disorder.	30	Doctors' ratings from live and video interviews, and nurses' ratings from ward behavior.
	31	Patients' reports of subjective state.

Note. Reprinted with permission of publisher from: Katz, M. M., Koslow, S. H., Berman, N., Secunda, S., Maas, J. W., Casper, R., Kocsis, J., & Stokes, P. A multi-vantaged approach to measurement of behavioral and affect states for clinical and psychobiological research. *Psychological Reports*, 1984, *55*, 619-671. Monograph Supplement 1 V55. Tables 3 and 4.

[a] Content of factors comprising the constructs of Positive Adaptation and Cognitive Impairment: Specific content in parentheses.

TABLE 10-4 Internal Consistencies of State Construct Subfactors: Parallel Model (Cronbach's Alpha)

State constructs	Factor		n	α
I. Depressed Mood	1	Subjective state	134	.93
	2	Interview behavior	195	.94
	3	Ward behavior	182	.91
II. Anxiety	4	Interview behavior	197	.82
	5	Ward behavior	182	.93
	6	Video interview behavior	150	.83
	7	Subjective state	219	.88
III. Retardation of Movement and Speech	8	Interview and video behavior	119	.92
	9	Psychomotor performance	214	.73
	10	Ward behavior	187	.83
IV. Agitation	11	Video interview behavior	151	.87
	12	Interview behavior	197	.68
	13	Ward behavior	182	.81
V. Hostility	14	Video interview behavior	151	.92
	15	Subjective state	170	.76
	16	Ward behavior	182	.83
VIII. Interpersonal Sensitivity	19	Subjective state	223	.88
	20	Ward and video interview behavior	114	.30
IX. Positive Adaptation	21	Video interview and ward behavior	114	.80
	22	Subjective state	222	.87
X. Cognitive Impairment	23	Confusion and lack of insight	113	.85
	24	Impaired concentration	137	.84

Note. Reprinted with permission of publisher from: Katz, M. M., Koslow, S. H., Berman, N., Secunda, S., Maas, J. W., Casper, R., Kocsis, J., & Stokes, P. A multi-vantaged approach to measurement of behavioral and affect states for clinical and psychobiological research. *Psychological Reports*, 1984, *55*, 619-671. Monograph Supplement 1 V55. Table 4.

In order to demonstrate how the constructs and vantages have been and are being applied to scientific and clinical issues in the NIMH Collaborative Program, the rest of this chapter describes the results of using them to examine several issues involving the effects of tricyclic drugs in depression.

THE TIMING AND SPECIFICITY OF THE ACTION OF TRICYCLIC DRUGS

After some 20 years of extensive study, there is little question about the overall efficacy of the tricyclic drugs in depression (Klerman & Cole, 1965). Despite the large number of such studies, however, certain issues relevant to an understanding of how the drugs work and to the prediction of their effects remain unresolved. Among the unresolved issues are the actual timing of the actions of the drugs, and on which aspects of behavior and affect they have their initial effects. Answers to such questions would contribute to understanding of their basic mechanisms of action. A second related set of issues, which has more direct application to the clinical situation, is that of the current limited capacity to predict their effects in the treatment of the various specific forms of the depressive disorders.

On the basis of prior evidence, it would be expected that some 66% of severely depressed patients will show marked improvement with adequate treatment within 4 weeks, and that approximately 50% of such patients will demonstrate full or nearly full recovery. Despite the extended history of research on these drugs, however, there remains (as noted) a lack of clarity concerning their speed of action, particularly in those patients who will actually recover with treatment. Furthermore, because of a lack of refined analysis of their effects on psychological functioning, the specificity of their initial actions on behavior, affect, and cognition is still unknown. The design of the Biological Studies component of the NIMH Collaborative Program was sufficiently detailed to provide new information on this set of problems.

Methods

In several earlier papers (Mass *et al.*, 1980; Secunda *et al.*, 1980), the design and methodology of this research program have been presented. It is useful to highlight a few of the most important characteristics here:

1. The total sample, drawn from six hospital centers, consisted of 132 hospitalized depressed patients (87 unipolars, 45 bipolars), 80 normals, and smaller samples of manic and schizophrenic patients. Diagnostic procedures utilizing the Schedule For Affective Disorders and Schizophrenia (SADS; Endicott & Spitzer, 1978) and the Research Diagnostic Criteria (RDC; Spitzer, Endicott, & Robins, 1978) were standardized across the six centers.
2. The average age of the patients was 49.2 years for the unipolar and 43.6 years for the bipolar depressives. Genders were balanced among the unipolars; however, as expected, males exceeded females by a ratio of 2:1 among the bipolars.
3. The design utilized a 2-week drug-free placebo period with assessments weekly and just prior to treatment, followed by a 4-week treatment period.
4. Patients whose depression was resolved or markedly decreased during the baseline period were removed from the treatment study. (Approximately 4% showed such change; the low rate of placebo response was attributed to the generally high level of severity of depression in this hospitalized sample.)
5. The drugs imipramine and amitriptyline were randomly assigned and administered in a double-blind design. A fixed dosage of 250 mg/day was achieved for both drugs by the end of the first week for 87% of the patients; the remaining patients were on 10-200 mg/day for the 4-week treatment period.
6. Steady-state and blood levels were measured; the data have been reported in a separate paper (Kocsis *et al.*, 1986).

If the drugs do have specific actions on affects and behavior that initiate the recovery process, it is necessary to search for the effects early in the treatment period (i.e., before the process of recovery begins to accelerate). Thus, detailed measurement of the potential actions of the drugs was initiated following the first week of treatment, and was conducted at approximately weekly intervals throughout the treatment period.

The design of this research program had certain advantages for the investigation of those effects of antidepressant drugs which are specifically associated with recovery, and for the study of differences in the actions of imipramine and amitriptyline. For example, the sample was large for such studies, making it possible to selectively investigate clearly recovered and clearly nonrecovered patients, the latter group usually being quite small in clinical trial studies.

Results

Assessing the Overall Clinical Efficacy of the Drugs over the 4-Week Treatment Period

In summary, through the use of a categorical system for determining "recovery" or "nonrecovery" based on multiple global measures of severity of the depressed state and extent of improvement, it was found following 4 weeks of treatment that (1) 66% of patients achieved marked improvement or complete recovery; and (2) the two drugs, amitriptyline and imipramine, did not differ in the proportion of recoveries effected or in the extent of overall improvement produced.

Analyzing the Timing and the Recovery-Related Actions of the Drugs during the Treatment Period

In the analysis of overall efficacy using a categorical system, it was determined that approximately 51% of patients achieved full or nearly complete recovery (i.e., greater than "marked improvement"), while 26% showed no improvement or the absolute minimum of progress over the 4-week treatment period. The remaining third category (23%), the "indeterminate," consisted of modestly to moderately improved patients. (The intermediate group was designated as "indeterminate," since their reaction to treatment beyond the 4 weeks would not be known. Some of the patients might, for example, recover within 6 to 8 weeks. Although we were not able to control treatment beyond the 4 weeks, it was not possible at that time to know the actual outcome for these patients over the extended treatment period.) The "indeterminate" group was not included in this analysis, in order to provide two qualitatively different groups for comparison.

The findings regarding the central issues in this study are now briefly summarized.

Differences at Baseline. It can be seen from the baseline values on the state constructs in Table 10-5 that there was a general tendency for those who would not show any sign of real improvement or recovery following 4 weeks of treatment to be more severely disturbed. This comparison was examined specifically through the use of the composite severity measures of Depressed State and General Psychopathology. These latter measures are called "outcome constructs"; they make use of summary or overall measures from, for instance, the HRSD and the Global Assessment Scale (GAS; Endicott, Spitzer, Fleiss, & Cohen, 1976). From these comparisons on the outcome constructs, we would draw the conclusion that the nonrecovered as a group were significantly more depressed and more ill generally than the recovered at baseline. (It is useful to keep in mind that the whole sample was by definition at the severe end of the continuum — i.e., a hospitalized patient sample.)

Furthermore, regarding the facets of the condition, the differences in the two groups were in Depressed Mood itself (the aspect of mood that reflects the subjective or experiential aspects of the state) and in Cognitive Impairment. It was a group of the more deeply psychologically depressed who failed to respond within the 4-week period of intensive treatment.

Differences in Amount of Change at 1 and at 2½ Weeks. Having identified distinguishing features at outset between the responders and nonresponders that appeared to have to do with the depth of the depressive state, we then examined the nature of changes that took place in these groups at 1 week following the initiation of drug treatment. In view of the already reported observation that the process of recovery in responders is rapid, once it begins, and that any specific actions the drugs may have are likely to be merged rather quickly in the process, the first week was considered to be the most significant assessment point. This was presumed both (1) from the standpoint of determining whether later effects could be predicted, and (2) in terms of identifying those actions of the drugs that appeared to be responsible for initiating the recovery process.

In Table 10-6, the differences in two groups at 1 week are examined

TABLE 10-5 Discriminating State and Outcome Constructs: Baseline Values by Outcome Group

Construct	Recovered	Indeterminate	Nonrecovered	p^a
State constructs				
Depressed Mood	4.46 ± 0.21 (54)	5.80 ± 0.29 (24)	5.29 ± 0.30 (26)	.001
Cognitive Impairment	2.60 ± 0.12 (50)	3.19 ± 0.22 (22)	3.23 ± 0.19 (24)	.009
Outcome construct				
Depressed State	3.01 ± 0.18 (49)	4.08 ± 0.26 (21)	3.93 ±0.27 (24)	.001

Note. Values for each group are given as mean ± *SE*. Sample sizes are shown in parentheses.

[a] *p*'s are from analyses of variance on the baseline means.

with respect to the ways in which each group changed. A T^2 multivariate analysis indicated that the two samples were representative of different patient populations. Of the 11 major aspects measured, one notes that the recovered group changed significantly more than the nonrecovered in 6: Depressed Mood, Anxiety, Distressed Expression, Hostility, Agitation, and Cognitive Impairment. The nonrecovered group showed little to no change at 1 week.

The phenomenon of accelerated recovery that is noted above can be seen most graphically when the effects distinguishing the groups after 2½ weeks of treatment are examined. On almost all of the constructs that were measured, the changes in the recovered group at this point were strong, while they were almost nonexistent for the nonresponders, except for Somatization and Sleep Disorder. (The distinction was so great between the two groups that, on the basis of a discriminant-function analysis, more than 80% of patients in the two groups could be accurately classified into those who would recover and those who would not following 4 weeks of treatment.)

Regarding the separate aspects of the depressed state, there were two or three important exceptions to the findings noted above. As mentioned, the nonrecovered changed almost as much as the recovered on the constructs of Sleep Disorder and Somatization. Changes in these latter areas, unlike the ones in the affect areas (identified as discriminators at 1 week), were therefore not necessarily associated with the recovery process itself.

Summary. To summarize the results, these analyses indicated the following:

1. When the tricyclic drugs were going to be effective in severe depression, they acted (when administered in adequate dosage) within the first week of administration.

TABLE 10-6 Recovered versus Nonrecovered Patient Groups: Significant Differences in Amount of Change at 1 Week of Drug Treatment

	Mean change from baseline		
Construct	Recovered	Nonrecovered	Difference in change[a]
Depressed Mood	0.99	0.22	0.77**
Anxiety	0.79	−0.08	0.87***
Agitation	0.32	−0.01	0.33**
Hostility	0.26	−0.09	0.35**
Distressed Expression	0.87	−0.13	1.00**
Cognitive Impairment	0.55	0.25	0.30**
Depressed State	0.82	0.22	0.42*

[a] Subjects in the two groups were compared on each construct using analysis of covariance with the baseline value as the covariate.

* $p < .05$.

** $p < .01$.

*** $p < .001$.

2. They acted on specific affects and behaviors in initiating the recovery process. The constructs of Anxiety, Depressed Mood, Hostility, and Cognitive Impairment showed improvement, as did the physical aspects of Distressed Expression and Agitation.

3. Of additional interest is the fact that relatively large changes could be detected after the first week in the constructs measuring somatic aspects, particularly in Sleep Disorder, but that these affects occured generally across patients and were not necessarily associated with the recovery process.

4. By the end of $2\frac{1}{2}$ weeks, improvement in those who would recover had taken on a "cascading" quality; any specifics of improvement that might be occuring could no longer be detected.

These results have some implications for our attempts to understand how the tricyclics bring about their effects in depression. For example, it appears that their so-called "lag" behind actions on neurochemistry is much shorter in time than was formerly believed. This finding should contribute to further understanding of the mechanisms of tricyclic drug actions (Frazer & Lucki, 1983).

Furthermore, the tricyclic drug effect in reducing sleep disorder makes it appear that this action is not in itself therapeutic. It leaves open the question of whether the efficacy of the tricyclics in depression can be traced to their sedative actions. It appears that their effects on anxiety and depressed mood, and on certain aspects of impaired cognitive functioning, are the more directly therapeutic actions of these agents. The "cascading" quality of the effect in some 50% of the severely depressed population also makes it appear that this "responder" group has some specific neurochemical dysfunction that is apparently partially resolved, directly or indirectly, by the tricyclics — a dysfunction not shared by the 25% of severe cases who show no response at all to the drugs.

PREDICTING RESPONSE IN THE CLINICAL SITUATION: THE "EFFECT SIZE" OF THE DIFFERENCES

As a follow-up to this examination of the important scientific issue of the timing and specificity of action of the tricyclic drugs, it was asked whether the differences reported between the recovered and nonrecovered patients were large enough to be useful in predicting response to treatment in the clinical situation.

Prior research on clinical predictors of tricyclic treatment, as reviewed by Bielski and Friedel (1976) and by Kessler (1978), has been disappointing. There is some evidence, although not confirmed, that the responders are likely to be of the endogenous type with associated somatic symptoms (Bielski & Friedel, 1976) and that the disorder of the responders is more "psychotic" in quality, more likely to include delusional symptomatology (Glassman, Kantor,

& Shostak, 1975). The evidence regarding other potential predictors of drug response is even more ambiguous.

In the Biological Studies, it was possible to examine the size of the differences between the group of patients who would recover in 4 weeks and the group who would not. (Since this was a predictive problem, the problem would be to determine whether those who would recover in 4 weeks could be distinguished from all other patients. "All others" would mean including the "indeterminate" group of responders with those patients who were classified as "nonrecovered.")

Furthermore, since the issue was whether the findings from the study of the timing and specificity of drug action were large enough to be useful in the clinical situation, doctors' ratings, nurses' ratings, and patients' self-reports would each be examined to determine whether these differences could be detected. That meant turning to the method factors or "vantages" described earlier, which comprise the constructs. Thus, we would be able to compare results from analyses from these different perspectives as to when and how the drugs would act in depressed patients.

At Baseline

In Table 10-7, the differences between the responders and nonresponders that were detected at baseline can be examined as they appeared to doctors, to nurses, and to the patients themselves. It will be recalled that the two groups differed markedly on the outcome construct of Depressed State at baseline. To assess the size of the difference, Cohen's (1969) measure of effect size was applied; it provides (in units of standard deviation) an estimate of whether the difference perceived between two groups is large enough to be "visible." Any effect size value equal to or greater than 0.50 is considered to be moderate in size, and thus visible. The difference between the responders and nonresponders on the Depressed State construct (in accord with Cohen's measure of effect size) was large at baseline. Although they can be distinguished best

TABLE 10-7 Recovered Group versus All Others: Baseline Values for Depressed State Construct, Clinical Rating Factors, and Self-Report Factors

Construct/factors	Recovered	All others	Difference[a]	Effect size
Depressed State	3.13 ± 0.18 (49)	4.10 ± 0.19 (45)	0.97**	0.77
Doctor ratings	3.35 ± 0.17 (54)	4.07 ± 0.18 (51)	0.72*	0.61
Self-reports	3.49 ± 0.29 (49)	4.80 ± 0.31 (45)	1.31*	0.64
Nurse ratings	2.69 ± 0.24 (54)	3.67 ± 0.26 (52)	0.98*	0.54

Note. Values for each group are given as mean ± *SE*. Sample sizes are shown in parentheses.
[a] Subjects in the two groups were compared using *t*-tests.
* $p < .01$.
** $p < .001$.

when all three vantages are combined, it can be seen in Table 10-7, that all three types of observers were able to significantly differentiate the groups at baseline (all effect sizes were greater than 0.50).

The next question to be considered was whether certain aspects of the Depressed State construct could be used to distinguish the responder and nonresponder groups in the clinical situation. Differences in Depressed Mood itself could apparently be detected through all three vantages (see Table 10-8). Furthermore, doctors saw greater Agitation at baseline in those who would not later respond to treatment. One aspect of Cognitive Impairment, severe impairment in the capacity to concentrate (in already severely depressed patients), also mitigated against response to tricyclic drugs.

Thus, differences in severity of depression between responders and all others, marked by intense Depressed Mood and certain forms of Cognitive Impairment, were large enough at baseline to be detectable by doctors, nurses, and patients. The strength of these findings speaks to the importance of these indications as predictors of response to tricyclic drugs.

After 1 and $2\frac{1}{2}$ Weeks of Drug Treatment

From the findings presented in Table 10-9, it can be seen that the doctors saw much change at 1 week in those patients who would eventually recover, and that these changes were for the most part also observed by the nurses in the patients' behavior on the ward. Thus, the doctors' view that the responders changed markedly by the end of the first week and were different from "all

TABLE 10-8 Recovered Group versus All Others: Baseline Values for State Constructs, Clinical Rating Factors, and Self-Report Factors

Constructs/factors	Recovered	All others	Difference[a]	Effect size
Depressed Mood	4.49 ± 0.21	5.68 ± 0.23	1.19***	0.77
Self-reports	4.34 ± 0.32	5.91 ± 0.35	1.56**	0.66
Doctor ratings	5.61 ± 0.21	6.68 ± 0.23	1.07**	0.69
Nurse ratings	3.58 ± 0.27	4.81 ± 0.29	1.23**	0.63
Agitation	2.19 ± 0.12	2.65 ± 0.13	0.46**	0.53
Doctor ratings	2.64 ± 0.16	3.25 ± 0.19	0.61*	0.50
Nurse ratings	1.84 ± 0.14	2.07 ± 0.14	0.23	0.23
Cognitive Impairment	2.68 ± 0.14	3.38 ± 0.18	0.70**	0.63
Confusion	0.98 ± 0.13	1.23 ± 0.17	0.25	0.24
Impaired concentration	4.47 ± 0.25	5.63 ± 0.25	1.16***	0.66

Note. Values for each group are given as mean ± *SE*. For recovered group, $n = 47\text{-}54$; for all others, $n = 43\text{-}52$.

[a] Subjects were compared using t-tests.

* $p < .05$

** $p < .01$.

*** $p < .001$.

TABLE 10-9 Recovered Group versus All Others: Comparisons of Changes on Global Severity Constructs, Clinical Rating Factors, and Self-Report Factors at 1 and 2½ weeks

	1 week		2½ weeks	
Constructs/factors	Differences in adjusted means[a]	Effect size	Differences in adjusted means[a]	Effect size
Depressed State	0.52*	0.58	1.30***	1.34
Doctor ratings	1.16***	0.97	1.84***	1.66
Nurse ratings	0.69*	0.53	1.35***	0.97
Patient self-reports	0.32	0.24	1.21***	0.85
General Psychopathology	0.35*	0.47	0.83***	1.12
Doctor and nurse ratings	0.40**	0.63	0.91***	6.54
Patient self-reports	0.47	0.37	0.90***	0.76

[a] Subjects in the two groups were compared on each construct using analysis of covariance with the baseline value as the covariate.
* $p < .05$.
** $p < .01$.
*** $p < .001$.

others" on Depressed State was supported by, if not as "visible" to, the nurses.

When the findings on the specifics of change are examined, it is clear that the doctors alone were able to detect major differences between the two response groups on Depressed Mood (effect size = 0.85), on Anxiety (0.76), and on Distressed Expression (0.80) (see Table 10-10). These findings were strongly supported in the first two cases by the nurses' observations and ratings. The responder group, however, did not report feeling very much better on Depressed Mood than did those who did not later respond to the drugs (see Table 10-8). This discrepancy in the reports of the doctors and the patients following the first week of treatment may in itself account for the disparate reports in the literature as to when the drugs actually begin to act in the treatment process (the so-called "lag" in clinical response).

On the other hand, the patients did report significant improvements at 1 week in Anxiety (0.69) and in Hostility (0.70). This would indicate that when the direct reports of patients are relied on for assessing changes related to drug treatment, these latter aspects are apparently the most sensitive in detecting positive changes.

Following 2½ weeks of treatment, the treatment effects were so large in all aspects of the depressed condition that they were apparent to almost all observers. These findings can be summarized as follows:

1. Differences between those who would recover and all others were large enough at baseline to be detectable by doctors, by nurses, or through patients' reports alone. Nonresponders were more severely ill in general; specifically, they showed more intense Depressed Mood and more Cognitive Impairment than those who would later respond.

TABLE 10-10 Recovered Group versus All Others: Comparisons of Changes on Constructs, Clinical Rating Factors, and Self-Report Factors at 1 and $2\frac{1}{2}$ weeks

	1 week		$2\frac{1}{2}$ weeks	
Constructs/factors	Differences in adjusted means[a]	Effect size	Differences in adjusted means[a]	Effect size
Depressed Mood	0.66*	0.58	1.96***	1.54
Doctor ratings	1.38***	0.85	2.62***	1.51
Nurse ratings	0.99**	0.65	1.94***	1.19
Patient self-reports	0.52	0.34	1.89***	1.04
Anxiety	0.97***	0.90	1.47***	1.34
Doctor ratings	1.16***	0.76	1.45***	0.99
Nurse ratings	0.95**	0.67	1.64***	1.04
Patient self-reports	1.05**	0.69	1.49***	0.98
Agitation	0.40*	0.54	0.59***	0.84
Doctor ratings	0.27	0.23	0.48*	0.44
Nurse ratings	0.48**	0.65	0.68***	0.82
Hostility	0.49*	0.51	0.88***	0.89
Nurse ratings	0.22	0.18	0.80***	0.70
Patient self-reports	0.81***	0.70	0.96**	0.68
Somatization	0.48**	0.56	0.91***	1.14
Distressed Expression	1.06***	0.80	1.44***	1.22
Interpersonal Sensitivity	0.63**	0.64	0.86***	0.75
Cognitive Impairment	0.63**	0.64	1.14***	1.46
Confusion	0.48**	0.57	0.69***	0.95
Impaired concentration	0.73*	0.50	1.78***	1.38

[a] Subjects in the two groups were compared on each construct using analysis of covariance with the baseline value as the covariate.

* $p < .05$.

** $p < .01$.

*** $p < .001$.

2. The finding that the tricyclic drugs acted as early as 1 week in those who would respond to the drugs was sufficiently strong to be useful in predicting treatment response in the clinical situation.

3. At 1 week, there was differential sensitivity among observers to the differences in amount of change between the responders and nonresponders. Doctors saw large and "visible" differences in the two groups on general severity (Depressed State), Depressed Mood, Anxiety, and constructs measuring physical and somatic expression (except Sleep Disorder). Most of these differences were supported through nurses' ward observations.

4. Patients, on the other hand, reported significant differences at 1 week on Anxiety and Hostility, but not on Depressed Mood.

5. All discrepancies between observer groups disappeared at $2\frac{1}{2}$ weeks, when the recovered group showed markedly greater change than the nonrecovered on almost all aspects of the depressed state.

CONCLUSION

These applications of the "multivantaged" approach have uncovered important findings about the timing of the action of antidepressant drugs and how the recovery process is initiated. Thus, we have potentially greater insight into the psychobiology of depression and the mechanisms of tricyclic drug action. The capacity to examine the state of depression through several vantages has significant practical value in assessing the extent to which certain aspects of the condition can be used to predict response to treatment. It has thus identified predictors of tricyclic drug response that are based on clinical observations, or on patient self-reports alone.

A question of prime interest now is whether this approach can further enlighten the field about the phenomenology or the nature of depression. Investigating the interrelationship of the "vantages" themselves, and the associations of the state constructs with significant neurochemical and neurohormonal systems, should move us further along in that direction.

Acknowledgment

The second part of this chapter was derived primarily from "The Timing, Specificity, and Clinical Prediction of Tricyclic Drug Effects in Depression" by M. M. Katz *et al.* (1987), *Psychological Medicine, 17*, 297-309. Reprinted by permission of Cambridge University Press.

References

Bielski, R. J., & Friedel, R. O. (1976). Prediction of tricyclic antidepressant response — a critical review. *Archives of General Psychiatry, 33*, 1479-1489.

Cohen, J. (1969). *Statistical power analysis for the behavioral sciences*. New York: Academic Press.

Endicott, J., & Spitzer, R. L. (1978). A diagnostic interview: The Schedule for Affective Disorders and Schizophrenia. *Archives of General Psychiatry, 35*, 837-844.

Endicott, J., Spitzer, R. L., Fleiss, J. L., & Cohen, J. (1976). The Global Assessment Scale, a procedure for measuring overall severity of psychiatric disturbance. *Archives of General Psychiatry, 33*, 766-771.

Frazer, A., & Lucki, I. (1983). Commentary: Problems with current catecholamine hypotheses of antidepressant agents. *Behavioral and Brain Sciences, 6*, 554-555.

Glassman, A. H., Kantor, S. J., & Shostak, M. (1975). Depression, delusions, and drug response. *American Journal of Psychiatry, 132*, 716-719.

Hamilton, M. (1960). A rating scale for depression. *Journal of Neurology, Neurosurgery and Psychiatry, 23*, 56-62.

Katz, M. M., Koslow, S., Berman, N., Secunda, S., Maas, J. W., Casper, R., Kocsis, J., & Stokes, P. (1984). A multivantaged approach to measurement of behavioral and affects states for clinical and psychobiological research. *Psychological Reports, 55*, 619-671.

Katz, M. M., Koslow, S., Maas, J., & Bowden, C. (1987). The timing, specificity, and clinical prediction of tricyclic drug effects in depression. *Psychological Medicine, 17*, 297-309.

Katz, M. M., Robins, E., Croughan, J., Secunda, S., & Swann, A. (1982). Behavioral measurement and drug response characteristics of unipolar and bipolar depression. *Psychological Medicine, 12*, 25-36.

Katz, M. M., Secunda, S., Hirschfeld, R. M., & Koslow, S. (1979). NIMH Clinical Research Branch Collaborative Program on the Psychobiology of Depression. *Archives of General Psychiatry, 36*, 765-811.

Kessler, K. A. (1978). Tricyclic antidepressants: Mode of action and clinical use. In M. A. Lipton, A. DiMascio, & K. F. Killam (Eds.), *Psychopharmacology: A generation of progress*. New York: Raven Press.

Klerman, G. L., & Cole, J. (1965). Clinical pharmacology of imipramine and related antidepressant compounds. *Pharmacological Review, 17*, 101-141.

Kocsis, J., Hanin, I., Bowden, C., Brunswick, D., Ramsey, A., & Butler, T. (1986). Imipramine and amitriptyline plasma concentration and clinical response in major depression. *British Journal of Psychiatry, 148*, 52-59.

Maas, J. W., Koslow, S. H., Davis, J., Katz, M. M., Mendels, J., Robins, E., Stokes, P., & Bowden, C. (1980). Biological component of the NIMH Clinical Research Branch Collaborative Program on the Psychobiology of Depression: I. Background and theoretical considerations. *Psychological Medicine, 10*, 759-776.

Redmond, D. E., Jr., Katz, M. M., Maas, J. W., Swann, A., Casper, R., & Davis, J. M. (1986). Cerebrospinal fluid amine metabolites. *Archives of General Psychiatry, 43*, 938-947.

Secunda, S., Koslow, S. H., Redmond, D. E., Garver, D., Ramsey, T. A., Croughan, J., Kocsis, J., Hanin, I., & Lieberman, K. (1980). Biological component of the NIMH Clinical Research Branch Collaborative Program on the Psychobiology of Depression: II. Methodology and data analysis. *Psychological Medicine, 10*, 777-793.

Spitzer, R. L., Endicott, J., & Robins, E. (1978). Research Diagnostic Criteria. *Archives of General Psychiatry, 35*, 713-782.

Swann, A., Koslow, S. H., Katz, M. M., Maas, J. W., Javaid, J., Secunda, S., & Robins, E. (1987). Lithium treatment of mania: CSF and urinary monoamine metabolites and treatment outcome. *Archives of General Psychiatry, 44*, 345-354.

SECTION IV

Psychosocial Measurement

CHAPTER 11

The Measurement of Personality in Depression

ROBERT M. A. HIRSCHFELD
National Institute of Mental Health
CHRISTINE K. CROSS
Group Operations, Inc.

INTRODUCTION

Hippocrates was among the first medical theorists who linked personality with depression. Four hundred years before the birth of Christ, he described four "humors," or basic bodily fluids, that determined temperament: blood, black bile, yellow bile, and phlegm. Black bile was associated with melancholic temperament, the substrate from which depression arose. In the intervening centuries many clinical theorists have attempted to improve upon the Hipprocratic formulation, and we summarize current approaches to personality and depression in this chapter.

This chapter presents a selected review of the literature on the role of personality in depression, focusing on the extent to which research findings support a relationship between specific traits and the development, nature, and course of depressive disorders.

Approaches to the Relationship between Personality and Depression

Predispositional Approach

The "predispositional approach" refers to the notion that certain personality characteristics are antecedent to depressive disorders and render the individual vulnerable to depression under certain conditions. This approach has predominated in both theory and research.

Subclinical Approach

The "subclinical approach" considers certain personality characteristics to be milder manifestations of affective disorders. According to this approach, such personality types and depressive syndromes are expressions of the same underlying genetic endowment. Thus, certain enduring behavioral patterns (e.g., cyclothymia) are considered to be part of a continuum that at one end does not differ perceivably from normality and at the other is the full-blown depressive syndrome. In contrast to the predispositional approach, which includes both inherited and acquired traits, the subclinical approach focuses only on inherited traits.

Pathoplasty Approach

The "pathoplasty approach" leaves pathogenesis aside, proposing instead that personality characteristics affect the symptomatic expression and course of the depressive episode. Thus, certain personality "types" may be associated with specific depressive symptom profiles and may influence outcome and course.

Complication Approach

A final view of the relationship between personality and depression is the "complication approach," perhaps the mirror image of the predisposition approach. According to the complication approach, the experience of depressive disorder influences personality. Changes in personality result from the experience of the depressive episode, particularly when the episode is severe and protracted. Such changes in personality may include changes in a person's perception of self and the environment, and/or in the person's style of interacting with others.

Note that, although differing in their emphases, these four approaches are not mutually exclusive. Nor do these views necessarily exhaust the range of ways in which personality and depression may relate to each other (Akiskal, Hirschfeld, & Yerevanian, 1983).

Methodological Issues

We are still far from a clear understanding of the nature of the relationship between personality and depression, despite the large volume of literature that has been amassed on the topic. This is largely due to several substantive methodological problems that characterize much of the research in the area. These problems, which compromise the reliability, validity, and generalizability of reported results, may be grouped into three general categories: specificity of patient samples; specificity of independent and dependent variables; and the effect of clinical state on assessment of personality.

Patient Characteristics

Clinical depression comprises a vast, heterogeneous group of mental disorders, with different etiologies, treatments, and clinical courses. Most clinical populations contain varying mixtures of these groups. Accordingly, the role of personality may differ substantially among different affective subtypes. In some, certain personality features may predispose individuals to the depression, while in others, personality features may be irrelevant. Unfortunately, our ability to differentiate among these subtypes is limited, and in much of the literature no attempt has been made to do so. This has resulted in combining of "apples and oranges," and consequently in inconsistent findings.

In this regard, while identification of such major subtypes as bipolar I and II, unipolar, melancholic, and the like has of late become standard practice in scientific reports, "double depression" is yet another category of depressive disorders that merits consideration in study samples for personality research. "Double depression" refers to a acute depressive episode superimposed on a pre-existing chronic depression. A recent study on the phenomenon suggests that patients with such disorders differ from those without in terms of their recovery and relapse rates (Keller & Shapiro, 1982). The relevance of the "double depression" diagnosis for the personality researcher lies in the heterogeneity of the category itself and the imprecision it may contribute to the study design. Within the framework of our four hypotheses, double depressions may be"predispositional" (depressive character predisposed to depressive episodes), "subclinical" (subaffective dysthymia vulnerable to depressive disorder), or a "complication" (personality modified by the experience). Unless premorbid personality assessments are available, this issue cannot be resolved, nor can an accurate determination of recovery status be made. Therefore, patients with such disorders are best either excluded from personality investigations or made the major focus of study.

Sex and age are two other characteristics whose distributions in patient samples have frequently been ignored. The results of personality studies may vary considerably if the sex ratios and age ranges of the research samples differ, since both of these factors affect personality attributes. Sound methodology requires not only that samples be adequately described with regard to these variables, but also that their influence be taken into account experimentally and/or statistically.

Assessment Issues

A second methodological problem area that has hampered personality research concerns the specificity with which the variables are defined and measured. Two issues are relevant: (1) the need for operational criteria to define both depressive disorders and personality characteristics; and (2) the need for objective and reliable measures of depressive disorders and personality characteristics.

A necessary first step in reducing unwanted variance and increasing homogeneity in research samples is to use operational criteria for defining all important variables. This is true for both depression and personality. Terms such as "neurotic depression," "orality," and "extraversion" mean different things to different people. Unless agreed-upon definitions for these and other variables are given operational formulation, study findings will be inconsistent and uninterpretable, and cross-study comparisons will be impossible.

Related to the need for operational criteria is the need for reliable measures of depressive disorders and personality characteristics, obtained under objective conditions. Reliable and standardized instruments to assess personality and to diagnose and subtype depression help to ensure replicability of research findings. Blind, independent ratings performed according to standard procedures minimize the possibility of biased, invalid assessment. Together, these elements of sound methodology facilitate the interpretation and understanding of study results by providing objective, reliable, and valid reflections of operationally defined variables.

Clinical Status

A final methodological problem that is related to the reliability and validity of assessments is the need for minimizing bias in personality assessment by reducing the influence of the depressive state on trait measurement. It has been well documented that depressed patients do not provide valid reports of their premorbid functioning but rather distort their views of themselves and their situation (Hirschfeld, Klerman, Clayton, Keller, MacDonald-Scott, *et al.*, 1983; Liebowitz, Stallone, Dunner, & Fieve, 1979). For example, in a recent study by Hirschfeld, Klerman, Clayton, Keller, MacDonald-Scott, *et al.* (1983), patients' scores on self-report personality inventories assessed during a depressive episode were compared with their scores on the same inventories after full recovery 1 year later. Clinical state was found to influence markedly personality scores reflecting emotional strength, interpersonal dependency, and extraversion. During the morbid period, patients rated themselves as significantly more neurotic, dependent, and introverted than they did when their depression had abated. These differences emerged despite test instructions to the patients while they were depressed that they respond according to their "usual" selves. Findings such as these underscore the need to obtain personality ratings from patients during an intermorbid, symptom-free period in order to ensure their reliability and validity.

PERSONALITY TRAITS

In the following pages, personality attributes are discussed that have received the greatest amount of attention from theorists and researchers. These include psychoanalytic personality patterns, interpersonal dependency, neuroticism, extraversion-introversion, social skills deficits, dysfunctional cognitive styles, cyclothymia, and dysthymic personality. The discussion of each trait includes a summary of its conceptual roots and a description of a representative sample of available measures for the trait. Because of the methodological issues that have been discussed, only studies that meet the following criteria are included: (1) clear delineation of the sample; (2) well-specified criteria for diagnosing depression; and (3) objective and reliable assessments of personality obtained during an intermorbid, symptom-free period.

Psychoanalytic Personality Patterns

Definition and Conceptual Roots

Much of the research on the role of personality in depression is an outgrowth of the psychoanalytic viewpoint that oral and obsessive personality patterns are the characterological underpinnings of depression.

The predispositional relationship of orality and obsessionality to depression was originally proposed by Abraham (1948). Although he stressed obsessionality in his early writings (likening the personalities of depressives to those of obsessional neurotics), a focus on oral characteristics emerged in his later papers. Abraham hypothesized that vulnerability to depression arose from emotional difficulties during the oral phase of psychosexual development. These difficulties generally took the form of withdrawal of maternal love from the infant. This led to a fixation of emotional development at the oral stage, and a resultant exaggeration of oral personality traits and marked susceptibility to depressive episodes following loss experiences.

The emphasis on orality in depression has been maintained by psychodynamic theorists. In gaining its predominance, however, the original psychosexual, libido-centered definition of "orality" has undergone modification. As currently used, the concept more broadly refers to exaggerated needs for affection and support coupled with excessive dependency on others for emotional gratification and maintenance of self-esteem (Chodoff, 1972).

Psychoanalytic personality patterns have also been linked to different depressive symptom patterns. Thus, an obsessional premorbid personality would lead to obsessional symptoms during depression (e.g., guilt, worry, anxiety), whereas an hysterical personality would be associated with histrionic symptoms (e.g., irritability, emotional lability).

Although psychodynamic theories have provided rich clinical descriptions of the personalities of depressives and have generated hypotheses concerning their psychogenic etiology, little systematic research has been conducted to test the validity of these theories. Most psychodynamic formulations, as well as the evidence offered as support for them, are based on unsystematic observations of limited samples of patients during their depressive illness.

Moreover, depression has most often been treated as a unitary entity in these reports.

Measures

The Lazare-Klerman-Armor Personality Inventory (LKA), developed in 1966, was designed to provide a reliable, valid, and efficient assessment of the traits associated with oral, obsessive, and hysterical personality patterns (Lazare, Klerman, & Armor, 1966). It is a self-report inventory composed of 139 items, which the respondent rates as "true" or "false" (see Table 11-1). When summed, these items yield scores on 20 factors. A short version comprising 60 items has been developed that also yields scores on the three patterns.

Research Findings

Two studies have been conducted that assess the role of psychoanalytic personality patterns in depression using the LKA. In the Clinical Studies component of the National Institute of Mental Health (NIMH) Collaborative Program on the Psychobiology of Depression, a battery of personality inventories, including the LKA, was administered to a group of carefully diagnosed primary nonbipolar depressed women when they were completely symptom-free (Hirschfeld, Klerman, Clayton, & Keller, 1983). Their personality scores were compared to those of two other groups: (1) female relatives who had also fully recovered from a depressive illness of the same type, and (2) other female relatives who had no history of psychiatric disorder ("never-ill" group). Both groups of recovered depressives scored signficantly higher on the LKA

TABLE 11-1 Scales Assessing Psychoanalytic Patterns and Interpersonal Dependency

Trait/scale name	Number of items	Item format	Name of inventory
LKA Inventory			
Orality	20	True-false	Lazare-Klerman-Armor Personality Inventory (LKA)
Obsessionality	20	True-false	LKA
Hysteria	20	True-false	LKA
IDI Inventory			
Emotional Reliance on Another Person	16	4-point Likert scale	Interpersonal Dependency Inventory (IDI)
Lack of Social Self-Confidence	16	4-point Likert scale	IDI
Assertion of Autonomy	16	4-point Likert scale	IDI

Orality subscale than did the never-ill group. No differences in obsessionality or hysteria were observed among the groups.

In a study designed to assess the relationship between personality characteristics and depressive symptoms, Paykel and his colleagues (Paykel, Klerman, & Prusoff, 1976) administered the LKA as well as other personality inventories to a large group of depressed patients after clinical improvement. Personality scores were compared to symptom ratings obtained during the depressive episode. It was found that a more neurotic, as opposed to endogenous, symptom picture was associated with higher Orality and lower Obsessionality scores. In addition, patients with higher Hysteria scores tended to be viewed as less severely depressed and tended to show greater irritability and less anxiety than patients with lower scores.

Interpersonal Dependency

Definition and Conceptual Roots

The concept of interpersonal dependency has been a major focus in predispositional theories of depression. "Interpersonal dependency" refers to a complex of thoughts, beliefs, feelings, and behaviors involving the need to form and maintain supportive attachments and to associate closely with valued others (Hirschfeld, Klerman, Chodoff, Korchin, & Barrett, 1976). This formulation has been influenced by three theories: (1) the psychoanalytic theory of object relations; (2) the ethological theory of attachment; and (3) the social learning theory's view of dependency as a learned drive.

Describing the role of dependency and attachment in infant development, the psychoanalytic theory of object relations postulates that the infant develops mental representations of the mother and other significant persons/objects. These mental representations constitute internalizations of the infant's attachment to these "objects." During periods of separation, the infant/child learns to call upon these internalizations for reassurance that the bond to the mother still exists (object constancy). These internalizations continue their supportive role throughout the period of emotional development and ultimately give meaning to objective reality, cue emotional responses, and provide emotional protection in later separations (Fenichel, 1945).

In ethological theory, the concept of "attachment" refers to the genetically based affectional bond that is formed between mother and infant and through which other social bonds to specific persons are formed. Attachment bonds provide the opportunity for learning, social communication, and group interactions (Bowlby, 1969).

From a standpoint of social learning theory, dependency is considered a class of help-seeking and affiliative behaviors acquired through early mother-infant experiences. Since these behaviors arise from the infant's need to satisfy primary drives (e.g., hunger, thirst), dependency becomes a secondary drive and subsequently generalizes to interpersonal relationships in general.

Excessive interpersonal dependency has been implicated in the predisposition to depression. Thus, depression-prone persons have been characterized as inordinately dependent on others for support and approval to maintain their self-esteem and obtain emotional gratification. According to this view, loss of support or approval leads to a fall in self-esteem and ensuing depression (Chodoff, 1972).

The "undue" interpersonal dependency thought to characterize the depression-prone person is generally considered to have its roots in the primary caretaker-infant relationship, whether this is described in psychoanalytic, ethological, or social learning theory terms. Within the framework of psychoanalytic theory, disruptions in the development of object constancy can lead to marked dependency on others for support, approval, and reassurance, and a predisposition to depression following (or when threatened by) "object loss." Similarly, in terms of ethological theory, early separations can cause disruptions in maternal-infant attachment bonding, in turn producing emotional and behavioral disruptions. Finally, according to the viewpoint of social learning theory, excessive dependency may result from any number of early experiences—for example, a high-ratio partial-reinforcement schedule (as in the case of the compulsive gambler), a high rate of success in obtaining reinforcement through dependency behavior, or a lack of alternative behaviors to secure reinforcement.

Measures

The Interpersonal Dependency Inventory (IDI) was specifically designed to measure interpersonal dependency in adults after a review of existing inventories revealed none to assess the concept fully and adequately (Hirschfeld *et al.*, 1977). The 48-item self-report instrument consists of three empirically derived scales reflecting different components of interpersonal dependency (see Table 11-1). The Emotional Reliance on Another Person scale reflects wishes for contact with and emotional support from specific other persons and a dread of loss of those persons. In addition, the scale reflects wishes for general approval and attention from others. The Lack of Social Self-Confidence scale assesses wishes for help in decision making, in social situations, and in taking initiative. Assertion of Autonomy, in contrast to the other two scales, reflects preferences for independent behavior and being alone, and the conviction that the person's self-esteem does not depend on approval from others.

Research Findings

In a comparison of IDI scores from recovered primary nonbipolar depressed women patients, recovered primary nonbipolar depressed women relatives, and never-ill women relatives, Hirschfeld, Klerman, Clayton, and Keller (1983) found Emotional Reliance on Another Person and Lack of Social Self-Confidence to differ significantly among the three groups. Both groups of recovered depressives had higher scores on Emotional Reliance on Another Person than did the never-ill group, whereas the recovered patient group had higher Lack of Social Self-Confidence scores than either relative group. No differences emerged on Assertion of Autonomy.

In a second study of interpersonal dependency, Pilowsky and Katsikitis (1983) compared the scores of nonendogenous depressives, endogenous depressives, and nondepressed psychiatric patients obtained at hospital discharge. Only Lack of Social Self-Confidence differentiated among the groups, with nonendogenous depressives scoring significantly higher on this scale than nondepressives. No differences were found between the two depressed groups on any of the scales.

Neuroticism and Introversion-Extraversion

Definition and Conceptual Roots

Although the concepts of orality and dependency have historically received primary emphasis in predispositional theories of depression, neuroticism and introversion-extraversion have been most frequently studied in personality research in depression. This may be due to the relatively long-standing availability of reliable measures of these traits — Eysenck's Maudsley Personality Inventory (MPI; Eysenck, 1962) and its revision, the Eysenck Personality Inventory (EPI; Eysenck & Eysenck, 1964).

According to Eysenck's general dimensions theory, "neuroticism" refers to emotional lability and overresponsivity. Individuals who are excessively neurotic tend to have a variety of somatic disturbances (e.g., headaches, insomnia, indigestion) and to be worrisome, anxious, and gloomy. Under stress such persons are prone to neurotic disorders, although high neuroticism is not necessarily indicative of inadequate functioning.

The concept of "introversion" derives from the work of C. G. Jung and others, and refers to a complex of "inner-directed" traits, including being reserved, introspective, cautious, serious, and controlled. The introverted person is likely to be quiet, to enjoy a well-ordered life, to be dependable and nonaggressive, and to place great value on maintaining high ethical standards. This behavioral pattern is in contrast to that of the extravert, who is outgoing, sociable, impulsive, and uninhibited. Extraverts enjoy taking part in social and group activites, tend to be risk takers, and are optimistic, aggressive, and quick-tempered.

The extraversion-introversion dimension is comprised of three components: sociability, restraint, and thoughtfulness. "Sociability" refers to an individual's predilection for and comfort with situations involving other people. "Restraint" refers to the degree that someone controls his or her impulses.

TABLE 11-2 Scales Assessing Emotional Strength and General Neuroticism

Scale name	Number of items	Item format	Name of inventory
Neuroticism	24	Yes-no	Maudsley Personality Inventory (MPI)
Neuroticism	24	Yes-no	Eysenck Personality Inventory (EPI)
Emotional Stability	30	Yes-no	Guilford-Zimmerman Temperament Survey (GZTS)
Ego Resiliency	40[a]	True-false	Minnesota Multiphasic Personality Inventory (MMPI)

[a] Two items overlap with the MMPI Ego Control scale.

"Thoughtfulness" refers to the degree of a person's reflectiveness and interest in other's motives.

As formulated by Eysenck (1964), neuroticism-stability and introversion-extraversion represent two general and orthogonal dimensions of personality that can be used to distinguish two different types of psychopathological individuals: "extraverted neurotics," who include hysterics and psychopaths; and "introverted neurotics," who include dysthymics, anxiety neurotics, and obssessive-compulsives. Thus, depressives would be expected to have premorbid personalities characterized by high levels of neuroticism and introversion.

Measures

Various inventories have been developed to measure neuroticism and introversion-extraversion (see Tables 11-2 and 11-3). The MPI is a 48-item self-report inventory developed by Eysenck to reflect his conceptualizations of the neuroticism-stability and introversion-extraversion dimensions. Each dimension is measured by 24-items, which are rated as true-false. Although viewed as orthogonal personality dimensions, subsequent research using the MPI revealed a slight negative correlation between the Neuroticism (N) and

TABLE 11-3 Scales Assessing Introversion-Extraversion

Scale name	Number of items	Item format	Name of inventory
Extraversion	24	Yes-no	MPI
Extraversion	24	Yes-no	EPI
Restraint	30	Yes-no	GZTS
Thoughtfulness	30	Yes-no	GZTS
Sociability	30	Yes-no	GZTS
Ego Control	32	True-false	MMPI

Extraversion (E) scales. This led to the construction of the EPI, a revised version of the MPI. The EPI's design and item number and content differ little from the earlier version. The EPI, however, includes a nine-item Lie scale, which reflects the extent to which a respondent is attempting to portray himself or herself in a good light rather than providing accurate information.

The Guilford-Zimmerman Temperament Survey (GZTS; Guilford & Zimmerman, 1949) predated the Eysenck inventories, and many of the Eysenck items are modifications of those in the GZTS. The GZTS is a self-report inventory consisting of 10 trait scales, each containing 30 items (300 items total). Items are rated yes-no and summed to yield a score for each trait. The Emotional Stability scale is virtually identical to the MPI N scale, although scored in the opposite direction (i.e., low scorces are indicative of neurotic tendencies). Items assess the evenness of moods, optimism, and composure. Three scales are generally reflective of introversion-extraversion. Items on the Sociability scale relate to having friends, enjoying social activities, and seeking contact with others. The Thoughtfulness scale measures reflectiveness, being an observer rather than a doer, and being inner-directed. Finally, the Restraint scale reflects serious-mindedness, self-control, and inhibition.

Neuroticism and introversion measures have also been derived for the Minnesota Multiphasic Personality Inventory (MMPI) by Block (1965). The Ego Resiliency scale consists of 40 items, rated true-false by the respondent, assessing general emotional health and adaptability. Low scores on this scale are indicative of rigidity, general maladjustment, and susceptibility to anxiety. The Ego Control scale is composed of 32 true-false items that reflect impulse control. High scores are indicative of impulsivity, inability to delay gratification, and emotional lability, whereas low scores reflect emotional constriction, inhibition, and aloofness.

Research Findings

Several recent studies have examined neuroticism and introversion in euthymic depressed patients, using one of Eysenck's inventories. Benjaminsen (1981) compared EPI scores in three groups of recovered depressed patients: primary endogenous, primary nonendogenous, and secondary with a primary diagnosis of neurotic disorder. Nonendogenous patients were found to have significantly higher N scores and lower E scores than endogenous patients. Secondary depressives were intermediate in introversion, differing significantly from neither of the other two groups, but were significantly more neurotic than either of the primary depressed groups.

The nonendogenous and, to some extent, the secondary depressives were more introverted than the norm. The endogenous depressives had scores very close to the norm on the E scale. The endogenous group again scored close to the norm for neuroticism on the N scale, whereas both the nonendogenous and secondary depressives scored within the neurotic range. Unipolar and bipolar endogenous depressives did not differ on either the N or the E scale.

The nonendogenous and secondary depressives were significantly more introverted than the bipolar but not the unipolar depressed patients. Secondary depressives were more neurotic than both endogenous groups but did not differ from them in introversion. The bipolar endogenous group scored within the normal range on both the N and the E scales, while endogenous unipolars were normal on the N scale but slightly introverted.

Bech *et al.* (1980) compared EPI scores in bipolar and nonbipolar melancholic patients. Consistent with Benjaminsen's results, Bech *et al.* found no difference on either N or E scores between the groups. The N scores of both groups were in the normal range. The nonbipolars, but not the bipolars, scored somewhat in the introverted range on the E scale.

Liebowitz *et al.* (1979) also assessed N and E scores in bipolar and nonbipolar endogenous patients using the MPI. As in the two studies just described, these investigators found no differences between the two groups on either measure. And, again, they obtained a pattern consistent with those of Benjaminsen (1981) and Bech *et al.* (1980) in normative comparisons.

Finally, Hirschfeld Klerman, Clayton, and Keller (1983) also compared MPI, GZTS, and MMPI scale scores in their three patient and relative groups, as previously described. Both groups of recovered nonbipolar depressed women scored significantly higher on all neuroticism measures and on the MPI and GZTS (Sociability) introversion measures than did their never-ill women relatives. In normative comparisons, however, it was found that neither of the previously depressed groups differed from the norm on the measures of neuroticism. Rather, the never-ill group scored significantly lower than the norm on these measures. On the measures of introversion, all three study groups scored above the norm, with the difference being most pronounced in the two groups of recovered depressives.

The MPI has also been used to study the relationship between neuroticism and introversion and the symptom pattern in and course of depressive episodes. Paykel *et al.* (1976), in their comparison of symptom ratings and MPI scores in a large groups of depressed patients, found that high N scores (obtained after clinical improvement) were associated with a more neurotic (as opposed to endogenous) symptom pattern.

In a study designed to investigate personality attributes as predictors of outcome, M. M. Weissman, Prusoff, and Klerman (1978) obtained symptom ratings and MPI scores in a group of nonmelancholic depressed women at 1, 8, 20, and 48 months following initiation of treatment. These investigators found 1-month MPI N scores to be the best predictor of outcome, as determined by symptom levels at each assessment period. Those patients who remained chronically symptomatic at follow-up had the highest initial N scores, while those considered asymptomatic for the entire follow-up period had the lowest initial N scores (these being in the normal range).

Social Skills Deficits: Definitions and Formulation

Although problems in interpersonal interactions are generally considered a key clinical feature in depressive disorders, Lewinsohn (1974) has proposed that such problems arise from the depressive's lack of social skills, and, moreover, that these deficits are an important antecedent condition in the disorder. "Social skills" refers to a class of behaviors involving social interactions that elicit reinforcement from others. Social skills deficits seen in depression include such characteristics as discomfort in social situations, a low rate of emitted positive responses, and heightened responsivity to negative responses from others.

Lewinsohn contends that a decrease in response-contingent positive reinforcement (i.e., a decrease in pleasant events or an increase in unpleasant events) leads to dysphoria and self-blame—two central aspects of depression. This being the case, an individual lacking in social skills would be at greater risk for depression, due to his or her already low rate of response-contingent reinforcement. Lewinsohn suggests further that once depressive behaviors occur, positive reinforcement in the form of sympathy, attention, and concern may lead them to escalate to the level of clinical depression. Youngren and Lewinsohn (1980) have conducted studies demonstrating that depressed persons are lacking in social skills, relative to nondepressed persons. However, since no studies have investigated social skills in remitted depressives, the antecedant or "trait" as opposed to "state" nature of these behaviors has yet to be shown.

Cognitive Style

According to cognitive theories of depression, depressive affect and behavior are secondary to dysfunctional cognitive style. That is, disturbances in thought content and processes are characteristics that predispose individuals to depression and are central to and typical of all depressive disorders. The two most prominant cognitive theories are Beck's theory of dysfunctional attitudes (e.g., Kovacs & Beck, 1978) and Seligman's reformulated learned helplessness model (e.g., Abramson, Seligman, & Teasdale, 1978).

Beck's Theory

Definitions and Formulation. Beck theorizes that depression results from the activation of specific cognitive schemas that are characteristic of depression-prone persons. "Schemas" are cognitive templates for screening, coding, assimilating, and responding to internal and external stimuli, and are derived from early experiences. "Depressogenic" schemas relate specifically to experiences concerning self-evaluation and interpersonal relationships. Once they have become activated by some stressor, these schemas lead depression-prone persons to an unrealistically negative and demeaning view of themselves, the world, and the future (the "negative cognitive triad"). These views, or "negative automatic thoughts," are associated with four systematic errors in logic:

1. Arbitrary inference — drawing conclusions in the absence of or contrary to the evidence.
2. Selective abstraction — focusing on those elements of a situation that are most consistent with the person's negative view of self and world, and ignoring other salient elements.
3. Magnification of negative events or faults and minimization of positive events, attributes, and accomplishments.
4. Overgeneralization — basing far-reaching conclusions on single, minor experiences or incidents.

Thus, according to Beck's theory, the thinking of a depression-prone person is characterized by erroneous and exaggerated negative views of self and experiences. These maladaptive attitudes — basic premises or "silent assumptions" — represent vulnerability factors for depression and are considered a facet of personality. Negative automatic thoughts, on the other hand, form part of the depressive symptom picture and are considered state characteristics.

Measures. Two questionnaires have been developed to assess aspects of cognitive style described by Beck (see Table 11-4). The Dysfunctional Attitude Scale (DAS) is a 40-item self-report inventory developed by A. N. Weissman (1979) in collaboration with Beck to provide a measure of the extent to which persons hold maladaptive beliefs specific to depression. The DAS contains statements that reflect both adaptive and dysfunctional attitudes, rated on a 7-point scale from "totally agree" to "totally disagree."

The Automatic Thoughts Questionnaire (ATQ; Hollon & Kendall, 1980). Is a 30-item self-report questionnaire that measures the frequency of occurence of negative self-statements (e.g., "I am worthless") associated with depression.

TABLE 11-4 Scales Assessing Cognitive Style

Trait/scale name	Number of items	Item format	Name of inventory
Dysfunctional Attitudes	40	7-point Likert scale based on agreement	Dysfunctional Attitude Scale (DAS)
Negative Automatic Thoughts	30	5-point scale based on frequency	Automatic Thoughts Questionnaire (ATQ)
Internality Stability Globality Importance	12 hypothetical situations, rated on each of the four scales	7-point Likert scale for degree of intensity	Attributional Style Questionnaire (ASQ)

Items are rated for occurrence during the preceding week on a 5-point scale ranging from "not at all" to "all the time". The ATQ score represents a summation of the 30 item ratings (range 30-150).

Research Findings. Although several outcome studies have been conducted that demonstrate the efficacy of the therapeutic techniques derived from Beck's theory, until recently no empirical evidence had been offered to support the predispositional validity of his model in asymptomatic, clinically depressed populations.

Two studies have recently appeared in the literature that have assessed dysfunctional attitudes in recovered depressed patients using the DAS. Eaves and Rush (1984) administered the DAS and the ATQ to groups of endogenous depressed and nonendogenous depressed patients and nondepressed control subjects. All three groups were tested at two time periods: the depressed groups when symptomatic and when recovered, and the matched controls at equivalently spaced time periods.

As expected, symptomatic patients had significantly more dysfunctional attitudes and more automatic negative thoughts than did control subjects and showed a significant reduction in these attitudes and thoughts with remission. Even in recovery, however, depressed patients continued to show more negatively biased attitudes than controls. Neither the DAS scores nor the ATQ scores of control subjects changed over time, nor did those of unrecovered depressed patients. Endogenous and nonendogenous depressives did not differ in their DAS or their ATQ scores, either when symptomatic or asymptomatic.

Silverman, Silverman, and Eardley (1984) compared the DAS scores of nonbipolar depressed outpatients when depressed and again when asymptomatic to those of recovered bipolar depressives, schizophrenics, schizoaffective patients, and other (nonorganic, nonpsychotic, nonaffective) psychiatric patients. In the nonbipolar depressives, recovery was associated with a significant reduction in DAS scores. When compared to the DAS "normative" sample, the depressed group actually had slightly lower DAS scores than the norm. Comparisons of the DAS scores of the five recovered psychiatric groups revealed the following low-to-high ranking: bipolar, nonbipolar, schizoaffective, other, and schizophrenic. The bipolar group had significantly fewer dysfunctional attitudes than any other group, while the nonbipolar group had significantly fewer such attitudes than both the other and the schizophrenic groups.

In a prospective study designed to determine whether dysfunctional attitudes — the "negative cognitive triad" — precede, accompany, and/or follow depressive episodes, Lewinsohn, Steinmetz, Larson, and Franklin (1981) measured depressive cognitions in a large community sample that was followed for 1 year. Subjects who were depressed at the time of initial assessment showed depressive cognitions as expected. Those subjects who were not depressed at the time of assessment but who became depressed during the follow-up period did not differ from nondepressed controls in cognitive style. Moreover, subjects who had a history of depression but who were not depressed at the time of assessment did not differ from nondepressed controls. Depressive cognitions were, however, somewhat predictive of course, in that depressed subjects with more depressed cognitions were more likely to remain depressed for the duration of the study period. This study did not use the DAS.

Learned Helplessness

Definitions and Formulations. As originally formulated, the learned helplessness theory of depression proposed that a variety of organisms show cognitive, motivational, and emotional deficits—which parallel the phenomenon of depression in humans—following experiences with uncontrollable events (Seligman, 1975). This model of depression was based on Seligman's laboratory experiments with dogs, in which the animals were exposed to inescapable electric shock. When subsequently put into a learning situation requiring the simple act of crossing a barrier to terminate electric shock, the dogs evidenced what Seligman termed "learned helplessness": They made few attempts to escape the shock (motivational deficit); were unlikely to repeat successful responses (cognitive deficit), and showed little overt reactivity to the shock (emotional deficit).

This phenomenon was interpreted by Seligman in cognitive terms. What the dogs learned in the shock exposure situation was that shocks (outcomes) were independent of responses, and this "expectation" of response-outcome independence generalized to novel situations, resulting in the "learned helplessness" deficits.

Although originally proposed in this form as a model for human depression, the learned helplessness theory has since been revised along attribution theory lines in order to account for the generality and chronicity of and self-esteem loss in depression (e.g., Abramson *et al.*, 1978). The reformulated learned helplessness theory proposes that the individual's interpretation of negative events determines whether the occurrence of such events will produce depression. According to the reformulation, particular causal explanations produce depression following negative events: (1) that the cause is internal (something about the person) rather than external (something about the situation); (2) that the cause is a factor that is stable (will persist over time) rather than unstable (transient); or (3) that the cause is global (affects a wide range of areas of living) rather than specific (limited to this certain event).

Each of these three causal dimensions is thought to affect a specific aspect of depressive symptomatology. Internal causal explanations produce a loss of self-esteem following the occurrence of bad events, whereas external explanations do not. Stable causal explanations produce chronic depressive symptoms following the occurrence of bad events, whereas unstable explanations produce short-lived depressive reactions. Global causal explanations produce pervasive depressive symptoms following bad events, whereas specific explanations produce circumscribed depressive symptoms.

Within the framework of this theory, the above-described explanatory style represents a risk factor for depression, not a sufficient cause. Rather, it is the expectation that no actions will affect future outcomes that is a sufficient condition for depressive symptoms (with the exception of loss of self-esteem). Because this expectation is influenced both by the individual's explanatory style and by the reality of the situation, depressive symptoms can occur and be pervasive and long-lasting without stable and global causal explanations. In such case, the consequences (outcomes) of the bad events are stable and global, although the causes may be unstable and specific. Thus, knowledge of an individual's explanatory style can predict depression in the face of bad events, but the occurrence of depression is not necessarily indicative of a person's explanatory style.

Measures. The Attributional Style Questionnaire (ASQ) was recently developed to measure differences in the use of internal versus external, stable versus unstable, and global versus specific causal explanations (Peterson *et al.*, 1982). The form consists of 12 hypothetical situations (6 good, 6 bad), each of which the subject is asked to imagine vividly and to state what its major cause would have been had it happened to him or her. The subject then rates the cause along internal, stable, and global dimensions. Scores for each dimension, as well as a composite, are computed separately for good and bad events by summing over items and taking the mean.

Research Findings. The use of internal, stable, and global causes to explain bad events, as assessed by the ASQ, has been found to correlate with levels of depressive symptoms in a college student population (e.g., Seligman, Abramson, Semmel, & von Baeyer, 1979). In addition, the use of such causes to explain bad events had been found to be characteristic of endogenous and nonendogenous depressed male patients, but not male medical-surgical or inpatient schizophrenic comparison groups; it has also been found to correlate with the duration and frequency of past depressive episodes (e.g., Raps, Peterson, Reinhard, Abramson, & Seligman, 1982).

Only one study to date, however, has used the ASQ to examine attributional style in asymptomatic depressed patients. Eaves and Rush (1984), in their study of endogenous and nonendogenous depressed patients and nondepressed control subjects, administered the ASQ to patients when symptomatic and when recovered and to matched controls at two equivalently spaced times. Both when symptomatic and when recovered, depressed patients used internal, stable, and global causes to explain bad events to a significantly greater degree than did control subjects. No change in ASQ scores were associated with recovery.

In their prospective longitudinal study of cognitive characteristics associated with depression, Lewinsohn *et al.* (1981) assessed internal attributional style in their community sample. As was the case for dysfunctional attitudes, an internal attributional style was found to be neither antecedent to nor a consequence of a depressive episode. Furthermore, no differences in attributional style were found in comparisions of depressed and nondepressed subjects. Again, however, it should be noted that no standard measure of attributional style was used.

Cyclothymia

Definition and Conceptual Roots

"Cyclothymia" refers to a behavioral pattern consisting of recurring and often alternating periods of elation and depression that do not appear to be accounted for by environmental circumstances. Elated periods are characterized by high energy, optimism, enthusiasm, sociability, impulsivity, and ambitious driveness. Depressed periods, in contrast, are characterized by low energy, pessimism, worry, withdrawal, and brooding. Cyclothymic temperament is generally considered to be an attenuated form of bipolar depressive disorder, as well as a predispositional factor in the disorder. That is, a trait-state continuum has been hypothesized to exist between the two, with both the temperament and the disorder representing expressions of the same genetic or constitutional factor.

Kraepelin (1921) was among the first writers to describe cyclothymia. He wrote of four affective personalities—depressive, manic, irritable (mixed), and cyclothymic (circular)—each of which was viewed as the temperamental basis for clinical forms of affective illness. Cyclothymia was considered by Kraepelin to be the temperamental substrate for manic-depressive psychosis. Kretschmer (1936) subsequently combined Kraepelin's four affective temperaments into a unitary cyclothymic personality, considered by him to be the precursor to manic-depressive illness as well. He proposed that within this type of temperament, balanced cycloids, hypomanic cycloids (predominantly elated), and depressed cycloids (predominantly depressed) could be identified on the basis of the pattern and frequency of elated versus depressive mood shifts.

Measures

The General Behavior Inventory (GBI) has recently been developed by Depue *et al.* (1981) as a first-stage screening instrument for cyclothymia (see Table 11-5). The design of the GBI is based on the continuity assumption. That is, cyclothymia is considered to be qualitatively similar to but quantitatively less severe than bipolar depressive disorder in terms of its episodic characteristics (intensity, duration, and rapid shifts) and core behaviors (e.g.,

TABLE 11-5 Scales Assessing Cyclothymia and Dysthymia

Trait	Scale name	Number of items	Item format	Name of inventory
Cyclothymia	Hypomanic	21	4-point scale	General Behavior Inventory (GBI)
	Biphasic	7	4-point scale	GBI
Dysthymia	Depressive	46	4-point scale	GBI

disturbances of mood, psychomotor, sleep, appetite, etc.). Items have been selected, therefore, to emphasize behavioral, somatic, and vegetative symptoms highly characteristic of and specific to bipolar disorder. These have been balanced for depressive-phase and hypomanic-phase behaviors.

Items are phrased to emphasize characteristics of the process of bipolar disorder in terms of the intensity, duration, and rapid shift of core behaviors. Finally, a 4-point item rating scale has been chosen to emphasize the frequency of occurrence of various symptoms, and, moreover, has been constructed to differentiate cases clearly from noncases (binomial model). That is, taking intensity, duration, and frequency into account, "normal" individuals can experience various items/symptoms "hardly ever" (a rating of 1) or "sometimes" (a rating of 2), but will be highly unlikely to experience them "often" (a rating of 3) or "very often" (a rating of 4). Only items rated 3 or 4 are included in the total score. Thus, the GBI rating represents the number of symptoms out of 69 possible endorsed by the respondent at a subsyndromal cyclothymic level. This ensures that the inclusion of false positives in the cyclothymic population identified by the GBI will be minimized.

Research Findings

Research on the relationship between cyclothymic temperament and depression differs in design from the studies of specific personality traits described previously. "Trait" investigations involve the measurement and comparison of specific characteristics in an identified depressed group and nondepressed controls (be they "normals" or psychiatric patients). Whether prospective or retrospective in nature, these studies are aimed at finding between-group differences in levels of the personality trait, such that the trait may be viewed as a predisposing factor in depression. Cyclothymia research, on the other hand, has generally focused on demonstrating similarities in characteristics between identified cyclothymic subjects and, most often, an identified bipolar depressed group in order to obtain support for a genetic continuum. Commonalities in such variables as family history of affective disorder, biochemical measures, clinical history, and manifestations are those most frequently reported.

Until recently, all investigations of cyclothymia have relied on a clinical interview and diagnosis for case identification (Akiskal, Djenderdejian, Rosenthal, & Khani, 1977; Akiskal, Khani, & Scott-Strauss, 1979). Since such samples are invariably drawn from psychiatric patient populations and are thus more extreme and impaired cases, results obtained in these studies may not be generalizable.

However, the results of several GBI validation studies conducted by Depue and his associates (1981) on both nonclinical and clinical populations both confirm and extend previous reports based on diagnosed cyclothymics, in that the diagnostic, clinical, familial, and biological characteristics associated with cyclothymia were found to resemble closely those of bipolar depressives. A relatively homogeneous symptom pattern, quite similar to the diagnostic criteria for hypomania and major depressive disorder set forth in the Research Diagnostic Criteria (RDC), was found in the cyclothymic cases. In addition, psychomotor retardation and hypersomnia, the best behavioral discriminators of bipolar depression, were highly characteristic of the cyclothymic subjects. Cyclothymic "cases" also evidenced interpersonal and social role impairment typical of bipolars, although not to the same clinically diagnosable level.

The clinical features found to characterize the nonpatient cyclothymic sample were consistent with those previously reported for more severe cyclothymic patients: an onset in early adolescence (average of 14 years), the frequency of episodes (ranging from two per year to one or more per month), and the duration of episodes (lasting from 2 to 6 days). Also consistent with previous reports was the finding that three types of cyclothymic courses could be identified — the balanced cyclothymic, in whom hypomanic and depressive episodes generally alternated and occured with similar frequency and duration (62% of the cases); the predominantly depressed cyclothymic, in whom depressive episodes occured on the average of five times more frequently than hypomanic (28% of the cases); and the predominantly hypomanic cyclothymic, in whom hypomanic episodes outnumbered depressive by an average of three to one (10% of the cases).

Fifty percent of the cyclothymic cases had a positive family history of depressive disorders, with 25% having bipolar family histories. This latter percentage corresponds closely to the percentage of bipolar family histories reported in bipolar I patients (26%) and cyclothymic patients (30%).

Dysthymia (Depressive Character)

Definition and Conceptual Roots

The term "dysthymia" refers to a behavioral pattern consisting of recurring or chronic mild depression. Dysthymic persons have been described as "habitually gloomy, introverted, brooding, overconscientious, incapable of fun, and preoccupied with personal inadequacy" (Akiskal, 1983, p. 11). As in the case of cyclothymia, Kraepelin (1921) was among the first writers to describe dysthymia as a type of affective personality and to consider it the temperamental substrate for melancholia. In addition to its possible role in depressive disorders, dysthymia may represent a complication (or chronic residue) of the depressive episode, as has been proposed by Klerman (1980).

Is dysthymia a subclinical form of affective disorder, a personality disorder, a residue of an incompletely recovered major depressive episode, or something else entirely? This question has been the source of considerable controversy. Akiskal (1983) has proposed a classification scheme that differentiates dysthymics into three subgroups. One of these consists of late-onset primary depressives in whom dysthymia represents residual chronicity (complication). A second group consists of persons in whom dysthymia occurs secondary to a pre-existing and incapacitating medical or nonaffective psychiatric disorder. The third group of dysthymics, termed "characterological depressives" by Akiskal, are those in whom dysthymia appears to be temperamental or characterological in nature, having an early and insidious developmental onset and fluctuating course.

Akiskal asserts that the characterological depressions can be further subdivided into character-spectrum disorders and subaffective dysthymic disorders on the basis of personality, family history, and biological criteria. According to his research findings on clinically diagnosed dysthymic patients (Akiskal, 1981; Akiskal *et al.*, 1980; Rosenthal, Akiskal, Scott-Strauss, Rosenthal, & David, 1981), character-spectrum disorders exhibit dependent, histrionic, or sociopathic personalities; have a family history of alcoholism; show normal sleep patterns; and are unresponsive to antidepressant medications. Subaffective dysthymics, on the other hand, evidence the classic "depressive" personality (e.g., nonassertive, pessimistic, self-critical, brooding, etc.); have family histories of affective disorder (both unipolar and bipolar); show the short rapid eye movement (REM) sleep latency characteristic of primary major depressives; and often respond to tricyclics or lithium carbonate. Since this dysthymic subgroup was found to have higher rates of familial bipolar disorder than are typical of unipolar depressives and to respond with hypomania to the tricyclic challenge, Akiskal has proposed that a continuum exists between dysthymia and cyclothymia, similar to that originally described by Kretschmer (1936).

Measures

To date, no assessment device is available to identify dysthymia specifically. Thus, past investigations have had to rely on clinical interview and diagnosis to define dysthymic cases. At this writing, Depue and his colleagues are incorporating a dysthymia measure into the GBI (see Table 11-5).

DISCUSSION

Up to this point, the evidence for a link between personality and depression has been examined by trait. But what of the *nature* of the link between these specific traits and depression? Based on the literature reviewed, the following summary presents our current knowledge concerning the nature of the relationship between personality and depression within the framework of the four hypotheses described earlier.

The predisposition approach proposes that personality characteristics are antecedent to and of etiological significance in depression. Support for a predispositional role exists for several traits. Perhaps most strongly implicated in the etiology of depression is social introversion, reported in virtually every study to measure it. In addition, modest levels of emotional instability (neuroticism) and interpersonal dependency also appear to characterize the premorbid personalities of depressives. Finally, there are some indications that maladaptive attitudes and an internal attributional style are cognitive features that precede clinical depression.

Rather than being universal to depression, however, these predisposing personality characteristics appear to differentiate major depressive subtypes. Whereas bipolar depressives, according to all recent reports, have relatively normal intermorbid personalities, major subtypes of unipolar depressives differ from normals in several respects. Primary melancholic unipolar depressives are characterized by moderate levels of introversion and dependency and by dysfunctional cognitive styles. Primary nonmelancholic unipolar depressives share all the personality features described for melancholics, but are somewhat more introverted and show some emotional instability as well. Although little is known about secondary depressives as compared to other subgroups, they have been found to be highly neurotic and slightly introverted.

The subclinical approach, which proposes that certain personality types represent attenuated forms of affective disorders, has received considerable support from recent research. Cyclothymics and some dysthymics have been found to share clinical, familial, and biological characteristics of bipolar and primary unipolar depressives.

Support for the pathoplasty approach, the view that the symptom picture and course of a depressive episode are influenced by personality, has been provided by studies that link premorbid neuroticism levels to a more chronic course of depression. Akiskal's work on character-spectrum dysthymia also provides indirect evidence of a connection between unstable personality and chronic depression.

Lastly, the complication approach, which proposes that personality may be affected by the experience of the depressive episode, has not been systematically tested by the necessary prospective studies. There are some indications that features of cognitive style are not affected by the experience of a depressive episode. However, this finding cannot be considered conclusive, since the observation is based on what may be inadequate assessments of attitudinal and attributional characteristics. Recent work on dysthymia is also relevant to the complication issue.

As Klerman (1980) points out, although most depressive episodes are relatively short-lived, with a return to the normal state typically following a time-limited period of symptomatology, "it has become increasingly recognized that a significant proportion of patients [some 15-20% of acute depressions] suffer from chronic affective disorders. . . . [Thus in some instances] dysthymic disorder probably represents the common clinical outcome of acute depressions of multiple causes" (p. 1332). This category of dysthymia corresponds to Akiskal's type 1 and 2 dysthymics and is supported by his research.

Although there are many unanswered questions concerning the relationship between personality and depression, recently developed personality measures and improvements in diagnostic assessment procedures should permit more definitive studies that address unresolved issues in the area to be conducted.

References

Abraham, K. (1948). *Selected papers on psychoanalysis*. London: Hogarth Press.

Abramson, L. Y., Seligman, M. E. P., & Teasdale, J. D. (1978). Learned helplessness in humans: Critique and reformulation. *Journal of Abnormal Psychology, 87*, 49-74.

Akiskal, H. S. (1981). Subaffective disorders: Dysthymic, cyclothymic, and bipolar II disorders in the "borderline" realm. *Psychiatric Clinics of North America, 4*, 25-46.

Akiskal, H. S. (1983). Dysthymic disorder: Psychopathology of proposed chronic depressive subtypes. *American Journal of Psychiatry, 140*, 11-20.

Akiskal, H. S., Djenderdejian, A. H., Rosenthal, K. H., & Khani, M. K. (1977). Cyclothymic disorder: Validating criteria for inclusion in the biopolar affective group. *American Journal of Psychiatry, 134*, 1227-1233.

Akiskal, H. S., Hirschfeld, R. M. A., & Yerevanian, B. I. (1983). The relationship of personality to affective disorders. *Archives of General Psychiatry, 40*, 801-810.

Akiskal, H. S., Khani, M. K., & Scott-Strauss, A. (1979). Cyclothymic temperamental disorders. *Psychiatric Clinics of North America, 2*, 527-554.

Akiskal, H. S., Rosenthal, T. L., Haykal, R. F., Lemmi, H., Rosenthal, R. H., & Scott-Strauss, A. (1980). Characterological depressions: Clinical and sleep EEG findings separating "subaffective dysthymias" from "character spectrum disorders." *Archives of General Psychiatry, 37*, 777-783.

Bech, P., Shapiro, R. W., Sihm, F., Nielsen, B. M., Sorensen, B., & Rafaelsen, O. J. (1980). Personality in unipolar and bipolar manic-melancholic patients. *Acta Psychiatrica Scandinavica, 62*, 245-257.

Benjaminsen, S. (1981). Primary non-endogenous depression and features attributed to reactive depression. *Journal of Affective Disorders, 3*, 245-259.

Block, J. (1965). *The challenge of response sets*. New York: Meredith.

Bowlby, J. (1969). *Attachment*. New York: Basic Books.

Chodoff, P, (1972). The depressive personality: A critical review. *Archives of General Psychiatry, 27*, 666-673.

Depue, R. A., Slater, J. F., Wolfstetter-Kausch, H., Klein, D., Goplerud, E., & Farr, D. (1981). Behavioral paradigm for identifying persons at risk for bipolar depressive disorder: A conceptual framework and five validation studies. *Journal of Abnormal Psychology, 90*, 381-437.

Eaves, G., & Rush, A. J. (1984). Cognitive patterns in symptomatic and remitted unipolar major depression. *Journal of Abnormal Psychology, 41*, 28-30.

Eysenck, H. J. (1962). *The Maudsley Personality Inventory*. San Diego: Educational and Industrial Testing Service.

Eysenck, H. J. (1964). Principles and methods of personality description, classification and diagnosis. *British Journal of Psychology, 55*, 284-294.

Eysenck, H. J., & Eysenck, S. B. G. (1964). *Manual of the Eysenck Personality Inventory*. London: University of London Press.

Fenichel, O. (1945). *The psychoanalytic theory of neurosis*. New York: Norton.

Guilford, J. P., & Zimmerman, W. S. (1949). *The Guilford-Zimmerman Temperament Survey: Manual of instructions and interpretations*. Beverly Hills, CA: Sheridan Supply.

Hirschfeld, R. M. A., Klerman, G. L., Chodoff, P., Korchin, S., & Barrett, J. (1976). Dependency-self-esteem-clinical depression. *Journal of the American Academy of Psychoanalysis, 4*, 373-388.

Hirschfeld, R. M. A., Klerman, G. L., Clayton, P. J., & Keller, M. B. (1983). Personality and depression: Empirical findings. *Archives of General Psychiatry, 40*, 993-998.

Hirschfeld, R. M. A., Klerman, G. L., Clayton, P. J., Keller, M. B., MacDonald-Scott, P., & Larkin, B. H. (1983). Assessing personality: Effects of the depressive state on trait measurement. *American Journal of Psychiatry, 140*, 695-699.

Hirschfeld, R. M. A., Klerman, G. L., Gough, H. G., Barrett, J., Korchin, S. J., & Chodoff, P. (1977). A measure of interpersonal dependency. *Journal of Personality Assessment, 41*, 610-618.

Hollon, S. D., & Kendall, P. C. (1980). Cognitive self-statements in depression: Development of an Automatic Thoughts Questionnaire. *Cognitive Therapy and Research, 4*, 383-395.

Keller, M. B., & Shapiro, A. W. (1982). "Double depression": Superimposition of acute depressive episodes on chronic depressive disorders. *American Journal of Psychiatry, 139*, 438-442.

Klerman, G. L. (1980). Other specific affective disorders. In H. I. Kaplan, A. M. Freedman, & B. J. Sadock (Eds.), *Comprehensive textbook of psychiatry* (3rd ed., Vol. 2, pp. 1332-1338). Baltimore: Williams & Wilkins.

Kovacs, M., & Beck, A. T. (1978). Maladaptive cognitive structures in depression. *American Journal of Psychiatry, 135*, 525-533.

Kraepelin, E. (1921). *Manic-depressive illness and paranoia*. Edinburgh: E. &. S. Livingstone.

Kretschmer, E. (1936). *Physique and character* (E. Miller, Trans.). London: Kegan, Paul, Trenck, Trubner.

Lazare, A., Klerman, G. L., & Armor, D. J. (1966). Oral, obsessive, and hysterical personality patterns: An investigation of psychoanalytic concepts by means of factor analysis. *Archives of General Psychiatry, 14*, 624-630.

Lewinsohn, P. M. (1974). A behavioral approach to depression. In R. Friedman & M. Katz (Eds.), *The psychology of depression: Contemporary theory and research* (pp. 157-185). New York: Wiley.

Lewinsohn, P. M., Steinmetz, J. L., Larson, D. W., & Franklin, J. (1981). Depression-related cognitions: Antecedent or consequences? *Journal of Abnormal Psychology, 90*, 213-219.

Liebowitz, M. R., Stallone, F., Dunner, D. L., & Fieve, R. F. (1979). Personality features of patients with primary affective disorder. *Acta Psychiatrica Scandinavica, 60*, 214-224.

Paykel, E. S., Klerman, G. L., & Prusoff, B. A. (1976). Personality and symptom pattern in depression. *British Journal of Psychiatry, 129*, 327-334.

Peterson, C., Semmel, A., von Baeyer, C. Abramson, L. Y., Metalsky, G. I., & Seligman, M. E. P. (1982). The Attributional Style Questionnaire. *Cognitive Therapy and Research, 6*, 287-300.

Pilowsky, I., & Katsikitis, M. (1983). Depressive illness and dependency. *Acta Psychiatrica Scandinavica, 68*, 11-14.

Raps, C. S., Peterson, C., Reinhard, K. E., Abramson, L. Y., & Seligman, M. E. P. (1982). Attributional style among depressed patients. *Journal of Abnormal Psychology, 91*, 102-108.

Rosenthal, T. L., Akiskal, H. S., Scott-Strauss, A., Rosenthal, R. H., & David, M. (1981). Familial and developmental factors in characterological depressions. *Journal of Affective Disorders, 3*, 183-192.

Seligman, M. E. P. (1975). *Helplessness: On depression, development, and death*. San Francisco: W. H. Freeman.

Seligman, M. E. P., Abramson, L. Y., Semmel, A., & von Baeyer, C. (1979). Depressive attributional style. *Journal of Abnormal Psychology, 88*, 242-247.

Silverman, J. S., Silverman, J. A., & Eardley, D. A. (1984). Do maladaptive attitudes cause depression? *Archives of General Psychiatry, 41*, 28-30.

Weissman, A. N. (1979). The Dysfunctional Attitude Scale: A validation study (Doctoral dissertation, University of Pennsylvania, 1979). *Dissertation Abstracts International, 40*, 1389B-1390B.

Weissman, M. M., Prusoff, B. A., & Klerman, G. L. (1978). Personality and the prediction of long-term outcome of depression. *American Journal of Psychiatry, 135*, 797-800.

Youngren, M. A., & Lewinsohn, P. M. (1980). The functional relationship between depression and problematic interpersonal behavior. *Journal of Abnormal Psychology, 89*, 333-341.

CHAPTER 12

The Familial and Psychosocial Measurement of Depression

KAREN JOHN
Yale University
MYRNA M. WEISSMAN
New York State Psychiatric Institute
College of Physicians and Surgeons, Columbia University

INTRODUCTION

Many psychosocial and familial factors are commonly associated with the onset, manifestation, course, and outcome of depressive illness. Negative childhood experiences such as parental loss, discord, and inadequacy have long been thought to predispose an individual to depression (Beck, 1967; Beck, Sethi, & Tuthill, 1963; Birtchnell, 1970; Orvaschel, Weissman, & Kidd, 1980). Psychological features or traits that are believed to be largely socially determined, such as low self-esteem, low perceived competence (Beck, 1967; Brown & Harris, 1978), inadequate coping skills (Lazarus, 1966), and learned helplessness (Seligman, 1975), have been suggested as factors that explain why certain individuals become depressed or are prone to recurrent depressions.

The absence of adequate social supports, including an intimate or confiding relationship, and inadequate physical or financial resources have been implicated in the onset, prolonged course, and poorer treatment outcome of depressive illness (Brown & Harris, 1978; Flaherty, Gaviria, & Pathak, 1983; Henderson, Byrne, & Duncan-Jones, 1981; Lin, Dean, & Ensel, 1981). The number and severity of stressful life events and long-standing social difficulties have been found to act as precipitators or provoking agents in the development of depression (Brown & Harris, 1978; Paykel *et al.*, 1969).

Individuals who are treated for depression have been found to evidence poorer social adjustment than their nondepressed neighbors, and to continue to function less adequately in certain areas long after their depressive symptoms have disappeared (Weissman & Paykel, 1974). Finally, recent studies suggest that birth cohort and family history of affective disorder are powerful factors associated with the development and severity of depressive illness (Weissman *et al.*, 1984).

How the measurement of these psychosocial and familial factors is approached depends on the complexity of the factor and the hypothesized relationship between the factor and the illness. Some factors, such as loss of one's parents or inadequate financial resources, are relatively easy to measure, but most require careful definition and operalization before any estimation of their importance in depression can be made. In depression, it is seldom clear whether a social factor causes or is a consequence of the disorder. Determination of the etiological role of a factor in the illness requires the development and testing of causal models. Indeed, the new generation of studies concerned with the etiology of depression and the lifelong characteristics of depressives have provided the field with some impressive new tools for the measurement of psychosocial and familial factors (e.g., Henderson *et al.*, 1981), as well as with models that attempt to account for the complex interactions among such factors (e.g., Brown & Harris, 1978) and for the relationship between social factors and genetic vulnerability (e.g., Kidd & Matthysse, 1978).

However, much of the interest and activity in the measurement of the psychosocial and familial aspects of depression has been stimulated by the need to develop methods appropriate for assessing the outcome of treatment (Gurland, Yorkston, Stone, Frank, & Fleiss, 1972; Weissman & Paykel, 1974). Those involved in treating depressed patients are particularly aware of the importance of social factors in the onset, course, and outcome of the illness. Typically, depressed patients report difficulties in their marital and other interpersonal relationships and impairment in their work performance; often they are dissatisfied with one or more aspects of their lives. Whether these problems are the result of the illness or predispose the individuals to the illness, they become a major focus of most therapies used to treat depressives. The rationale for this focus is that positive changes in the psychosocial world of a patient will promote a reduction in symptoms and perhaps protect the individual from further illness (Klerman, Weissman, Rounsaville, & Chevron, 1984). A wide variety of scales have been used or devised to detect and characterize these changes (Katschnig, 1983; Weissman, 1975; Weissman, Sholomskas, & John, 1981).

The measurement techniques to be reviewed in this chapter come from two kinds of depression research. One kind primarily focuses on the psychosocial and familial factors believed to play an etiological or causal role in depressive illness, and requires careful separation of factors that predate the illness from factors that may be concomitants of the illness. Such studies measure and estimate the importance of social risk factors in depression. Studies of the other kind are concerned with the psychosocial and familial concomitants or consequences of depression, regardless of their potential etiological role in the illness, and require that the social functioning and relationships of depressives be assessed over time. Such studies measure and/or monitor changes in social adjustment.

While there is often overlap in the concepts that underlie measures of social risk factors and measures of social adjustment, the different purposes of the studies for which they were developed provide a convenient way to organize a review of the instruments. Therefore, we first present an overview and review of assessment techniques used to measures psychosocial and familial risk factors (specifically, those that have demanded conceptualization, operationalizing, and testing), and then we review a variety of scales that are suitable for the assessment of social adjustment in depressed persons.

THE MEASUREMENT OF PSYCHOSOCIAL RISK FACTORS IN DEPRESSION

Differences in how risk factors are measured often appear to explain differences in findings across studies. Even seemingly straightforward measurement tasks can be approached in a variety of ways — for example, how "social class" is determined; whether "loss of parent" includes loss by death and by separation; or what is regarded as an "intimate relationship." When an investigator is considering the measurement of such factors in depression, careful attention to what has already been found and an appreciation for the potential power of distinctions seem prudent. When more complex factors are being considered, the measurement issues become even more complicated. Parental inadequacy, stressful life events, and an absence of adequate social supports are factors believed to increase the risk of depressive illness, but how they are measured depends on how they are conceptualized.

Measurement of Parental Characteristics

The Child Report of Parent Behavior Inventory

Beck (1967), among others, has suggested that the negative attitudes of the depression-prone individual are acquired during early life and influenced by interactions between parent and child. However, of five early studies linking depression in adulthood to negative parental behavior in childhood (Abrahams & Whitlock, 1969; Jacobson, Fasman, & DiMascio, 1975; Munro, 1966; Perris, 1966; Raskin, Boothe, Reatig, Schulterbrandt, & Odle, 1971), only the Raskin *et al.* study used a measure of demonstrated validity and reliability to assess the parental characteristics that were examined.

In consultation with the author of the 192-item Child Report of Parent Behavior Inventory (CRPBI; Schaefer, 1963, 1965), Raskin and his colleagues (1971) shortened the CRPBI to 90 items before administering it to the depressives and normals in their sample. They found that two dimensions of the self-administered instrument differentiated the parents of the depressed patients from those of normals: (1) "rejection," and (2) "psychological control." A subsequent, more carefully designed study comparing the 90-item CRPBI among depressives and normals was conducted by Crook, Raskin, and

Eliot (1981). In this study, (1) only patients with clincial depression were included; (2) to reduce possible bias, patients did not complete the CRPBI until 5 weeks after discharge, when their depressive symptoms had remitted; and (3) judgments of parental behavior during childhood were made by social workers based on sources other than subjects' reports, to provide an independent (if not blind) assessment of the major parental dimensions believed likely to emerge. The parents, particularly the mothers, of depressives were reported to have been much more rejecting and controlling through derision, debasement, withdrawal of affection, and manipulation through guilt and anxiety than the parents of normal controls. The judgments of the social workers, for the most part, confirmed these findings.

The Parental Bonding Instrument

Parker, Tupling, and Brown (1979) sought to operationalize Bowlby's (1969) concepts of parental bonding. Beginning with a list of 114 parental behaviors and attitudes thought to characterize the principal dimensions of parental bonding, the authors conducted a series of studies and factor analyses from which they derived the 25 items that comprise the two scales of the self-administered Parental Bonding Instrument (PBI): Care (i.e., "care" vs. "indifference/rejection") and Overprotection (i.e., "overprotection" vs. "allowance of autonomy/independence"). Together, the two scales permit five types of parental bonding to be examined: (1) high Care-low Overprotection (conceptualized as optimal bonding); (2) low Care-low Overprotection (conceptualized as absent or weak bonding); (3) high Care-high Overprotection (conceptualized as affectionate constraint); (4) low Care-high Overprotection (conceptualized as affectionless control); and (5) average (defined statistically by norms). In an impressive program of research, Parker has found the following:

1. Lower parental Care and higher parental Overprotection scores on the PBI differentiated subjects with either trait or clinical depession from those who were not depressed and those who suffered from bipolar depression (Parker, 1979a, 1979b).
2. Depressives' mothers rated themselves on the PBI in much the same way as the depressives did — that is, as low in Care and high in Overprotection. This suggests that depressives' recall of past parental behavior is not biased by their depressed state (Parker, 1981).
3. The same associations between PBI scores and depressive symptoms existed among adoptees who had never lived with their biological parents, providing support for the causal influence of parental characteristics on mood levels in the absence of hereditary influence that might otherwise explain the associations between PBI scores and symptoms (Parker, 1982).

G. Parker and K. Wilhelm (personal communication, December 14, 1983) found that "care" and "control" dimensions accounted for and explained the variance in a pool of items selected to assess marital and other intimate adult relationships. From their preliminary work they have devised a 24-item self-administered report measure, which, when reliability and validity studies are completed, will provide the field with a new tool to examine marital bonding along the same dimensions as parental bonding. Empirical research comparing the behaviors of depressives' parents with the behaviors of the depressives' spouses could contribute considerably to our understanding of the link between the childhood and adult bonding patterns in depression.

The Measurement of Expressed Emotion

Brown, Birley, and Wing (1972) and Vaughn and Leff (1976a) provided empirical evidence that deleterious aspects of the family environment could be specified and measured with standardized procedures. Their work on expressed emotion (EE) revealed that measures of overinvolvement, hostility, and critical comments by schizophrenic patients' relatives at the time of hospital admission possessed powerful prognostic information about the likelihood of relapse (Goldstein & Doane, 1982).

Until recently, the methods used to assess EE in families have been quite complicated and time-consuming, and thus more appropriate for researchers with small inpatient populations. But Goldstein and Doane (1982) have devised a sort method for assessing EE, which involves obtaining a 5-minute audio-recorded description of the patient from a parent or other close relative. From the speech sample, a straightforward scoring of EE content can be made. EE scores from the 5-minute audiotapes have been found to agree highly with scores from the traditional 1½-hour video-recorded family sessions among schizophrenic adolescents (M. Goldstein, personal communication, October 30, 1983).

Using the lengthy family interview method, Vaughn and Leff (1976b) found that there was a relationship between relatives' high EE scores and relapses among neurotic depressives. In contrast to schizophrenics, the depressives were found to be more sensitive to criticism and were not protected against relapse by drug treatment or by reduced contact with relatives. In addition, factors similar to high EE *scores* have been found by others to differentiate parents of depressives from parents of normal controls (Crook *et al.*, 1981; Parker, 1979a, 1979b), and such relationships between EE and the development and course of depression will probably be found when 5-minute audiotape methods are employed. Furthermore, an alternative to the self-administered report measures of parental behaviors and attitudes is sorely needed, if only to strengthen the findings from family interview and self-administered measures. This new brief technique for obtaining EE scores now makes it possible to assess this important dimension of parental behavior in large outpatient samples.

Measurement of Stressful Life Events

A considerable amount has already been written about approaches to the assessment of stressful life events. Most recently, Dohrenwend and Dohrenwend (1981) edited a comprehensive volume in which they suggested guidelines for the selection and measurement of events when etiological questions concerning events and illness are being investigated. It seems more useful to provide a summary of their recommendations than to attempt a review of the many scales that have been devised to assess life events.

Stressful life events are those that are proximate to rather than remote from the disorder. Only if the investigator can date the onset of the event in relation to the onset of pathology, and learn whether the event was within or outside the control of the subject, can relatively unambiguous inferences about the etiological role of such events be made. There are at least three types of events that should be kept distinct when considering their causal relationship to the illness: (1) events that may be confounded with the subject's condition; (2) events consisting of physical illnesses and injuries to the subject; and (3) events whose occurrences are independent of the subject's physical and psychiatric condition.

Post hoc personal measures of the stressfulness of particular life events should be avoided. On the other hand, if group norms are used to assign weights to events, they should be determined for the group and time studied. Finally, quantitative estimates of the relationships between various aspects of life events and different kinds of health changes should be developed, and the nature of these relationships should be expanded in terms of a life stress process composed of life events and the psychological and social contexts in which they occur (Dohrenwend & Dohrenwend, 1981, pp. 3-23). For example, Brown and Harris (1978) found that "provoking agents — defined as stressful life events and ongoing difficulites — were several times more likely to produce depression when the working-class women in their sample had one or more vulnerability factors (i.e., loss of mother before age 11, the presence of three or more children aged 14 or under at home, lack of paid employment, and lack of an intimate or confiding relationship). Such studies go beyond the simple question "Does the event increase the risk of depression?" and help to delineate the contexts in which events will be most likely to produce illness.

Measurement of Social Support

The concept of social support has become a focal point in research for its potential contribution to the epidemiological explanation of depression, particularly because social supports may serve as mediating or buffering factors between stressors and illness (Lin *et al.*, 1981). Social support is defined as "support accessible to an individual through social ties to other individuals, groups, and the larger community" (Lin, Simeone, Ensel, & Kuo, 1979, p. 109). Since there is conceptual overlap between scales that measure social support and those that measure the broader construct of social adjustment, a review of measures of social support is included in the next portion of this chapter. However, it should be noted here that in the Brown and Harris (1978) study and in a number of subsequent studies (Campbell, Cope, & Teasdale, 1983; Costello, 1982; Roy, 1978, 1981; Solomon & Bromet, 1982) the absence of an intimate or confiding relationship, simply and directly assessed, was found to be a powerful risk factor in the development of depression.

THE MEASUREMENT OF SOCIAL ADJUSTMENT IN DEPRESSION

The separation of measures of social adjustment in depression from measures of psychosocial and familial risk factors in depression is somewhat arbitrary, since social adjustment might easily be conceptualized and measured as a risk factor. However, there are several reasons why we have divided the review in this way.

First, most research in depression has involved the study of persons once they are already ill. And while studies have found that social adjustment and symptoms may by partially independent (Strauss & Carpenter, 1972; Weissman, Klerman, Paykel, Prusoff, & Hanson, 1974), impairment in social adjustment is expected to be a concomitant feature of depression. Only in prospective studies of persons who may already be at risk for depression (e.g., by virtue of depressive illness in a parent) can social adjustment be assessed as a risk factor — possibly conceptualized as a component of personality. With the exception of the Henderson *et al.* (1981) study of neurosis and social supports, we know of no published study in which social adjustment per se has been considered as a risk factor in depression.

Second, because of the practical need for measures of social adjustment in planning treatment and assessing treatment efficacy, many more scales have been developed to assess social adjustment than other psychosocial and familial factors in depression. Finally, social adjustment has been broadly conceptualized, and as a result, nearly every imaginable psychosocial and familial variable has been assessed by one scale or another. While the newer scales tend to measure more unitary concepts, many of the most commonly used and studied instruments comprehensively assess social adjustment. The large number and variety of scales available for use require that they be reviewed together, compared, and evaluated.

The remainder of the chapter provides an historical overview of this active area of measurement; alerts the reader to the controversies in, and operational and practical approaches to, the measurement of social adjustment; and reviews 16 scales that are suitable for use with depressed patients.

Historical Overview of Social Adjustment Measurement

Over the past three decades, there has been an unprecedented interest in the community adjustment of psychiatric patients, and this recently has expanded to include medically ill patients. In psychiatry, interest in patients' community adjustment has been a natural outgrowth of the treatment trend from custodial to outpatient care. This trend gained momentum in the United States with the opening of community mental health centers in the 1960s and further accelerated in the 1970s when it became apparent that deinstitutionalized patients with chronic disorders were having problems in the community.

The expansion of interest into the social world of the patient required the addition of new measures of disturbances — ones that were distinct from those assessing symptoms or abnormalities of thought. Several scales were developed for the assessment of social adjustment. The first scales in psychiatry, which appeared in the 1950s and 1960s, were used to evaluate the posthospital adjustment of schizophrenic patients discharged on regimens of the new major tranquilizers or to assess psychotherapy outcome in selected outpatient populations. In the 1970s, systematic assessment of patients' social functioning became a part of the evaluation of their initial state as well as of their treatment outcome.

The first review of available social adjustment scales appeared in 1975 (Weissman, 1975); it described 15 scales that met criteria of reliability, validity, and utility. Criteria for evaluating scales with regard to content, methods for obtaining information, sources of information, and psychometric properties were established. Other factors involved in scale selection were described, such as time period assessed, length of time required to administer, scoring, and training. Scales that were limited in scope, underdeveloped, or developed for one particular study were not included. Most of the 15 scales in the review sufficiently met selection criteria, but three early scales were included because of their historical interest and because later scales were derived from them.

In 1981, a second review appeared (Weissman *et al.*, 1981), in which 12 new social adjustment scales were described. Some of the scales covered had been adapted from pre-existing scales for use with new patient populations; some had been designed with medically ill patients in mind; and some offered new approaches to the problem of how "best" to assess social adjustment. Thus, by 1981 at least 27 social adjustment scales that met criteria of reliability, validity, and utility were available.

Definition and Components of Social Adjustment

"Social adjustment" is neither a unitary nor a global concept. Broadly defined, it is the interplay between the individual and the social environment. In practice, the concept primarily involves the evaluation of an individual's functioning in different roles that are commonly accepted as appropriate. Normally, an adult will function in most of the following roles: occupational; marital, as spouse and parent; within an extended family, with parents, siblings, and other close relatives; and in the community, with friends, acquaintances, and groups. Within each role, functioning may be further divided into instrumental performance and affect, or behavior and attitude in roles. Typically, the individual is evaluated in terms of the way his or her role performance conforms to the norms of his or her referent group.

Theoretically, a discrepancy in the person-environment fit may result from a disability on the side of the individual or from disturbances in the social environment (Katschnig, 1983). Katschnig identified 21 different terms used to describe social adjustment or some aspect of it; of these, seven were positive (e.g., "social attainment," "social competence"), six were neutral (e.g., "social performance," "adaptive functioning"), and eight were negative (e.g., "social maladjustment," "social impairment"). The length of the list and diversity of the terms provide some hint of the multidimensional nature of the concept and of the theoretical biases of the investigators who study social adjustment.

Controversies in the Concepts and Measurement of Social Adjustment

Symptoms and Social Adjustment

The early social adjustment scales were designed to provide broad and extensive coverage of discharged psychiatric inpatients' social functioning in the community. Many of these scales included measures of symptomatic behavior believed likely to impair the patients' interpersonal relations and performance of instrumental tasks. With such assessments, an estimation of the burden a patient represented to his or her family and community could be ascertained. Authors of later scales — designed primarily for use with treated outpatient populations — tended to avoid the inclusion of symptoms per se, seeking to separate the measurement of social functioning from psychopathology. They reasoned that while an overlap between symptoms and social adjustment is often found, they may be quite independent: For example, some persons may function reasonably well although symptomatic, and others may function poorly although asymptomatic (Strauss & Carpenter, 1972; Weissman *et al.*, 1974). Furthermore, treatment may have differential effects on symptoms and social functioning. Symptoms are primarily a reflection of internal psychological and physical states that may have consequences in social relations. On the other hand, social adjustment is a reflection of the patient's interactions with others and of his or her performance and attitudes in roles, all of which are likely to be modified by previous personality and by familial and cultural expectations.

A resolution of the question of the independence of symptoms and social adjustment requires that they be measured separately and as accurately as possible. Investigators who employ social adjustment scales that assess satisfaction and feelings in social roles, both of which are likely to overlap with the symptoms of depression, should separate those items from the more objective performance items when they calculate role or overall social adjustment. In this way, subgroups of patients in whom the relationship between symptoms and social adjustment may differ can be identified. Such subgroups may be found to require different therapeutic intervention.

Operational Approaches to the Assessment of Social Adjustment

Recent developers of social adjustment scales have been critical of the use of ideal standards and the reliance on normative data in the assessment of social adjustment (Clare & Cairns, 1978; Platt, Weyman, Hirsch, & Hewett, 1980; Remington & Tyrer, 1979). Their scales instead assess the patient by making use of his or her own social context and by concentrating on more objective indicators of the patient's functioning within that context. At this stage, the merits of the less value-laden approaches to the assessment of social adjustment cannot be fully evaluated. Only when a substantial body of data on both patient and nonpatient groups becomes available can full appraisal of their usefulness in this measurement area be determined.

Methods of Obtaining Information and Informants

Methods of Obtaining Information

The methods available for obtaining information on patients' social adjustment have been described in detail by Weissman (1975). In general, written self-administered report inventories are the least expensive to administer. Their disadvantages are as follows: (1) Illiterate informants require that someone read the inventory to them; (2) psychotic and delusional patients may underreport their impairments; (3) very disturbed patients may be unable to complete or understand the intent of the task; and (4) some respondents falsify their responses. In-person interviews have the advantage of providing the most complete information, in that both respondent and interviewer ratings are typically made. Other advantages are that the interviewer may be able to calm a patient who might otherwise be unable to participate, can detect the tendency to underreport or falsify, and can make efforts to encourage the subject to give accurate information. The main disadvantages are the costs of training and employing skilled interviewers.

Informants

The patient is the most direct and available source of information in outpatient studies. Depressives can be quite reliable informants, although they have been found to rate themselves as more impaired than an interviewer rates them (Weissman & Bothwell, 1976). Significant others — usually a spouse or someone who is in close contact with a patient — can also provide the information. Both patients and significant others are likely to be somewhat biased in their reports. However, studies that have compared the ratings of patients and their significant others have found impressively high rates of agreement and no particular pattern in the discrepancies between them (Glazer, Aaronson, Prusoff, & Williams, 1980; Weissman & Bothwell, 1976).

Selecting a Scale

Table 12-1 describes the properties of 16 scales that we review in this chapter. There are a number of concepts underlying social adjustment, which are measured with varying emphasis in the different scales. Apart from the practical issues involved in choosing a scale, the major consideration should be how well it measures the concepts that are of particular interest in the study for which it is intended. This will require an examination of both the qualitative and quantitative properties of the instrument.

The scales included for review here are those that seem particularly suited for studies of depressed patients. They represent a variety of approaches to the conceptualization and measurement of social adjustment. The scales are grouped in the following manner:

1. *Functioning in roles.* Included are 11 scales that broadly assess adjustment in a variety of social roles and areas.
2. *Functioning in circumscribed roles.* Included are 2 scales, the first of which comprehensively covers the adult roles in which women have traditionally functioned, and the second of which provides extensive coverage of the marital role.
3. *Available social supports.* Included are 3 scales, each of which primarily assesses the practical and emotional support available to the patient.

Within the groups, the scales are arranged as they became available chronologically over the past 20 years.

Functioning in Roles

The Katz Adjustment Scale — Relative's Form. Katz and Lyerly (1963) and Hogarty and Katz (1971) developed the Katz Adjustment Scale —

TABLE 12-1 Detailed Characteristics of Social Adjustment Scales Suitable for Depressed Patients

Scale	Informant	Method	Content	Original use	Target populations	Populations studied	Psychometric properties	Number of items	Period assessed	Completion time
				Functioning in roles						
Katz Adjustment Scale — Relative's Form	Significant other (patient/ subject optional)	Written self-administered	Occupational; community/ social; marital family; assessment of psychiatric symptoms	Establishment of community norms of social adjustment; identification of candidates for treatment	Inpatients and outpatients after psychiatric treatment; community residents	Community outpatients and normals; schizophrenics and DEPRESSIVES	Reliability; validity; sensitivity; scoring system	205	3 weeks	25-40 minutes
Personality and Social Network Scale	Patient/ subject (significant other optional)	Written self-administered	Occupational; community/ social; marital family; extended family	Assessment of effects of inpatient and outpatient psychiatric treatment	Psychiatric inpatients and outpatients	Psychiatric inpatients and outpatients	Reliability; validity; sensitivity; scoring system	17	Present	Est. 10 minutes
Community Adaptation Schedule	Patient/ subject	Written self-administered	Occupational; community/ social; marital; parental; extended family; economic; physical environment; utilization of health facilities	Multitreatment evaluation	Psychiatric inpatients and outpatients	Psychiatric inpatients and outpatients	Reliability; validity; sensitivity; scoring system	217	Present	30-60 minutes
Structured and Scaled Interview to Assess Maladjustment	Patient/ subject	Interview	Occupational; community/social; marital; parental; marital family; extended family	Outpatient psychotherapy outcome study	Psychiatric outpatients	Psychiatric outpatients; DEPRESSIVES	Reliability; validity; sensitivity; scoring system	60	Past month	1 hour

(*continued*)

Table 12-1 (cont'd)

Scale	Informant	Method	Content	Original use	Target populations	Populations studied	Psychometric properties	Number of items	Period assessed	Completion time
Social Adjustment Scale	Patient/ subject	Interview	Occupational; community/social; marital; parental; extended family; economic	Outcome study of pharmaco-therapy and psychotherapy in depressed outpatient women	Outpatient depressives	Community residents; substance abusers; sucide attempters; unipolar and bipolar DEPRESSIVES	Reliability; validity; sensitivity; scoring system	48	Past 2 months	45-60 minutes
Social Adjustment Scale — Self-Report	Patient/ subject; significant other	Written self-administered	Occupational; community/social; marital; parental; extended family; economic	Assessment of treatment outcome among depressed outpatients	Depressed outpatients	Psychiatric outpatients; community residents; DEPRESSIVES	Reliability; validity; sensitivity; scoring system	42	Past 2 weeks	15-20 minutes
Self-Assessment Guide	Patient/ subject	Written self-administered	Occupational; community/social; marital; extended family; physical health-illness; assessment of psychiatric symptoms	Assessment of treatment outcome among psychiatric inpatients	Discharged psychiatric inpatients	Discharged psychiatric inpatients; community residents	Reliability; validity; sensitivity; scoring system	55	Past 3 months	20 minutes
Social Maladjustment Schedule	Patient/ subject; significant other	Interview	Occupational; community/social; marital; parental; extended family; economic; physical environment; assessment of psychiatric symptoms	Assesment of social maladjustment	General medical patients; community residents	General medical patients; chronic neurotic outpatients	Reliability; partial validity; scoring system	41	Present	1 hour
Social Problem Questionnaire	Patient/ subject	Written self-administered	Occupational; community/social; marital; parental; extended family; economic; physical environment; legal matters	Assessment of social maladjustment	General medical patients; psychiatric outpatients	Neurotic outpatients	Reliability; partial validity; sensitivity; scoring system	41	Present	5-10 minutes

Social Behavior Assessment Schedule	Significant other	Interview	Occupational; community/social; marital household; physical environment; physical health-illness; utilization of health facilities; assessment of psychiatric symptoms	Measurement of impact of illness on significant others	Discharged psychiatric or medical patients	Discharged psychiatric and medical patients	Reliability; validity; sensitivity; scoring system	239	Past 1 month; past 3 months	45-90 minutes
Social Functioning Schedule	Patient/ subject; significant ofter	Interview	Occupational; community/social; marital; parental; economic; self-care	Assessment of social role functioning of psychiatric day patients and outpatients	Psychiatric day patients and outpatients	Neurotic and character-disordered outpatients; psychiatric inpatients; DEPRESSIVES	Reliability; validity; sensitivity; scoring system	16	Past month	10-20 minutes
Functioning in circumscribed roles										
Social Role Adjustment Instrument	Patient/ subject	Interview	Occupational (homemaker); community/social; marital; parental; extended family	Measurement of women's adjustment to adult roles	Normal community residents; psychiatrically ill mothers	Normal community women; psychiatrically ill mothers; DEPRESSIVES	Reliability; validity; sensitivity; scoring system	200	Present	1-2 hours
KDS-15 Marital Questionnaire	Patient/ subject; significant other	Written self-administered	Occupational; community/social; marital; parental; extended family (history); physical health-illness; sexual dysfunction	Assessment of pretreatment marital adjustment	Couples entering therapy	Patient and nonpatient couples; DEPRESSIVES	Reliability; validity; sensitivity; scoring system	Approx. 80	Varies	30-60 minutes

(*continued*)

Table 12-1 (cont'd)

Scale	Informant	Method	Content	Original use	Target populations	Populations studied	Psychometric properties	Number of items	Period assessed	Completion time
					Available social supports					
Personal Resources Inventory	Patient/ subject	Interview	Occupational; community/social; marital; parental; extended family; economic; physical environment (the instrument refers to each of these factors as a support system)	Pretreatment assessment of social support system	Psychiatric inpatients	DEPRESSED inpatients and outpatients	Scoring system	41	Last 6 or 12 months	20 minutes
Interview Schedule for Social Interaction	Patient/ subject	Interview	Occupational; community/social; marital; parental; extended family (the instrument refers to each of these factors as a support system)	Longitudinal epidemiological study	Normal community residents; nonpsychotic neurotic persons	Normal community residents; non-psychotic neurotic persons	Reliability; partial validity; scoring system	52	Present	1 hour
Social Support Network Inventory	Patient/ subject	Written self-administered	Occupational; community/social; marital; parental; extended family (the instrument refers to each of these factors as a support system)	Assessment of social support received by psychiatric outpatients	Psychiatric outpatients	DEPRESSED outpatients; residents of urban community and religious commune	Reliability; validity; sensitivity; scoring system	55	Present	15-30 minutes

Relative's Form (KAS-R) to assess symptomatic behavior and life situation adjustment of patients in the community. The KAS-R is a self-report inventory; 205 items are rated on a 4-point global scale by a close family member who has recently interacted with the patient. Items are clearly stated and require only a sixth-grade reading level. From 25 to 45 minutes are required for completion. A 3-week time period is assessed.

The scale contains the following five sections: a 127-item rating of symptoms and social behavior; a 16-item rating of performance at socially expected tasks; a 16-item rating of the relative's expectation for the performance of these tasks; a 23-item rating of free-time activities; and a 23-item rating of the relative's satisfaction with the patient's performance of free-time activities. One of the earliest scales, the KAS-R has been widely used over the past 20 years in a variety of settings, and with heterogeneous diagnostic and nonpatient populations. There are considerable data available on reliability, validity, sensitivity, and norms, as well as instructional material with a color movie film for training purposes.

This scale provides an excellent assessment of the former inpatient's symptomatic behavior and instrumental performance within the family, and of his or her recreational participation. Marital, parental, and extended-family relations have less coverage.

The cooperation of relatives has been reported to be good, and the extensive development and use of this scale make it an attractive relative-as-informant inventory. The KAS-R is currently being completed by both patients and significant others in a 5-hospital study of depressed patients in the National Institute of Mental Health (NIMH) Collaborative Program on the Psychobiology of Depression (P. Clayton, personal communication, January 26, 1984). Thus, considerable KAS-R and KAS-S information will be available on depressed patients in the near future.

Personality and Social Network Adjustment Scale. Broad areas of the patient's adjustment and satisfaction with himself or herself in society, work, and in associational and family groups are assessed in Clark's (1967, 1968) Personality and Social Network Adjustment Scale. This is a self-report inventory, in which 17 globally defined items are rated on a 5-point scale by the patient. The form has been used as a mail questionnaire; however, an early study using relative informants was unsuccessful because too few forms were returned. Some test — retest reliability data and evidence for validity have been presented. The scale has been used primarily to evaluate the treatment effects of inpatient and outpatient communities. The time period assessed is "at present." The scale is simple and quick to complete and requires no training. There is a scoring system, but the form is not precoded.

When the scale was employed to evaluate the effects of treatment in a therapeutic community, it was found that adjustment improved from admission to discharge, deteriorated in the first 6 months after discharge, but returned to the level at discharge in the following 6 months. This level was maintained 18 months after leaving the hospital. Adjustment assessed during a 3-year follow-up showed that patients who were part of the therapeutic community maintained their improvement 5 years after discharge.

The Personality and Social Network Adjustment Scale was used by Frank as an outcome assessment in psychotherapy, and he reported that it correlated highly with the global ratings of the Structured and Scaled Interview to Assess Maladjustment (Gurland *et al.*, 1972; see below). He has found the scale useful in outcome assessment because of its brevity and simplicity (J. Frank, personal communication, February 8, 1977).

This scale is brief and economical. However, information on specific roles is limited, with no specific assessment of marital and parental roles. Individual assessments and response points are global.

Community Adaptation Schedule. The Community Adaptation Schedule (CAS; Burnes & Roen, 1967; Cook & Josephs, 1970; Roen & Burnes, 1968) assesses behavior, affect, and cognition in the work, family (marital and parental), and social (larger commerical and professional) communities. It is a 217-item self-administered report inventory, completed by the patient and rated on a 6-point scale. The time period assessed is "at the present time." Data on reliability, validity, internal consistency, and instructional material are available. The scale takes 30-60 minutes to complete and requires sixth-grade reading ability. Norms for various patient and nonpatient groups are published in a manual, and the scoring system and templates are available.

The most definitive application of the scale has been in multitreatment studies of aftercare, including psychotherapy. The scale has broad coverage of roles and includes both instrumental and affective performance. Items included present a mixture of lifelong characterological behavior and measures of current behavior during the past year, making it potentially less sensitive for evaluative research.

Structured and Scaled Interview to Assess Maladjustment. The Structured and Scaled Interview to Assess Maladjustment (SSIAM; Gurland *et al.*, 1972) assesses subjective distress, deviant behavior, and friction with others in five roles: work (as worker, housewife, or student), social, family, marital, and sex. Objective behavior in a given social context and subjective reactions in that context are included. Rater's global assessments and a general prognostic measurement are made. Sixty items are rated on an 11-point scale, with anchoring definitions for 5 of the 11 point. Information is collected during a structured interview with the patient, which is conducted by a trained professional with clinical experience; the scale takes about 30 minutes to administer. Specific instructions for the structuring of the interview are printed on the interview schedule. The time period assessed varies, but "the past month" is the most usual. Reliability, validity, scoring, results of factor analysis, and instructional material are available. The current form is not precoded.

This is one of the few structured social adjustment interviews. The interview structuring, anchoring definitions, and guiding explanations reduce ambiguity and provide precision. The items operationalize the assessments of aspects of behavior in a detailed fashion. The coverage is broad, and areas are tapped that are particularly relevant to outpatient populations. The scale was designed as an outcome measure for psychotherapy, and therefore the quantitative or instrumental aspects of behavior have less coverage and may require supplementation. These limitations are minor, and this scale has much to recommend it.

The Social Adjustment Scale. Instrumental and affective performance in work (as worker, housewife, or student), social and leisure activities, relationships with the extended family, marital and parental adjustment, and economic independence are assessed by the Social Adjustment Scale (SAS; Paykel, Weissman, Prusoff, & Tonks, 1971; Weissman *et al.*, 1974; Weissman & Paykel, 1974; Weissman, Paykel, Siegel, & Klerman, 1971). Global evaluations are made by the rater. Each role area includes assessments of performance at tasks, interpersonal relations, friction, and satisfaction in roles. The scale was modified from the previously described SSIAM, with revisions of core items and changes in anchor points for scoring. However, many of the items are directly comparable.

Forty-eight operationally defined items are rated on a 5-point scale. Information is obtained through a semistructured interview with the patient, which takes 45-60 minutes and is conducted by a trained bachelor's-degree-level rater. Initial questions are specified on the interview format. A 2-month period is assessed. Data on reliability, validity, sensitivity, and results of factor analysis are available, as are a video training tape and an instructional manual. The scoring sheet in precoded.

The scale was designed for a maintenance trial of antidepressants and psychotherapy in outpatient women. It has been used to assess nonpsychiatric community populations, suicide attempters, and methadone-maintained patients.

The SAS — Self-Report. A written self-administered version of the SAS, the SAS — Self-Report (SAS-SR; Weissman & Bothwell, 1976; Weissman, Prusoff, & Thompson, 1978) is comparable with the SAS in that it contains 42 questions that measure affective and instrumental performance in occupational role, social and leisure activities, relationship with extended family, marital role, parental role, family unit, and economic independence. The SAS-SR is completed in 15 to 20 minutes, ideally in the presence of a research assistant who instructs the patient about format, answers questions, and checks for completeness of responses. The period assessed is 2 weeks, in order to facilitate recall and accurate reporting of behavior. The form is precoded and is scored on a 5-point scale, from which role-area means and overall score and/or factorially derived dimensions can be obtained. Higher scores indicate greater impairment.

Agreement between results from the SAS-SR and the SAS interview was examined in 76 depressed outpatients receiving pharmacological treatment and was found to be excellent. Agreement among the patients' self-reports, the significant others' self-report ratings of the patients, and the interviewers' assessments of the patients' condition was good.

The SAS-SR is sensitive to change in depressed patients; improvement in the patients' social adjustment was found to be concomitant with clinical recovery. High internal consistency and test-retest stability across two time periods were found (Edwards, Yarvis, Mueller, Zingale, & Wagman, 1978). The SAS-SR discriminates between patient and nonpatient populations, with patient groups yielding poorer adjustment scores. Norms are available for nonpatient community sample populations, acutely ill and recovered depressed outpatients, schizophrenics, alcoholics, and methadone-maintained opiate addicts.

The Self-Assessment Guide. The Self-Assessment Guide (Willer & Biggin, 1974, 1976) is a written self-administered scale and was developed using factors identified by long-term follow-up studies as those associated with discharged patients' successful community adjustment. Most of the items are based on factor-analytic findings that were found to differentiate patient and nonpatient social functioning. Other items are based on the consensus of a number of professionals in the mental health care field, or relatives of patients regarding what constitutes community adjustment.

The complete questionnaire contains 55 items that cover the following seven areas: physical health, general affect, inter-personal skills, personal relations, use of leisure time, control of aggression, and financial support (employment). The Self-Assessment Guide is to be completed at admission and at some specified time following discharge. It is designed for evaluation of treatment outcome (and thus is intended to be responsive to changes in patients' behavior) and to predict community tenure.

Studies of test-retest reliability and split-half comparison demonstrated that the Self-Assessment Guide is reliable. A comparison of patients and nonpatients using an earlier version of the guide indicated that the scale differentiated between the two groups. The questions included in the final version do not differ substantially form those in the earlier version.

The Self-Assessment Guide was intended to provide information for a goal-directed approach to treatment. The Guide and a computerized scoring system have been designed to identify and print out a list of the patient's social adjustment problems prior to hospitalization. These are used to establish treatment goals relevant to the patient's future community adjustment.

Social Maladjustment Schedule. The Social Maladjustment Schedule (Clare & Cairns, 1978) was developed with the primary goal of operationalizing and standardizing criteria for social maladjustment. The authors' additional goals were that the scale be easy to administer and score, and be generally applicable for use in medical and community settings.

Marital and family relationships, other social relationships and activities, housing, occupation, leisure, and income are assessed. The unique aspect of this scale is that it measures three general categories that are relevant to and cut across all of the domains. They are "material conditions," "social management," and "satisfaction"; independent assessment ratings are determined for each of these categories.

In their attempt to establish objective criteria by which social adjustment and satisfaction could be measured, the authors standardized ways of measuring "material conditions." The importance of these criteria is that to realistically assess a person's social functioning and satisfaction, a yardstick of basic requirements for living must be established. This approach minimizes the impact of subjective report, and the person's subjective report may be compared with the objective criteria.

The category of "social management" and the assessment of functioning therein are extricated less easily from subjective report. However, the authors explicitly define functioning in this category in terms of leisure time and social and familial relationships. The "satisfaction" category takes into account the person's subjective report and measures the degree of satisfaction reported.

The semistructured interview is administered in about 1 hour by a trained interviewer. Forty-one ratings are made on a 4-point scale that indicates absence or degree of maladjustment. The schedule is easy to score and may be analyzed by component analysis. A manual contains a detailed glossary, sample probes, and suggestions for handling problems.

Interrater reliability was demonstrated by several methods. The overall percentage of agreement between raters was measured with respect to how frequently the raters agreed or disagreed on the presence or absence of maladjustment. There were lower percentages of agreement among raters when indicating the presence rather than absence of maladjustment, but general agreement was good. Weighted kappa values were high for eight interrater reliabilities. For 3 of the 17 items analyzed, a significant difference among raters was reported (household care, leisure opportunities, and number of leisure activities).

Partial validity has been established for the Social Maladjustment Schedule. The scale has been used in a number of studies of psychosocial morbidity in the community and in general practice in the United States, the United Kingdom, and Europe.

Social Problem Questionnaire. Corney, Clare and Fry (1982) felt the need for an easy-to-complete, short, and reliable self-administered report for use in primary care, social work, and psychiatry settings, and none had been developed or validated in Britain. The Social Problem Questionnaire (SPQ), which they developed, is essentially a self-administered report version of the Social Maladjustment Schedule (Clare & Cairns, 1978), described above. Although they attempted to assess the adequacy of the patients' circumstances, the "material conditions" component of the interview could not be covered as fully in the questionnaire. However, the "social management" and "satisfaction" components are directly comparable with the interview, as are the areas covered. Four items were added to determine the presence or absence of legal problems, problems associated with disability in the family, quality of interaction with friends, and other unspecified problems. The SPQ item ratings are the same as those used with the interview: A 4-point scale indicates the absence or severity of the problem.

The SPQ has been found to be simple to administer and readily acceptable to patients in general practice. The 41-items take about 5-10 minutes to complete. When compared with the social workers' assessments in preliminary testing and general practitioners' assessment in the pilot study, only 1 patient's problems out of 22 patients identified were not selected by the questionnaire. Agreement between the interview schedule and the SPQ was generally good; however, there was some degree of discrepancy between ratings.

As the authors assert, the pilot version of the SPQ appears to be a useful screening device to detect social problems among general practice and community patients. However, they intend to do additional work comparing the questionnaire with the Social Maladjustment Schedule, conducting test-retest reliability studies, and devising and testing alternative response scales.

The Social Behavior Assessment Schedule. The Social Behavior Assessment Schedule (SBAS; Platt, Hirsch, & Knights, 1981; Platt *et al.*, 1980) was designed to evaluate both objective changes due to the patient's mental or physical illness and subjective distress experienced by the family as a result of to these changes. The informant is a significant other, and guidelines for choosing the appropriate informant (e.g., face-to-face contact, lives in the same household, assumes responsibility for the patient) have been delineated by the authors. To quantify the impact of the illness, items assessing the patients' disturbed behavior, his or her limited social performance, and the adverse effects of the patient's behavior on the household are included, as well as item measuring the distress to the informant arising from these factors.

The interview is administered by a trained interviewer and consists of 239 items administered in a semistructured format; it takes about 60 to 90 minutes to complete. The interview consists of six sections, five of which cover the past month, and one of which covers the past 3 months. Rated in the sections are the following: (1) background information collected about the patient's illness, his or her behavior, and its effect on the family in view of the patient's recent social history; (2) the patient's behavior, which is rated in terms of onset, severity, and distress experienced by the informant as a result of the patient's behavior; (3) the patient's social performance, health, and employment history; (4) the objective consequences of the patient's behavior for the informant and the household, as well as the "reported distress" or the emotional consequence of each symptom, and the date of onset of the adverse effects; (5) serious concomitant life events experienced by the informant or by his or her household; and (6) support systems available to the informant, which are assessed in terms of help from friends, relatives, and social services, and housing situation. The interview manual defines the anchor points for ratings.

Several studies have been designed to measure the scale's validity. A total of 127 significant others were interviewed at the time of patients' hospitalizations and after 16 weeks. In one analysis, the relationship between the patients' symptomatic behavior and the extent of the informants' distress was examined. With the severity of the illness held constant, a divergence was found in the relationship between severity of objective symptoms and the extent of informant's distress. The data suggest that informants differ in their distress responses to the same symptoms and lend validity to the concept that subjective and objective aspects of "burden" should be considered separately.

Interrater reliability was established by four raters of diverse professional backgrounds. Agreement between pairs of raters on the total score of the six sections of the SBAS, the objective ratings of behavior, and ratings of reported distress was excellent.

The SBAS is an impressive scale. The interview manual and guidelines provide excellent examples of operationalizing and defining ratings. Further work on the scale's validity and sensitivity are forthcoming. The initial data have shown that the scale discriminates objective from subjective burden and accurately measures the impact of physical or psychiatric illness on a patient's household.

Social Functioning Schedule. The Social Functioning Schedule (SFS; Remington & Tyrer, 1979; Remington, Tyrer, Newson-Smith, & Cicchetti, 1979) is a brief, semistructured interview schedule designed for use with outpatients or day patients, which can be administered to a patient or to an informant. The authors developed the SFS because existing scales assumed either that there is some universally agreed-upon optimal functioning or that normative data are available. With the SFS "norms are decided by the patient or informant, not imposed from outside" (Remington & Tyrer, 1979, p. 152). They chose an interview format because it is most appropriate for use in clinical practice; it has been demonstrated to be more reliable than self-reports; and it offers the interviewer flexibility in determining how the *patient* feels he or she is functioning.

The SFS is structured around 12 sections that incorporate functioning both within and outside the home: (1) employment; (2) household chores; (3)

money; (4) self-care; (5) marital relationships; (6) child care; (7) patient-child relationships; (8) patient-parent relationships; (9) household relationships; (10) extramarital relationships; (11) social contacts; and (12) hobbies and spare-time activities. The 12 areas of functioning were chosen to give a reasonably comprehensive coverage of life situations for a variety of individuals. Some sections, such as the one on social contacts, apply to all individuals; others, such as the ones on employment and marital relationships, apply to large segments of the populations; and still others, such as the one on household relationships, apply only to a few individuals who reside with friends, acquaintances, or relatives other than parents, spouse, or children. The sections on employment, household chores, money, and spare-time activities are divided into "behavior" and "stress" subsections. Under "behavior," the patient's report of his or her own performance is rated; under "stress," the patient's description of his or her feelings, such as strain or worry, is rated. The sections and subsections make 16 potential areas for questions and rating. Within each section and subsection a group of questions is asked, but the semistructured nature of the instrument permits the interviewer to adapt or add to questions in order to elicit an adequate report. The patient's reports are then summarized by rating on an analogue scale, ranging from "no difficulties" at one extreme to "severe breakdown" at the other extreme, with no other defined anchor points. The interviewer makes his or her rating of reported problems by intersecting the scale at the appropriate point with a vertical line. Administration of the full schedule requires 10-20 minutes, depending on the range and severity of the problems. Patients are asked about, and ratings are made of, problems occurring in the past month, but the schedule can be adapted to cover other time periods.

Interrater and interinformant agreement was assessed and found to be satisfactory. The SFS was found to discriminate among personality-disordered and non-personality-disordered patients and a nonpatient group. Analysis of data collected on day patient and outpatient neurotics prior to treatment and after 4 and 8 months of treatment indicated that the SFS is sensitive to change over time.

The SFS provides a quick and quite reliable means to collect data on social functioning in the major role areas. Interviewers should be experienced clinicians, although some training with efforts made to reduce rater bias seems to be required for successful use of the schedule.

Functioning in Circumscribed Roles

Social Role Adjustment Instrument. The Social Role Adjustment Instrument (SRAI; Cohler, Grunebaum, Weiss, Gallant, & Abernethy, 1974; Cohler *et al.*, 1975) was developed because its authors could find no instrument that was suited to measure the conflict women experience in adapting to adult roles. Designed for a study of women's adjustment to motherhood, this scale assesses how successfully a woman has adjusted to her major adult roles. It provides separate measures of the degree of contact maintained with others in a specific role and her adaptation to that role.

The instrument consists of 25 9-point scales and approximately 200 items, which are administered in a semistructured 1 to 2-hour interview. A high score indicates satisfactory performance. The present form of the SRAI is a modification and revision of an earlier instrument developed by Shader, Kellam, and Durrell (1967).

A woman is asked to rate her performance as a homemaker, friend, wife, mother, and daughter. For each role, separate ratings are made on the frequency of contact with the other or others involved in the particular role relationship, the degree of conflict experienced with regard to that role, the depth of investment or involvement with the other or others, and overall adaptation to that role.

For three of the specified roles, additional scales are scored and are included in determining overall ratings of adjustment. For the role of wife, a separate rating is completed on the degree of sexual satisfaction experienced in marriage. For the maternal role, a separate rating is made on the degree of satisfaction that a woman derives from motherhood. For the role of daughter, a separate rating is made on the extent to which a woman can achieve appropriate and flexible autonomy from her own parents.

For a woman's performance as a housewife, a rating is made on the extent to which she can carry out the associated tasks of cooking, cleaning, managing the household budget, and supervising the children's activities when her husband is not present; a rating also is made on her degree of involvement in a hobby or other form of recreation. As a result of these more specific data, four summary adjustment scales are rated, including global social affiliation, overall investment in interpersonal relationships, overall inner discomfort, and overall psychiatric disturbance.

Shader *et al.* (1967) reported excellent interrater reliability correlations. Test-retest interviews conducted 18 months apart with a nonpatient sample showed stability over time in ratings, suggesting that the interviewer was able to code these interviews in a reliable manner.

The SRAI is appropriate for, and has been shown to discriminate between patient and nonpatient populations. Its focus is limited to the traditional roles of women, but it provides a thorough evaluation of a woman's adjustment to those roles.

KDS-15 Marital Questionnaire. The KDS-15 (Frank, Anderson, & Kupfer, 1976; Kupfer & Detre, 1974) is an 80-item self-administered questionnaire designed to assess marital relationships. Each marital partner is asked to privately complete the scale, which elicits both fixed-choice and essay-type responses. Completion time is unspecified; however, we estimate 30-60 minutes. Forms are to be returned to the researcher clinician without partners' discussing their responses.

The informant is asked to provide sociodemographic information about himself or herself and each of his or her parents and a developmental and psychosocial history that focuses on the marital relationship of his or her parents. The informant's current marital relationship is assessed through questions about courtship patterns, attitudes of extended family toward marriage, current living situation, makeup of household (including children), expression of affection, expression of disagreements between the couple, and satisfaction and dissatisfaction in all of these areas. Questions about the informant's specific sexual dysfunctions and those of his or her spouse are assessed for the following two time spans: "most of marriage" and "only recently." Items on parenting inquire about attitudes toward children, factors contributing to the decision to have children, attitudes toward child rearing, and effects of children on the couple's relationship. Finally, work, social activities, medical and psychiatric history, and opinions about sex-role division of responsibility in the household are assessed. Attitudes toward divorce, changing women's role, open marriages, and the like are elicited in essay form, and the informant is asked to offer any additional information that may provide insight into the marriage. Individual items are scored.

Reliability was tested using a nonpatient population and was found to be good. The scale discriminated between couples who were entering sexual therapy and those who were not, and between nonpatient and patient groups on items dealing with satisfaction in a sexual relationship. In a study of depressed inpatients and their spouses compared to normal couples, depressed couples reported significantly poorer functioning in all marital areas (Merikangas, Prusoff, Kupfer, & Frank, 1985).

The KDS-15 appears to be quite suitable for use with both patient and nonpatient populations. Whether it is applicable for use with persons who may have difficulty with the essay-type questions requires further testing. It is currently being used in a large-scale clinical trial of drugs and interpersonal psychotherapy in the maintenance treatment of recurrent depression.

Available Social Supports

Personal Resources Inventory. The Personal Resources Inventory (PRI; Clayton & Hirschfeld, 1977) was developed to assess the resources or social supports available to a person during his or her "most well" period of functioning in a defined 1-year period. The PRI is composed of 41 items administered in a structured interview with the patient on admission to a psychiatric treatment facility. A manual with specific probes, anchor points, and a predefined rating system for the items is available. Specific guidelines for defining the 12-month period to be assessed also are provided in the manual and are those delineated in the Research Diagnostic Criteria (RDC). Overall and specific ratings are obtained for the following potential sources of social support: current marriage, dating relationships, family, friends, neighbors, job or work role, financial resources, social contacts, living situation (safety and physical aspects), and other resources (e.g., religion, organizations, recreation, and pets). The interviewer asks the patient to make specific and global assessments of the social supports available prior to the onset of the current illness. A trained research assistant can administer the scale, since interviewer assessment of the patient is not required, and the interviewer is instructed to score "what the patient says."

Despite the fact that reliability and validity studies are not yet complete, this new scale is very promising because it provides a means for collecting data on another dimension of a person's social environment. It may prove useful for comparing differences in the resources available to various patient and nonpatient populations. A computerized scoring system is being developed, but a precoded data summary sheet is now available. The scale is being used in the NIMH Collaborative Program on the Psychobiology of Depression and in other ongoing studies of depressives (P. Clayton, M.D., personal communications, 1977, 1980, 1984).

Interview Schedule for Social Interaction. The Interview Schedule for Social Interaction (ISSI; Henderson *et al.*, 1981; Henderson, Byrne, Duncan-Jones, Scott, & Adcock, 1980; Henderson, Duncan-Jones, Byrne, & Scott, 1980) was developed by Henderson and Duncan-Jones to assess a person's current social-interactional system and, within that system, to measure the availability, and adequacy, as perceived by the person, of social supports. It was intended to provide a descriptive representation of social relationships and the basis for the development of a "causal model of interrelationships." The authors hypothesized a model that assumes that supportive social relationships act as a buffer is times of stress, and perhaps offset the development of psychiatric illness.

The conceptual structure of the ISSI is based on Weiss's theoretical model in which social relationships are defined by the following six dimensions: (1) attachment; (2) social integration; (3) taking responsibility for another; (4) reassurance of worth; (5) reliable alliance; and (6) obtaining guidance.

The ISSI consists of 52 items in a semistructured interview that takes approximately 1 hour to administer. A precoded interview, an interview guide manual in which each of the 52 items is operationalized, and directions for data analysis are available.

Designed for use in a longitudinal epidemiological study of nonpsychotic or neurotic disorders, the ISSI was administered to a random sample of 756 adults in Canberra, Australia. Data from the first wave of the study were analyzed; they supported the construct validity and reliability of the scale. A detailed description of the data analysis and the development of ISSI items can be obtained.

Correlation matrices were calculated, and 24 variables measuring the availability of social supports and 29 variables measuring the adequacy of social supports were isolated. The authors state that the ISSI items correspond well to Weiss's structural model. The reliability of the 52 items was tested on a subsample of 282 persons and was found to be acceptable. The ISSI is potentially suitable for use with various adult populations, including normal persons, psychiatrically ill persons, and the elderly, but this has not yet been demonstrated. Its well-developed approach to the assessment of social relationships makes it ideal for studies that focus on that aspect of social functioning.

Social Support Network Inventory. The Social Support Network Inventory (SSNI; Flaherty, Gaviria, Black, Altman, & Mitchell, 1983; Flaherty, Gaviria, & Pathak, 1983) is a written self-administered scale developed to assess the amount of social support received by psychiatric outpatients from their five closest social network members (e.g., relatives, friends, associates). Eleven items are rated for each of the five network members listed. The items cover four important aspects of support: availability, emotional support, practical support, and specific event-related support. Each item is rated from 1 to 5, with higher scores indicating greater support. Additional information is obtained with the SSNI: basic demographics, including whether any children live in the geographic area; a list of *all* network members, which is elicited before respondents are asked to choose their closest five; and data on age, sex, relationship with, and number of years each of the persons has been known to the respondent. Although these data are not incorporated into the scale's scoring, they are of use for detailed network analysis.

Clinicians' global ratings of the strength of 22 unipolar depressed patients' support systems were compared with the patients' SSNI scores, and support for the convergent validity of the instrument was found. To examine concurrent validity, mean SSNI scores were compared for 32 members of a religious commune and a pair-matched group of 32 from an urban neighborhood. As predicted, the respondents from the religious commune reported significantly greater social support, compared with the urban dwellers.

Forty-Four outpatients with unipolar depression were assessed on the SSNI, the Hamilton Rating Scale for Depression (HRSD), and the SAS-SR. The high-social-support group was found to have far lower mean HRSD scores (i.e., to be much less depressed) than the low-social-support group, and to have much lower SAS-SR scores (i.e., to be much better adjusted).

The SSNI is an attractive scale. It is easily administered, takes only 15-30 minutes to complete, has a straightforward scoring system, and elicits off-scale data that are potentially useful for additional social support or network analyses.

COMMENT ON THE MEASUREMENT OF SOCIAL ADJUSTMENT

While we have reviewed only 16 scales — those deemed suitable for use with depressives — there are currently at least 30 published scales that measure various aspects of social adjustment. Although the scales reviewed here represent a range of approaches to the measurement of social adjustment, there are still at least two major limitations in the available methodology. These limitations are both practical and conceptual. On a practical level, the scales have been tested on, and are applicable to, only adult populations; there is a lack of scales designed specifically for children, adolescents, or the elderly. Moreover, many of the scales cannot be adapted to reflect changes in traditional roles, especially among women.

On the conceptual level, the scales often include overlapping and unspecified concepts. A number of conceptual areas underlie the notion of "social adjustment"; typically, two or three areas are measured with varying emphasis, depending on the scale. For example, a scale designed to measure functioning in roles may also measure availability of supports and capacity for intimacy. Since dysfunctioning in each of these areas may have considerably different implications for intervention, a fruitful task for future development would be the explication and measurement of more unitary concepts. An additional impetus for the clarification of these conceptual areas is that impairment in social functioning has emerged as an integral part of the *Diagnostic and Statistical Manual of Mental Disorders*, third edition (DSM-III), multiaxial diagnostic system. Specificity in diagnostic criteria, which has been a major achievement of DSM-III, suggests that social adjustment should ultimately be approached in a similar manner.

Acknowledgment

Work on this chapter was supported in part by the Yale Mental Health Clinical Research Center (Grant No. MH 30929), and by the John P. and Catherine T. MacArthur Foundation Network on Risk and Protective Factors in the Major Mental Disorders.

References

Abrahams, M. J., & Whitlock, F. A. (1969). Childhood experience and depression. *British Journal of Psychiatry, 115*, 883-888.

Beck, A. T. (1967). *Depression: Clinical, experimental and theoretical aspects*. London: Staples Press.

Beck, A. T., Sethi, B. B., & Tuthill, R. W. (1963). Childhood bereavement and adult depression. *Archives of General Psychiatry, 9*, 295-302.

Birtchnell, J. (1970). Depression in relation to early and recent parent death. *British Journal of Psychiatry, 116*, 299-306.

Bowlby, J. (1969). *Attachment and loss* (Vol. 1). London: Hogarth Press.

Brown, G. W., Birley, J. L. T., & Wing, J. F. (1972). Influence of family life on the course of schizophrenic disorders: A replication. *British Journal of Psychiatry, 121*, 241-258.

Brown, G. W., & Harris, T. (1978). *Social origins of depression: A study of psychiatric disorder in women*. London: Tavistock.

Burnes, A. J., & Roen, S. R. (1967). Social roles and adaptation to the community. *Community Mental Health Journal, 3*, 153-158.

Campbell, E. A., Cope, S. J., & Teasdale, J. D. (1983). Social factors and affective disorders: An investigation of Brown and Harris's model. *British Journal of Psychiatry, 143*, 548-553.

Clare, A. W., & Cairns, V. E. (1978). Design, development and use of a standardized interview to assess social maladjustment and dysfunction in community studies. *Psychological Medicine, 8*, 589-604.

Clark, A. W. (1967). Conditions influencing patient response to treatment in a therapeutic community. *Social Science and Medicine, 1*, 309-319.

Clark, A. W. (1968). The Personality and Social Network Adjustment Scale. *Human Relations, 21*, 85-96.

Clayton, P., & Hirschfeld, R. M. A. (1977). *Personal Resources Inventory (PRI)*. Unpublished interview, Washington University School of Medicine.

Cohler, B. J., Grunebaum, H. U., Weiss, J. L., Gallant, D. H., & Abernethy, V. (1974). Social role performance and psychopathology among recently hospitalized mothers. *Journal of Nervous and Mental Disease, 159*, 81-90.

Cohler, B. J., Robbins, D. M., Shader, R. I., Grunebaum, H. U., Gallant, D. H., & Weiss, J. L. (1975). Social adjustment and psychopathology among formerly hospitalized and nonhospitalized mothers: I. Development of the Social Role Adjustment Instrument. *Journal of Psychiatric Research, 12*, 1-18.

Cook, P., & Josephs, P. (1970). The Community Adaptation Schedule and the California Psychological Inventory: A validational study with college students. *Community Mental Health Journal, 6*, 366-370.

Corney, R. H., Clare, A. W., & Fry, J. (1982). The development of a self-report questionnaire to identify social problems — a pilot study. *Psychological Medicine, 12*, 903-909.

Costello, C. G. (1982). Social factors associated with depression: A retrospective community study. *Psychological Medicine, 12*, 329-339.

Crook, T., Raskin, A., & Eliot, J. (1981). Parent-child relationships and adult depression. *Child Development, 52*, 950-957.

Dohrenwend, B. S., & Dohrenwend, B. P. (1981). Life stress and illness: Formulation of issues. In B. S. Dohrenwend & B. P. Dohrenwend (Eds.), *Stressful life events and their contexts* (pp. 1-27). New York: Prodist.

Edwards, D. W., Yarvis, R. M., Mueller, D. P., Zingale, H. C., & Wagman, W. J. (1978). Test-taking and the stability of adjustment scales: Can we assess patient deterioration? *Evaluation Quarterly, 2*, 275-291.

Flaherty, J. A., Gaviria, F. M., Black, E. M., Altman, E., & Mitchell, T. (1983). The role of social support in the functioning of patients with unipolar depression. *American Journal of Psychiatry, 140*, 473-476.

Flaherty, J. A., Gaviria, F. M., & Pathak, D. S. (1983). The measurement of social support: The Social Support Network Inventory. *Comprehensive Psychiatry, 24*, 521-529.

Frank, E., Anderson, C., & Kupfer, D. J. (1976). Profiles of couples seeking sex therapy and marital therapy. *American Journal of Psychiatry, 133*, 559-562.

Glazer, W., Aaronson, H. S., Prusoff, B. A., & Williams, D. H. (1980). Assessment of social adjustment in chronic ambulatory schizophrenic outpatients. *Journal of Nervous and Mental Disease, 168*, 493-497.

Goldstein, M. J., & Doane, J. A. (1982). Family factors in the onset, course, and treatment of schizophrenic spectrum disorders: An update on current research. *Journal of Nervous and Mental Disease, 170*, 692-700.

Gurland, B. J., Yorkston, N. J., Stone, A. R., Frank, J. D., & Fleiss, J. L. (1972). The Structured and Scaled Interview to Assess Maladjustment (SSIAM). *Archives of General Psychiatry, 27*, 259-267.

Henderson, S., Byrne, D. G., & Duncan-Jones, P. (1981). *Neurosis and the social environment*. Sydney, Australia: Academic Press.

Henderson, S., Byrne, D. G., Duncan-Jones, P., Scott, R., & Adcock, S. (1980). Social relationships, adversity and neurosis: A study of associations in a general population sample. *British Journal of Psychiatry, 136*, 574-583.

Henderson, S., Duncan-Jones, P., Byrne, D. G., & Scott, R. (1980). Measuring social relationships: The Interview Schedule for Social Interactions. *Psychological Medicine, 10*, 723-734.

Hogarty, G. E., & Katz, M. M. (1971). Norms of adjustment and social behavior. *Archives of General Psychiatry, 25*, 470-480.

Jacobson, S., Fasman, J., & DiMascio, A. (1975). Deprivation in the childhood of depressed women. *Journal of Nervous and Mental Disease, 160*, 5-14.

Katschnig, H. (1983). Methods for measuring social adjustment. In T. Helgason (Ed.), *Methodology in evaluation of psychiatric treatment* (pp. 205-218). New York: Cambridge University Press.

Katz, M. M., & Lyerly, S. B. (1963). Methods of measuring adjustment and social behavior in the community: I. Rationale, description, discriminative validity and scale development. *Psychological Reports, 13*, 503-535.

Kidd, K. K., & Matthysse, S. (1978). Research design for the study of gene-environment interactions in psychiatric disorders: Report of an FFRP panel. *Archives of General Psychiatry, 35*, 925-932.

Klerman, G. L., Weissman, M. M., Rounsaville, B. J., & Chevron, E. S. (1984). *Interpersonal psychotherapy of depression*. New York: Basic Books.

Kupfer, D. J., & Detre, T. P. (1974). *KDS: A modern mental health charting system*. Unpublished manuscript, University of Pittsburgh.

Lazarus, R. S. (1966). *Psychological stress and the coping process*. New York: McGraw-Hill.

Lin, N., Dean, A., & Ensel, W. (1981). Social support scales: A methodologic note. *Schizophrenia Bulletin, 7*(1), 73-88.

Lin, N., Simeone, R. S., Ensel, W. M., & Kuo, W. (1979). Social support, stressful life events and illness: A model and an empirical test. *Journal of Health and Social Behavior, 20*, 108-119.

Merikangas, K. R., Prusoff, B. A., Kupfer, D. J., & Frank, E. (1985). Marital adjustment in major depression. *Journal of Affective Disorders, 9*, 5-11.

Munro, A. (1966). Parental deprivation in depressive patients. *British Journal of Psychiatry, 112*, 443-457.

Orvaschel, H., Weissman, M. M., & Kidd, K. K. (1980). Children and depression: The children of depressed parents; the childhood of depressed patients; depression in children. *Journal of Affective Disorders, 2*, 1-16.

Parker, G. (1979a). Parental characteristics in relation to depressive disorders. *British Journal of Psychiatry, 134*, 138-147.

Parker, G. (1979b). Reported parental characteristics in relation to trait depression and anxiety levels in a nonclinical group. *Australian and New Zealand Journal of Psychiatry, 13*, 260-264.

Parker, G. (1981). Parental reports of depressives: An investigation of several explanations. *Journal of Affective Disorders, 3*, 131-140.

Parker, G. (1982). Parental representations and affective symptoms: Examination for an hereditary link. *British Journal of Medical Psychology, 55*(1), 57-61.

Parker, G. Tupling, H., & Brown, L. B. (1979). A parental bonding instrument. *British Journal of Medical Psychiatry, 52*, 1-10.

Paykel, E. S., Myers, J. K., Diendelt, M. N. Klerman, G. L., Lindenthal, J. J., & Pepper, M. P. (1969). Life events and depression: A controlled study. *Archives of General Psychiatry, 21*, 753-760.

Paykel, E. S. Weissman, M. M., Prusoff, B. A., & Tonks, M. B. (1971). Dimensions of social adjustment. *Journal of Nervous and Mental Disease, 152*, 158-172.

Perris, C. A. (1966). A study of bipolar (manic-depressive) and unipolar recurrent depressive psychoses, Part 2 (Childhood environment and precipitating factors). *Acta Psychiatrica Scandinavica, 42*(Suppl. 194), 45-57.

Platt, S. D., Hirsch, S. R., & Knights, A. C. (1981). Effects of brief hospitalization on psychiatric patients' behaviour and social functioning. *Acta Psychiatrica Scandinavica, 63*, 117-128.

Platt, S. D., Weyman, A., Hirsch, S., & Hewett, S. (1980). The Social Behavior Assessment Schedule (SBAS): Rationale, contents, scoring and reliability of a new interview schedule. *Social Psychiatry, 15*, 43-55.

Raskin, A., Boothe, H. H., Reatig, N. A., Schulterbrandt, J. G., & Odle, D. (1971). Factor analyses of normal and depressed patients' memories of parental behavior. *Psychological Reports, 29*, 871-879.

Remington, M., & Tyrer, P. (1979). The Social Functioning Schedule — a brief semi-structured interview. *Social Psychiatry, 14*, 151-157.

Remington, M., Tyrer, P. J., Newson-Smith, J., & Cicchetti, D. V. (1979). Comparative reliability of categorical and analogue rating scales in the assessment of psychiatric symptomatology. *Psychological Medicine, 9*, 765-770.

Roen, S. R., & Burnes, A. J. (1968). *Community Adaptation Schedule preliminary manual*. New York: Behavioral Publications.

Roy, A. (1978). Vulnerability factors and depression in women. *British Journal of Psychiatry, 113*, 106-110.

Roy, A. (1981). Risk factors and depression in Canadian women. *Journal of Affective Disorders, 3*, 65-70.

Schaefer, E. S. (1963). Children's reports of parental behavior: An inventory. *Child Development, 36*, 413-424.

Schaefer, E. S. (1965). A configurational analysis of children's reports of parent behavior. *Journal of Consulting Psychology, 29*, 552-557.

Seligman, M. E. P. (1975). *Helplessness: On depression, development and death*. San Francisco: W. H. Freeman.

Shader, R., Kellam, S., & Durrell, J. (1967). Social field events during the first week of hospitalization as predictors of treatment outcome for psychotic patients. *Journal of Nervous and Mental Disease, 145*, 142-153.

Solomon, Z., & Bromet, E. (1982). The role of social factors in affective disorder: An assessment of the vulnerability model of Brown and his colleagues. *Psychological Medicine 12*, 123-130.

Strauss, J. S., & Carpenter, W. T., Jr. (1972). The prediction of outcome in schizophrenia: I. Characteristics of outcome. *Archives of General Psychiatry, 27*, 739-746.

Vaughn, C., & Leff, J. P. (1976a). The measurement of expressed emotion in the families of psychiatric patients. *British Journal of Social and Clinical Psychology, 15*, 157-165.

Vaughn, C., & Leff, J. P. (1976b). The influence of family and social factors on the course of psychiatric illness: A comparison of schizophrenic and depressed neurotic patients. *British Journal of Psychiatry, 129*, 125-137.

Weissman, M. M. (1975). The assessment of social adjustment: A review of techniques. *Archives of General Psychiatry, 32*, 357-365.

Weissman, M. M., & Bothwell, S. (1976). The assessment of social adjustment by patient self-report. *Archives of General Psychiatry, 33*, 1111-1115.

Weissman, M. M., Klerman, G. L., Paykel, E. S., Prusoff, B. A., & Hanson, B. (1974). Treatment effects on the social adjustment of depressed patients. *Archives of General Psychiatry, 30*, 771-778.

Weissman, M. M., & Paykel, E. S. (1974). *The depressed woman: A study of social relationships*. Chicago: University of Chicago Press.

Weissman, M. M., Paykel, E. S., Siegel, R., & Klerman, G. L. (1971). The social role performance of depressed women: Comparisons with a normal group. *American Journal of Orthopsychiatry, 41*, 390-405.

Weissman, M. M., Prusoff, B. A., & Thompson, W. E. (1978). Social adjustment by self-report in a community sample and in psychiatric outpatients. *Journal of Nervous and Mental Disease, 166*, 317-326.

Weissman, M. M., Sholomskas, D., & John, K. (1981). The assessment of social adjustment: An update. *Archives of General Psychiatry, 38*, 1250-1258.

Weissman, M. M., Wickramaratne, P., Merikangas, K. R., Leckman, J. F., Prusoff, B. A., Caruso, K. A., Kidd, K. K., & Gammon, G. D. (1984). Onset of major depression in early adulthood: Increased familial loading and specificity. *Archives of General Psychiatry, 41*, 1136-1143.

Willer, B., & Biggin, P. (1974). *Self Assessment Guide: Rationale, development and evaluation.* Unpublished manuscript, Lakeshore Psychiatric Hospital, Toronto.

Willer, B., & Biggin, P. (1976). Comparison of rehospitalized and non-hospitalized psychiatric patients on community adjustment: Self-Assessment Guide. *Psychiatry, 39*, 239-244.

CHAPTER 13

The Measurement of Depressive Experience and Disorder across Cultures

ANTHONY J. MARSELLA
University of Hawaii
The Queen's Medical Center, Honolulu

INTRODUCTION

Current conceptions of the evolution of life acknowledge the reciprocal relationships between life forms and their environment. For many primitive and immobile life forms, the physical environment is the only context to which they must adapt. A profound change in the physical environment can result in the extinction of the life form because of its inability to adapt to the demands of the change.

However, for higher forms of life, especially human beings, adaptation to the environment is complicated by several factors, including the presence of culture. A behavior-oriented definition of culture is "shared learned behaviors that are transmitted from one generation to another for purposes of adjustment and adaptation" (adapted from Linton, 1945, p. 32). In this definition, culture becomes a resource for promoting human growth and development, as well as a source of environmental demands.

For human beings, genetic potential is tested against the changing demands of a physical and cultural environment. Both of these forces are potent determinants of adaptation via the responses we call behavior. In recent decades, there has been a growing awareness among scientists and professionals that normal and abnormal behavior must be construed as the outcome of many forces both within and external to the human organism. The relationship among these forces has been termed "ecological," a word referring to the systematic relationships that develop between organisms and their life milieu (Marsella, 1984).

It is puzzling that most theories of human behavior focus on only limited segments of the spectrum of behavioral determinants. Virtually all contemporary theories of behavior endorse either biological or psychological determinants of human functioning while ignoring or giving only passive attention to the determinants within the cultural and the physical environment. This is true for theories of both normal and disordered human functioning.

In my opinion, if we are to progress in our understanding, control, and prediction of human behavior, both normal and disordered, it will be necessary for us to reconceptualize our existing theories to incorporate a broader spectrum of the determinants of human behavior and their relationship to one another. Figure 13-1 displays a framework that acknowledges the interaction of external and internal determinants of human behavior. The premise of Figure 13-1 is that the different forces find themselves represented in one another in the process of adaptation. What we are biologically (i.e., our biochemical functioning, our sensory processes) is determined in part by psychological, physical, and cultural forces. Similarly, what we are psychologically is determined in part by our biological, cultural, and physical environments.

Too often, we speak of health and illness from the limited perspectives of only one of these levels of conceptualization. We focus on content, but we forget the process by which content is changed or maintained. Hormone levels change in response to genetic programs; however, they also change in response to cultural contexts that constitute threats to organismic adjustment.

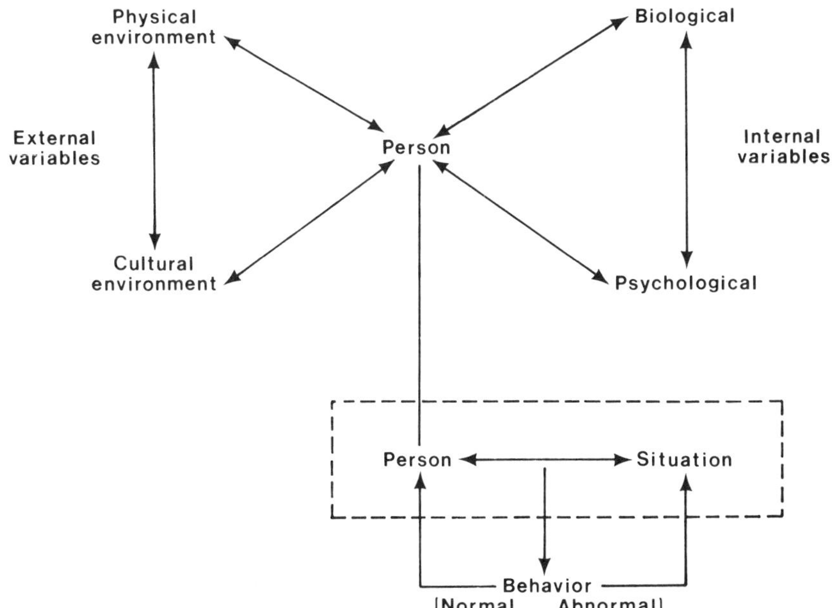

FIGURE 13-1 General interactional model of human behavior.

Indeed, the very perception of a threat that elicits the hormonal change is determined by culturally conditioned perceptions.

Table 13-1 displays the hierarchy of determinants in which human beings are embedded. These range from large, macrosocial levels to biopsychosocial levels that include cells, chemistry, and other physiological systems. Although we often separate the different levels, it is important to acknowledge that each level incorporates the others and represents them within its own expressive modes (e.g., a culturally induced stressor may be represented as an increase in norepinephrine levels in the neural synapse).

The purpose of this chapter is to discuss the measurement of depressive disorders from a cross-cultural perspective, and the reader may well question the reason for this prologue. The answer is quite simple. Of all the determinants of human behavior, especially psychopathology, cultural determinants have received the least attention and credence. It is natural that this should be the case, since mental disorders have been largely the purview of psychiatrists and clinical psychologists, and these professions are based on biomedical and psychological premises that only minimally incorporate sociocultural knowledge. But if we are to understand disordered behavior, especially problems such as depression, it is necessary that we attend to the full spectrum of determinants of human behavior. Cultural determinants constitute the context in which biological and psychological processes are embedded. They can serve as formative, precipitative, exacerbative, and maintenance causes of depressive disorders. The approach to multicausality is displayed in Figure 13-2.

TABLE 13-1 Hierarchical Systems in Human Adaptation and Psychopathology

Systems level	Typical variables
I. Macrosocial (political, social, economic)	I. Westernization, industrialization, sociotechnical change, poverty
↓ ↑	
II. Microsocial (family, schools, work)	II. Family relations, general social relations, social networks
↓ ↑	
III. Psychosocial (personality, situations)	III. Psychological needs and motives, stressors
↓ ↑	
IV. Biobehavioral (individual functioning)	IV. Basic sensory-motor functions, cognitive processes (attention, memory)
↓ ↑	
V. Biopsychosocial (cells, chemistry, organs)	V. Neurotransmitters, immune systems, hormones, structures

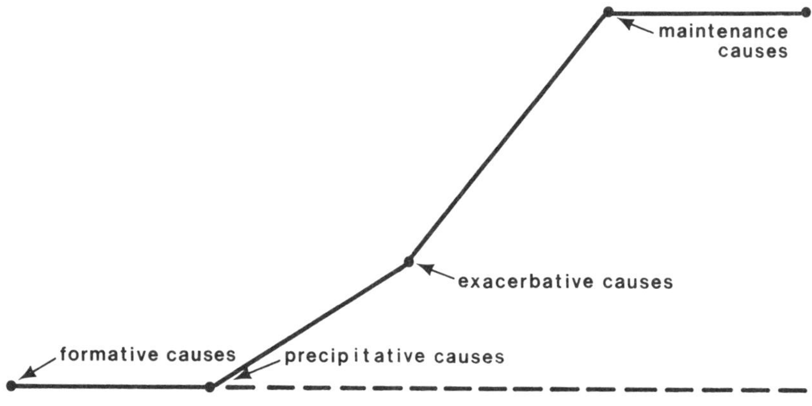

FIGURE 13-2 Multicausality model.

Perhaps if we consider the role of context and milieu in something as fundamental as the evolution of life, it will be easier to acknowledge the importance of these factors in our everyday behavior, which is the foundation of adaptation. I am not promoting a cultural theory of psychopathology, but rather an interactional model in which cultural factors are given credence along with biological, psychological, and physical determinants. Clinical research designs can then be conceptualized as multilevel and multidimensional, as displayed in Table 13-2. If the importance of cultural factors is accepted, then the purposes of this chapter will be clearer and more powerful, and the issues raised and addressed will achieve the position of respect they deserve.

CULTURE AND PSYCHOPATHOLOGY

Statement of the Problem

The problems associated with the measurement of depressive disorders assume new levels of complexity when we cross ethnocultural boundaries of human experience. At this point, we are faced with numerous problems regarding the meaning, expression, and psychosocial correlates of depressive disorders. This fact has only recently gained acceptance among researchers and professionals (Marsella, 1981). The particular purpose of this chapter is to discuss the issues, methods, and unresolved questions associated with the measurement of depression among people from non-European cultural traditions.

Within the northern European cultural traditions from which our current conceptions of depression are derived, depressive disorders comprise a spectrum

TABLE 13-2 Multilevel and Multidimensional Clinical Research Design

Hierarchical level	Clinical parameters				
	Onset	Symptoms	Course	Outcome	Diagnosis
Macrosocial					
Microsocial					
Psychosocial					
Biopsychosocial					

of dysfunctions varying from mild, transient mood disruptions to severe, chronic impairments that embrace somatic, psychological, and interpersonal functioning. Among the severe depressive disorders, individuals may suffer complete emotional and physical retardation, with accompanying hallucinations, delusions, and bizarre behavior.

Within the Western world, depression is considered one of the most important dimensions of human experience, and there are numerous disorders that are concerned with it. We speak of depression as a mood, as a symptom, and as a syndrome that involves cognitive, affective, existential, interpersonal, and somatic functioning. However, there is growing evidence that the experience, expression, and correlates of depressive disorders as they are construed in the West are not universal, but rather vary as a function of ethnocultural experience. To the extent that ethnocultural traditions are similar to those of the northern European cultures, similarities across these aspects of depressive disorder are found; however, as the differences in ethnocultural traditions increase, variations also grow (Marsella, 1981).

That this is the case should not be surprising, for ethnocultural experience constitutes an important determinant of human behavior, especially in the areas of perception, thought, emotion, motivation, social behavior, and health ideologies and treatments. Indeed, the influences of ethnocultural traditions extend far beyond even these processes and content into basic epistemological and ontological levels. It is not only the content of human experience and behavior that varies across ethnocultural boundaries, but the very foundations by which people come to know and organize the world. This approach is displayed in Figure 13-3. Our language, self-structure, and representation mode mediate depressive experience.

The Concept of Culture

There are many definitions of the term "culture." Kluckhohn and Kroeber (1952) reviewed more than 150 of these definitions and point out the problems associated with efforts to define the concept. Culture is represented in both external and internal dimensions of human behavior.

At an external level, culture is represented in various artifacts, architectural and expressive forms, institutions, and role and behavioral patterns. But culture is also represented internally, in the values, attitudes, beliefs, cognitive styles, and patterns of consciousness of an individual. As such, it is the primary mediator or filter for interacting with the world; it is the lens by which we experience and define reality and orient ourselves to others, to the unknown, and to our subjective experience.

What I am contending is that ethnocultural experience ultimately influences our biological, psychological, social, and spiritual functioning. When we encounter a person from a different ethnocultural tradition, we are encountering a person whose reality is different from our own. The differences exceed the language and physical variations between us. They involve basic human experience.

Many researchers and professionals have been unwilling to accept the reality of ethnocultural variations and their implications for disordered human behavior. Often, this unwillingness has been predicated on the assumption that the perception of human differences represents racism sexism, or ageism, which are untenable on both religious and moral grounds. Yet it may well be that these grounds are the basis of many of the pernicious effects of ethnocentricity that come to characterize our efforts in mental health research and service, including erroneous diagnoses, treatment failures, clinical abuses, and service deprivations.

Quite simply, psychopathology is as much influenced by ethnocultural factors as is normal human behavior. To the extend that physical factors are involved in any disorder, the range of variation may narrow; however, it is never nonexistent, even when exact neurological sites are implicated among patients from different cultural traditions. This premise is displayed in Figure 13-4. As this figure indicates, variation is greatest among normal behavior and more focused as neurological substrates become involved. But even given similar neurological substrates (e.g., epinephrine levels, cell vacuoles), the individual must still interpret this condition, translate it into a behavioral

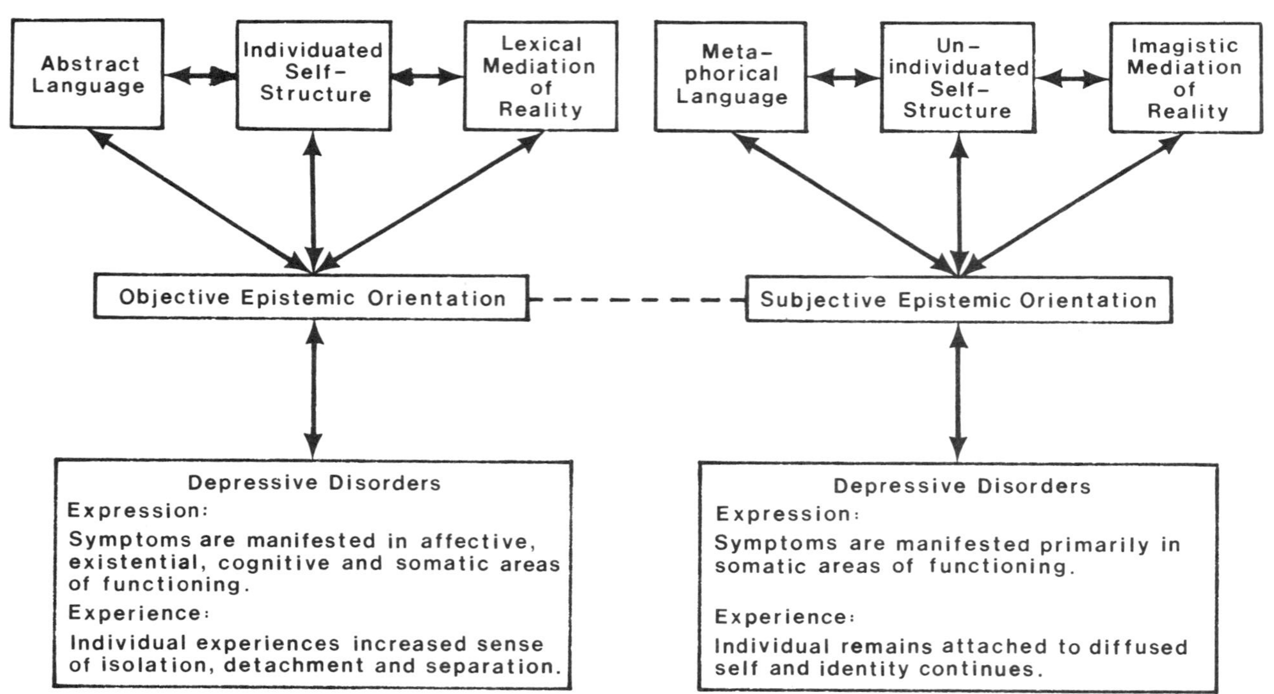

FIGURE 13-3 Continuum of objective versus subjective epistemological orientations.

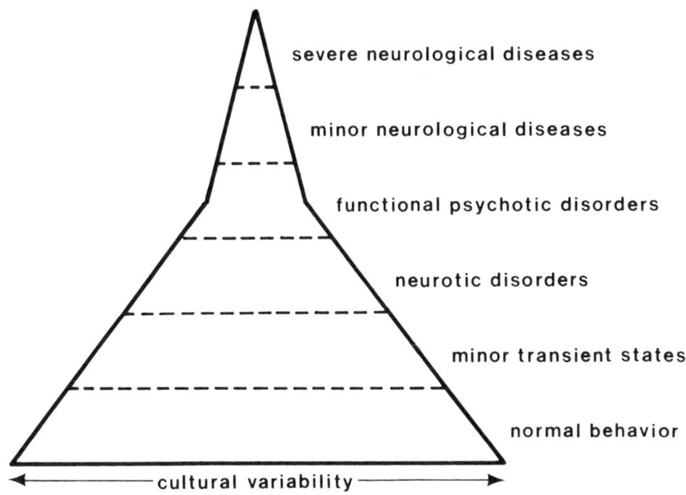

FIGURE 13-4 Symptom variability across normal behavior-neurological disease spectrums.

repertoire, and experience the social response to this display. All of the latter are culturally determined phenomena.

Cultural factors are capable of mediating psychopathology in a number of ways (Leighton & Murphy, 1959; Marsella, 1982):

1. Culture helps determine the types and parameters of physical and psychosocial stressors.
2. Culture determines the types and parameters of coping mechanisms and resources used to mediate stressors.
3. Culture determines basic personality patterns. These include, but are not limited to, the self-structure, self-concept, and need/motivational systems.
4. Culture determines the language system of an individual, and it is language that assists us in the perception, classification, and organization of responses to reality.
5. Culture helps determine the standards of normality, deviance, and health of an individual and society. It influences health ideology and attitudes, as well as treatment orientations and practices.
6. Culture determines classification patterns for various disorders and diseases. In this respect, all mental disorders are culture-specific, and not simply those designated by Western professionals as exotic disorders.
7. Culture determines the patterns of experience and expression of psychopathology, including such factors as onset, manifestation, course, and outcome.

Within this conceptual framework, it is incumbent that all researchers and professionals interested in depressive disorders consider the range of cultural factors that may be acting upon a depressive episode. Let us briefly examine some of the relevant research literature on the topic of culture and depressive experience and disorder.

CULTURE AND DEPRESSIVE EXPERIENCE AND DISORDER

In 1904, Emil Kraepelin, the father of our modern Western psychiatric classification systems, visited a number of non-Western societies as part of an international lecture tour. In many non-Western settings, he found himself puzzled by the forms of psychopathology. During the course of his stay in Indonesia, he noted that there appeared to be an absence of depressive disorders — a fact that he attributed to diet and climate, rather than to life styles and patterns of human experience.

In the eight decades since Kraepelin first registered his observations, there has been a considerable interest in the study of depressive disorders among non-Western people. These studies have been reviewed by several writers (Fabrega, 1974, 1975; Kiev, 1972; Marsella, 1981; Marsella, Sartorius, Jablensky, & Fenton, 1985; Prince, 1968; Pfeiffer, 1970; Sartorius, 1973; Singer, 1975). As a group, these publications have examined the epidemiology, phenomenology, correlates, and etiological dimensions of depressive disorders across cultures. The range of actual research on the topic has involved clinical, psychometric, field, and laboratory studies. Based on an overview of this literature, and with proper regard for research limitations, the following conclusions emerge:

1. Western European concepts of depressive disorders are not universally shared. Many cultures have no equivalent concepts or terms for depression as viewed in the West.
2. Because of problems in measurement, including the definition and identification of a case, it is difficult to determine cultural variations in the epidemiology of depressive disorders.
3. The phenomenology and manifestation of depressive disorders appear to vary across cultures. In many non-Western cultures, there is an absence of psychological dimensions to the problem (i.e., self-denigration and abasement, guilt, suicidal thoughts and impulses, sadness); however, somatic dimensions seem to be present (i.e., sleep difficulties, fatigue and weakness, eating disorders). It may be that culture determines the psychological content and processes associated with depressive disorders.
4. The measurement of depressive disorders across cultures is characterized by problems in translation; by lack of equivalence in norms and reference groups, concepts, and scales; and by different dietary and disease history factors.

5. The personality correlates of depressive disorders differ across cultural boundaries. Low self-esteem, self-concept discrepancy, guilt, obsessions, and defense systems are not universally present.

Cross-cultural research represents a methodology for comparing differences in groups of individuals who belong to different ethnocultural traditions. It offers the opportunity to examine both similarities and differences in human behavior that may be attributed to acquired experience and the interactions of acquired experience with genetic factors. Cross-cultural research on depressive disorders indicates that the way we construe this range of problems in the Western world may be a function of historical and cultural forces. If this is the case, cross-cultural research may help us escape the confines of our current notions and may open up alternative perspectives that will lead to new avenues for research and clinical practice. However, first, we must address the problems associated with cross-cultural measurement.

CROSS-CULTURAL MEASUREMENT: ISSUES AND METHODS

Within the last two decades, there has been a growing awareness that cross-cultural studies require methods designed to limit ethnocentric bias. For many years, researchers assumed that research instruments and methods developed in one culture could readily be applied to other cultures, with only minor adjustments for translation. Gradually, and at a high cost of misinformation, researchers came to recognize that cross-cultural measurement demands careful attention to the problems of translation, conceptual equivalence, and scale equivalence. These problems are addressed here in order.

Translation

For many researchers, the use of a test, interview schedule, or rating scale across cultures simply involves its translation into the appropriate language. To accomplish this, they may turn the instrument over to a friend in a language department and then pick it up a few days later in its new form. This approach has led to serious problems.

To correct for the limitations involved in simple translation, cross-cultural research requires the use of "back translation" methods (Brislin, Lonner, & Thorndike, 1973; Lonner, 1979; Werner & Campbell, 1970). "Back translation" requires that material translated into a different language be retranslated into the original language for comparison purposes. Thus, the following paradigm is used:

Language A → Language B → Language A

This cycle can be repeated a number of times, using individual or group translation routines, to guarantee that the original denotative and connotative meaning is not lost.

There are many other procedures that can be used in conjunction with back translation, involving the use of bilingual individuals, pilot efforts, semantic analyses, and so forth. All of these procedures are designed to increase the accuracy of the translation. The problem, of course, is that many words and concepts do not have similar connotative meanings even when similar denotative meanings are present. A camel is not a camel in all cultures. This problem is compounded when we seek to study abstractions such as emotions, needs, and disorders. This leads to problems of conceptual equivalence.

Conceptual Equivalence

It is cruical for cross-cultural researchers to understand that concepts do not possess equivalent meanings in different cultures (Sears, 1961). For example, in traditional Anglo-American culture, a premium is placed on being independent, autonomous, and individualistic. Dependency is associated with immaturity and psychopathology. However, in Japanese culture, *amae*, which is the closest equivalent term to "dependency" in the English language, is highly valued and encouraged. Not only is *amae* acceptable, it is actively fostered. This is because Japanese culture has long prized group cohesion and solidarity over individualistic effort or personal aggrandizement (Doi, 1973). Thus, if we as Anglo-Americans study dependency in Japan, we are likely to conclude that the entire society is immature and childish from our point of view because personal independence is devalued. This would be an unfortunate mistake, as Sony, Toyota, Nikon, Ricoh, and Benihana restaurants have proved.

Procedures to establish conceptual equivalence have been developed in several fields, including cognitive anthropology and cross-cultural psychology (Spradley, 1979; Triandis, 1972; Triandis & Berry, 1980). These procedures include (1) defining the domain, (2) determining the domain's organization, (3) analyzing meanings, and (4) analyzing behavior. In addition to these procedures, data analysis methods such as factor anlaysis have been used to compare factorial structures of different scales across cultures (e.g., Johnson & Marsella, 1978; Kuo & Marsella, 1977). These procedures are presented in Table 13-3.

Procedures to establish conceptual equivalence are not complex, but they do require that proper research begin with basic cultural studies. For example, when a Japanese colleague and I sought to investigate depression in Japanese culture, we found the closest equivalent term to be *yuutsu*. When we asked Japanese and American subjects to word-associate to the words *yuutsu* and "depression," respectively, the association patterns were very different (Tanaka-Matsumi & Marsella, 1976). In the same study, a comparison of the semantic differential profiles for the two words also differed (Tanaka-

TABLE 13-3 Methods for the Study of Subjective Experience across Cultures

1. Domain definition
   A. Domain elicitation interviews
   B. Analysis of ethnographies
2. Organization
   A. Categorization and sorting
   B. Ranking
   C. Scaling
3. Meaning
   A. Work associations
   B. Antecedents-consequences
   C. Triadic contrasts
   D. Semantic differential
   E. Implication grids
   F. Attribute interviews
4. Behavior
   A. Behavioral differential
   B. Behavior observation and analysis
   C. Behavior baselines (frequency, intensity, duration)

Matsumi & Marsella, 1976). Japanese psychiatrists interested in Western depression concepts are forced to use the term *melanchorii*, a bastardization of "melancholy," because an equivalent term does not exist. Even the Japanese word for sadness, *kanashi*, has a more positive connotation, because traditional Japanese values emphasize the positive virtues of suffering and the nobility of failure.

The use of the antecedent-consequent method involves the use of sentence completion tasks that seek both the antecedents and consequences of different states or behaviors. For example, one might ask subjects from different cultures to complete the following sentences: "When Juan is sad, Juan —" or "Some of the things that make Juan sad are —." By content-analyzing the responses from individuals from different cultural groups, researchers can gain a better understanding of the conceptual equivalence of an emotion, a disorder, or a personality construct.

Scale Equivalence

Even if efforts are made to establish accurate translations and conceptual equivalence, researchers must still deal with the problem of scale formats as used in psychiatric rating scales, self-report questionnaires, and personality and performance measures. Virtually everyone in Western society is exposed to Likert scales, Thurstone scales, true-false ratings, and other efforts to quantify life experiences, opinions, attitudes, and behavior patterns.

When one conducts cross-cultural research, however, it cannot be assumed that all ethnocultural groups will understand different scale formats or that they will be valid indicators of behavior. For example, when I was studying life satisfaction among different socioeconomic classes in the Philippines, I asked subjects to rate their life satisfaction on the basis of a "simple" scale composed of five steps. I told one subject, "Juan, the man at the top of the stairs is very satisfied with his life, while the man at the bottom of the stairs is very dissatisfied with his life. On what step would you place yourself, Juan?" The Filipino man, Juan, thought at considerable length about his answers; he stared at the card on which the stairs and figures were displayed, he stroked his chin, and he scratched his head. Then he said, "I would place myself on the bottom stair." I was quite happy with Juan's response, as it seemed to validate Juan's life circumstances, which involved living in a slum, earning no money, and having no food for his family. But when I asked Juan to say why he placed himself on the bottom stairs, Juan replied, "Because I do not wish to fall down the stairs and hurt myself, Doctor." A scale is not a scale everywhere in the world!

In a similar vein, I once had a difficult time using a semantic differential scale in Sarawak (a 7-point bipolar adjustive scale), because the subjects said that "fast" and "slow" may be 7 points apart, but "good" and "bad" are much more widely spaced. Even true-false items may be difficult, because some cultural groups do not respond well to the Western willingness to give generalized statements that are far removed from actual situations. For example, subjects might be asked to respond true or false to the statement, "I find myself feeling angry much of the time." An Iban will struggle with this statement and say, "Sometimes I am angered by my wife when she does not cook, but I forgive her. I was angry when my spear was lost by my brother," and so forth. But he will have difficulty saying "true" or "false," and if he does, the validity may be questionable.

Increasingly, cross-cultural researchers are recognizing the need to engage in good ethnocultural interviews and ethnographies before beginning cross-cultural research. It should be pointed out that this advice is useful not only for strange and exotic cultures, but also for those of urban minorities an rural communities in Western societies. The goal, of course, is acquiring an understanding of the people under study so that accuracy can be increased. For almost two decades, it has become fashionable in cross-cultural research to use the terms "emic" and "etic" (Pike, 1966) to refer to understanding a culture from an imposed set of terms. The "emic" view is the internal perspective, while the "etic" view is the external perspective. What is at stake is valid understanding of why people behave as they do. When seen from a foreign point of view, a culture's practices may appear strange, bizarre, and even crazy. But from its own point of view, the culture's practices may to very rational.

In brief, cross-cultural research requires investigators to acknowledge that cultures constitute different realities and that efforts to measure normal and abnormal behavior within the context of these different realities must consider problems of translation, conceptual equivalence, and scale equivalence. This does not mean that one cannot apply measures from one culture to another, but that there must be an awareness of the risks involved and efforts to control them.

THE MEASUREMENT OF DEPRESSIVE EXPERIENCE AND DISORDER ACROSS CULTURES

Epidemiology

Numerous reviews of the epidemiology of depressive disorders both within cultures (e.g., Bebbington, 1978; Boyd & Weissman, 1982) and across cultures (Marsella, 1978; Sartorius, 1973) have been published. Cross-cultural studies have posed particular difficulties for comparison purposes because of several factors, including cultural variations in the definition of depression, differences in case-finding and sampling procedures, diagnostic reliability problems, and failure to consider indigenous definitions. As a result, in spite of the scores of community and treated prevalence-incidence studies that have been conducted, it is difficult to determine whether rates of depression actually vary across cultures.

If this situation is to be improved, it may be necessary to develop a new epidemiological research strategy for cross-cultural studies. This strategy should involve (1) the use of both Western and indigenous definitions of depressive disorder; (2) the use of similar case identification and sampling methods in the different cultures; (3) the establishment of frequency, severity, and duration baselines of symptomatology; and (4) the identification and examination of illness and sick role meanings in a given culture to assist in case counting.

Instrumentation

Self-Report Measures

One of the most popular approaches to the measurement of depressive disorders in Western psychiatry has been the self-report instrument, in which subjects are asked to report on the frequency or severity of their symptoms or mood states. Some of the more popular instruments include the Beck Depression Inventory (BDI), which requires subjects to report the severity of 20 symptoms; the Zung Self-Rating Depression Scale (SDS), which requires subjects to report the frequency of 20 symptoms; and the Center for Epidemiologic Studies Depression Scale (CES-D), which also requires subjects to report the frequency of 20 symptoms in a given time period. The first two scales have been used extensively in cross-cultural research, and the third will probably increase in popularity as more foreign translations of it are made.

Another type of self-report measure of depression is the mood scale, one of the best-known of which is the Depression Adjective Check List (DACL; Zuckerman & Lubin, 1975). Mood scales require subjects to endorse adjectives associated with depressive moods.

In some instances, self-report scales for assessing depressive disorders have been derived from personality inventories. In many of these, subjects are asked to respond true or false to indicator items (e.g., "I like mechanics magazines"); a good example of this is the Minnesota Multiphasic Personality Inventory (MMPI) Depression (*D*) Scale.

All of these self-report scales have been used in cross-cultural depression research with varying degress of validity. For example, we (Marsella, Kameoka, Shizuru, & Brennan, 1975) compared the scores of Chinese, Japanese, and Caucasian subjects on the MMPI *D*, BDI, SDS, and DACL. We found that the scores showed high cross-correlations for the Caucasian samples but not for the other groups. The use of different measuring formats influenced the subjects' reports. Some ethnic groups find it difficult to use mood adjectives; in addition, some groups find it unacceptable to report the severity of problems, because group members are expected to endure in the face of adversity. Scale format is very important in cross-cultural studies of depressive disorders.

In addition to scale format, another major problem is scale content. The popular scales tend to sample symptoms that conform to the prototypical Western depression syndrome. These include somatic, cognitive, existential, affective, and interpersonal symptoms. But many non-Western ethnocultural groups do not present their problems in these terms. For example, Ebigno (1982) identified a number of complaints among depressed Nigerian patients that would have been highly unusual among Westerners:

1. Heaviness in the head.
2. Heat in the head.
3. Crawling sensation in the legs.
4. Burning sensation in the body and belly.
5. Feeling as if the belly is bloated with water and it moves around the body.
6. Crawling sensation in the head.

If one relies solely on a Western-style presentation of symptoms and complaints, it is possible that many cases will be misdiagnosed. This is because Western depression involves existential complaints. We (Marsella, Kinzie, & Gordon, 1973) examined depressive symptoms among normal and depressed Japanese, Chinese, and Caucasian subjects. We found that the Japanese presented depression as interpersonal complaints, the Chinese as somatic complaints, and the Caucasians as existential complaints. The results were interpreted as representations of the ways different ethnocultural groups define the self:

> What emerges is the possibility of interpreting depression complaints . . . as reflections of self perceived as somatic functioning, as interaction, . . . and as an existential process. . . . In all these instances, the complaints come to reflect an extension of self which is perceived to be disordered, limited impaired, or generally inadequate. (Marsella, Kinzie, & Gordon, 1973, p. 449)

Depressive disorders are filtered through ethnocultural experience, and this produces variations in the way the dysfunctions are presented, understood, experienced, and treated. To the extent that cultures differ in their concepts of personhood, causality, and disease, differences should be expected.

Scores of empirical studies have pointed out that the standard symptoms of depressive disorders in the Western world are not present or are present only minimally in non-Western people. For example, Kleinman (1982), in an extensive study of depression in the People's Republic of China, found that anhedonia, helplessness, hopelessness, guilt, memory impairments, suicidal thoughts, and worthlessness were not found in the majority of cases. The World Health Organization (WHO) five-country study of depression reported broad variations in the presentation of depression in Iran, Japan, Switzerland, and Canada (WHO, 1983). Similar results have been reported by Sechrest (1963), Murphy, Wittkower, and Chance (1967), Kimura (1965), and Pfeiffer (1970). Reviews of these studies are available (Marsella, 1981; Marsella *et al.*, 1985).

It is important to recognize that problems in measurement have profound treatment implications. We cannot ignore cultural variations in symptomatology without risking iatrogenic consequences. Efforts must be made to incorporate indigenous terminology and conceptualizations in our scales. Elsewhere, I have stated:

> Depressed somatic functioning does not have to have psychological implications! . . . Without psychological representation, it is conceivable that somatic problems may pass more quickly. . . . It is when the psychological representation occurs that the somatic experience of depression assumes completely different consequences and implications. . . . (Marsella, 1981, p. 261)

Rating Scales and Interview Schedules

Many of the problems associated with self-report scales are present in rating scales and interview schedules. The Hamilton Rating Scale for Depression, the Bech-Refaelsen Melancholia Scale, the Newcastle Scale, the Schedule for Affective Disorders and Schizophrenia, and the WHO Schedule for the Standardized Assessment of Depressive Disorders are all based on Western assumptions about the nature of depression (Bech, 1981). In addition, they have the added problem that the evaluations are made by professional observers who may not be familiar with patients' ethnocultural tradition. When research studies have been conducted "through the eyes of the beholder," interesting variations have emerged.

If the validity of clinical studies of cross-cultural depression studies is to be increased, it is necessary that efforts be made to deal with issues such as indigenous symptoms and complaints, cultural variations in illness ideologies and roles, scale format problems, and perceptual baselines and biases of raters. These issues require that a research initiative be launched to address the problem. Failure to resolve these issues can only result in higher personal, social, and economic costs.

Personality and Depression

"Personality" is a widely used term and concept in Western psychiatry and psychology. It is an abstraction that embraces the total organized functioning of the individual, especially the individual's unique style of adjustment. Western theorists have developed scores of personality theories that emphasize different determinants and conceptual frameworks (see Corsini & Marsella, 1983, for a review and evaluation). However, at issue in cross-cultural depression research are (1) the perceived nature of the person and the concept of personality, and (2) the cultural equivalence of the constructs.

Hsu (1985) has challenged the Western notion of personality as ethnocentric. He argues that personality itself is a Western creation that does not fit the perceived nature of personhood in non-Western cultures. He asserts that the term "personality" emerges from an epistemology that separates person from context, and that this idea is alien to non-Western people. Several volumes examine the question of culture and self among Japanese, Chinese, and Indian cultures and their contrasts to Western ideas (Marsella, DeVos, & Hsu, 1985; Nakamura, 1964).

Differences in the conceptualization of personality do not prevent cross-cultural comparisons, but they do encourage greater care than has been used in the past. For example, if personality concepts associated with depressive disorders in the Western world are to be investigated in non-Western cultures, conceptual equivalence must be examined. "Aggression," "dependency," "locus of control," "anxiety," and "obsessiveness" are Western terms that may not have comparable meanings or implications in other cultures.

In addition, there are questions of norms for Western tests of personality. If the MMPI norms were developed on people in Minnesota, the use of the same cutoff points for people in Nigeria, Japan, and India is problematic. A case in point is the conclusion reached by Christie and Geis (1970). They contended that the Chinese were more manipulative and exploitive of others because of higher scores on the Machiavellianism Scale. But when a Chinese colleague and I (Kuo & Marsella, 1977) investigated the conceptual equivalence of the concept among Chinese, we found that the Machiavellianism Scale measured different things. What is "obsessiveness" to a Japanese? What is "hysteria" to a Cuban? What is "aggression" to a Samoan?

An interesting research strategy would be to diagnose patterns of depressive disorders among patients from different ethnic groups, using both Western and indigenous criteria, and then to elicit personality descriptors associated with these conditions to determine accompanying configurations of personal and social qualities. For example, using a similar definition of depression, we (Marsella, Walker, & Johnson, 1973) found that self-concept discrepancies (real vs. ideal) were a correlate of depression in Caucasian and Chinese but not in Japanese females. We concluded that the normal ritualistic tendency to abase and denigrate oneself among the Japanese made it nonpredictive of depressive conditions.

Ethnocultural Identity

A critical and long overlooked issue in cross-cultural research is ethnic identity. Most cross-cultural research is in fact a comparison of national groups or racial subtypes rather than cultural groups. This is the case because studies do not examine ethnic identity levels of their subjects. Rather, they sample members of different ethnic groups without any awareness of their attachment or affiliation to a particular cultural tradition. For example, if a research is comparing Puerto Ricans and Caucasians, the researcher needs to assess the extent of the subjects' identification with particular ways of life that constitute the different cultures. Some Puerto Rican people may be more "Anglo" than a Vermont farmer in their behavior patterns, values, and way of life. Measurement of ethnic identity may emphasize attitudinal, behavioral, or experiential criteria. For example, Meredith (1967) created an ethnic identity scale based on attitudes for measuring the degree of "Japaneseness" of an individual. But ethnic identity scales seldom find their way into cross-cultural studies of psychopathology. As a result, large studies such as the International Pilot Study of Schizophrenia and the WHO depressive disorders study (WHO, 1983) are, in fact, cross-national studies. If we are to study the effects of ethnocultural factors on depression, ethnocultural affiliation must be assessed via ethnic identity measures.

Culture, Biology, and the Measurement of Depressive Disorders

The preceding sections have discussed current knowledge on the measurement of clinical and phenomenological dimensions of depressive disorders. Another approach to the measurement of depressive disorders involves the use of biological measures, such as central nervous system (CNS) metabolites in urine and cerebrospinal fluid (CSF), and psychophysiological indices. At the present time, WHO is engaged in an ethnopsychopharmacological study in six countries; however, no data are yet available. Studies are being conducted on neurotransmitter precursors and metabolites in CSF in a number of non-

Western countries, but the studies are not being conducted for the purpose of analyzing ethnocultural variations. A study of this type would require careful control of diet, health histories, and other source of individual variability to determine the effects of distinct acquired behavior patterns and stressors associated with particular cultures.

In contrast to psychopharmacology, there have been many cross-cultural studies of psychophysiology. The earliest studies in this area were conducted almost 50 years ago (e.g., Stratton & Henry, 1938, 1943). Their studies compared electrodermal and respiratory responses of Caucasian, Japanese, and Chinese students. In the interim, a number of other psychophysiological response systems have been studied across different ethnocultural groups (see Marsella, Sine & Foiles, 1984, and Shapiro & Schwartz, 1970, for overviews).

We (Marsella *et al.*, 1984) compared the electrodermal response patterns of Japanese and northern European females under conditions of depressed and anxious states and traits. We found no ethnocultural differences in the absolute amounts of (1) tonic levels, (2) amplitude levels, (3) response latency speed, (4) recruitment speed, or (5) recovery speed. However, there was a

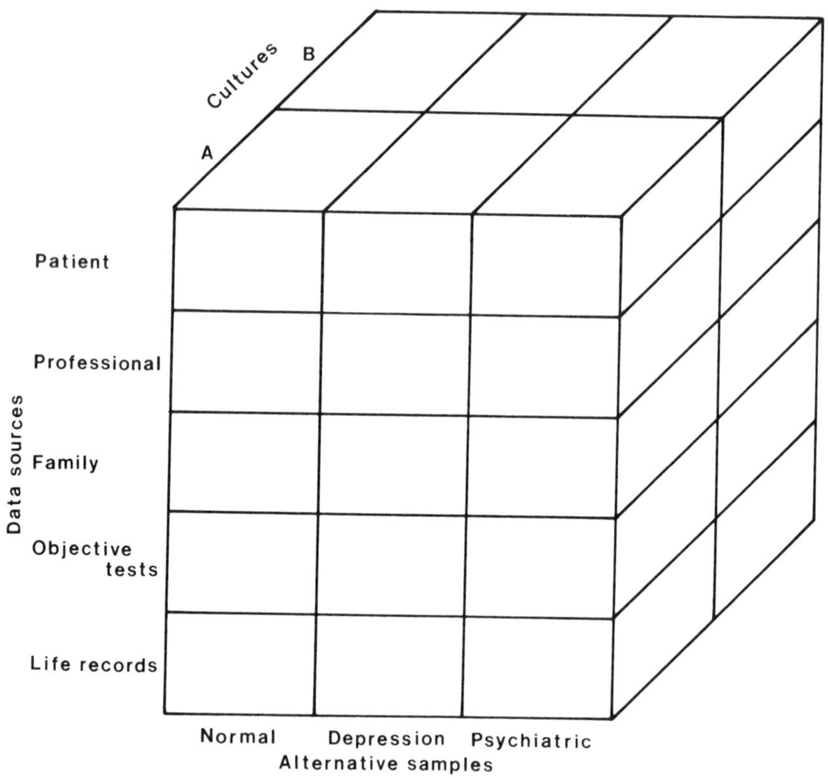

FIGURE 13-5 Research paradigm for cross-cultural clinical studies of depressive disorders.

relationship among ethnocultural group, affective measures, and electrodermal response measures. Specifically, the higher the depressed state and trait scores among the Japanese subjects, the more rapid the half-time recovery speed. It was speculated that Japanese culture may condition this phenomenon by child-rearing practices that encourage the suppression of emotional responses. Much effort and energy are expended in Japanese culture on acquiring and maintaining emotional "control." Is it possible that these controls become represented physiologically in a more rapid recovery rate of the electrodermal response when depression increases?

The relationship among culture, biology, and depressive disorders is still not well developed in the research literature; however, this area has promise for explaining ethnocultural variations in clinical and phenomenological dimensions of depressive disorders. Many of the problems associated with self-reports and rating scales in the measurement of depression across cultures could be reduced by using the more "objective" approaches associated with biological functioning.

Figure 13-5 displays a research strategy for cross-cultural depressive studies. This strategy acknowledges the importance of the data source. It advocates the use of patient, professional, family/peer, objective (e.g., performance, biological assay), and life record approaches.

References

Bebbington, P. (1978). The epidemiology of depressive disorders. *Culture, Medicine and Psychiatry* 2, 297-341.

Bech, P. (1981). Rating scales for affective disorders: Their validity and consistency. *Acta Psychiatrica Scandinavica, 64*(Suppl.), 295.

Boyd, J., & Weissman, M. (1982). Epidemiology. In E. Paykel (Ed.), *Handbook of affective disorders* (pp. 109-125). New York: Guilford Press.

Brislin, R., Lonner, W., & Thorndike, R. (1973). *Cross-cultural research methods*. New York; Wiley-Interscience.

Christie, R., & Geis, F. (1970). *Studies in Machiavellianism*. New York: Academic Press.

Corsini, R., & Marsella, A. J. (1983). *Personality theories, research, and assessment*. Itasca, Ill: F. E. Peacock.

Doi, T. (1973). *The anatomy of dependency*. Tokyo: Kodansha International Press.

Ebigno, P. (1982). Development of a culture specific screening scale of somatic complaints indicating psychiatric disturbance. *Culture, Medicine, and Psychiatry, 6*, 29-43.

Fabrega, H. (1974). Problems implicit in the cultural and social study of depression. *Psychosomatic Medicine, 36*, 377-398.

Fabrega, H. (1975). Cultural and social factors in depression. In E. Anthony & T. Benedek (Eds.), *Depression and human existence*. Boston: Little, Brown.

Hsu, F. (1985). The self in cross-cultural perspective. In A. J. Marsella, G. DeVos, & F. Hsu (Eds.), *Culture and self: Western and Asian perspectives*. London: Tavistock.

Johnson, F., & Marsella, A. J. (1978). Attitudes toward verbal behavior in Japanese-American and Caucasian-American males and females. *Genetic Psychology Monographs, 97*, 43-76.

Kiev, A. (1972). *Transcultural psychiatry*. New York: Free Press.

Kimura, B. (1965). Vergleichende untersuchungen über Depressive Erkrankungen in Japan und in Deutschland. *Fortschritte der Neurologie und Psychiatrie, 33*, 202-215.

Kleinman, A. (1982). Neurasthenia and depression: A study of somatization and culture in China. *Culture, Medicine, and Psychiatry, 6*, 117-190.

Kluckhohn, C., & Kroeber, A. (1952). *Culture*. New York: Vintage Press.

Kraepelin, E. (1904). Vergleichende Psychiatrie. *Zentralblatt für Nervenherlkande und Psychiatrie, 15*, 433-437.

Kuo, H., & Marsella, A. J. (1977). The meaning and measurement of Machiavellianism in Chinese and Americans. *Journal of Social Psychology, 101*, 165-173.

Leighton, A., & Murphy, J. (1959). Cultures as causative of mental disorder. In *Causes of mental disorders: A review of epidemiological knowledge*. New York: Milbank Memorial Fund.

Linton, R. (1945). *The cultural background of personality*. New York: Appleton-Century. Crofts.

Lonner, W. (1979). Issues in cross-cultural psychology. In A. Marsella, R. Tharp, & T. Ciborowski (Eds.), *Perspectives on cross-cultural psychology*. New York: Academic Press.

Marsella, A. J. (1978). A note on cross-cultural aspects of the epidemiology of depression. *Culture, Medicine, and Psychiatry, 2*, 343-357.

Marsella, A. J. (1981). Depressive experience and disorder across cultures. In H. Triandis & J. Draguns (Eds.), *Handbook of cross-cultural psychology. Vol. 6. Psychopathology*. Boston: Allyn & Bacon.

Marsella, A. J. (1982). Culture and mental health: An overview. In A. J. Marsella & G. White (Eds.), *Cultural conceptions of mental health and therapy*. Hingham, MA: G. Reidel.

Marsella, A. J. (1984). An interactional theory of psychopathology. In B. Lubin & W. Connor (Eds.), *Ecological models in clinical and community psychology*. New York: Wiley.

Marsella, A. J., DeVos, G., & Hsu, F. (Eds.). (1985). *Culture and self: Asian and Western perspectives*. London: Tavistock.

Marsella, A. J., Kameoka, V., Shizuru, L., & Brennan, J. (1975). Cross-validation of self-report measures of depression among normal populations of Japanese, Chinese, and Caucasian ancestry. *Journal of Clinical Psychology, 31*, 281-287.

Marsella, A. J., Kinzie, D., & Gordon, P. (1973). Ethnocultual variations in the expression of depression. *Journal of Cross-Cultural Psychology, 4*, 435-458.

Marsella, A. J., Sartorius, N., Jablensky, A., & Fenton, F. (1985). Depression across cultures. In A. Kleinman & B. Good (Eds.), *Culture and depression*. Berkeley: University of California Press.

Marsella, A. J., Sine, L., & Foiles, S. (1984). *Ethnocultural variations in electrodermal correlates of trait and state depression and anxiety*. Unpublished manuscript, University of Hawaii.

Marsella, A. J., Walker, E., & Johnson, F. (1973). Personality correlates of depression in female college students of different ethnic groups. *International Journal of Social Psychiatry, 19*, 77-82.

Meredith, G. (1967). Ethnic identity questionnaire: A study in transgenerational communication patterns. *Pacific Speech Quarterly, 2*, 63-67.

Murphy, H. B., Wittkower, E., & Chance, R. (1967). Cross-cultural inquiry into the symptomatology of depression. *International Journal of Psychiatry, 3*, 6-15.

Nakamura, H. (1964). *Ways of thinking of Eastern people*. Honolulu: East-West Center Press.

Pfeiffer, W. (1970). *Traskulturelle psychiatrie: Ergebnisse und problime*. Stuttgart, West Germany: Georg Thieme.

Pike, E. (1966). *Language in relation to a unified theory of the structure of human behavior*. The Hague, Netherlands: Mouton.

Prince, R. (1968). The changing picture of depressive syndromes in Africa: Is it fact or diagnostic fashion. *Canadian Journal of African Studies, 1*, 177-192.

Sartorius, N. (1973). Culture and the epidemiology of depression. *Psychiatria, Neurologia, et Neurochirugia, 76*, 479-487.

Sears, R. (1961). Transcultural variables and conceptual equivalence. In B. Kaplan (Ed.), *Studying personality cross-culturally*. New York: Harper & Row.

Sechrest, L. (1963). Symptoms of mental disorder in the Philippines. *Philippine Sociological Review, 7*, 189-206.

Shapiro, D., & Schwartz, G. (1970). Psychophysiological contributions to social psychology. *Annual Review of Psychology*, 87-112.

Singer, K. (1975). Depressive disorders from a transcultural perspective. *Social Science and Medicine, 9*, 289-301.

Spradley, J. (1979). *The ethnographic interview*. New York: Holt, Rinehart & Winston.

Stratton, G., & Henry, F. (1938). Mongolians and Caucasians: Psychophysiological reactions to emotional stimuli. *Psychological Bulletin*, 1938, *35*, 66.

Stratton, G., & Henry, F. (1943). Emotion in Chinese, Japanese, and Whites: Racial and national differences and likeness in physiological reactions to an emotional stimulus. *American Journal of Psychology, 56*, 161-180.

Tanaka-Matsumi, J., & Marsella, A. J. (1976). Ethnocultural variations in the phenomenology of depression: I. Word association studies. *Journal of Cross-Cultural Psychology, 7*, 379-396.

Triandis, H. (1972). *The analysis of subjective culture*. New York: Wiley-Interscience.

Triandis, H., & Berry, J. (1980). *Handbook of cross-cultural psychology: Vol. 2. Methodology*. Boston: Allyn & Bacon.

Werner, O., & Campbell, D. (1970). Translating, working through interpreters and the problem of decentering. In R. Naroll & R. Cohen (Eds.), *A handbook of method in cultural anthropology*, New York: American Museum of Natural History.

WHO (World Health Organization). (1983). *Depressive disorders in different cultures*. Geneva, Switzerland: Author.

Zuckerman, M., & Lubin, B. (1975). *Manual for the Depression Adjective Check List*. San Diego: Educational and Industrial Testing Service.

Index

Acetylcholine
    depression mechanism, 127, 128
    interactive systems, 143-145
Acquaintance method, 93
ACTH, 181, 182
Activity level
    assessment, 202, 216, 224
    electronic device, 224
Activity schedules, 230-232
Adaptation, and normal depression, 4-8
Adenyl cyclase system, 117-119
Adjustment (*see* Social adjustment)
Adjustment disorder with mood disturbance, 25
Adjustment reaction, 12
Adoption studies, 90, 92
Adrenocorticotropic hormone, 181, 182
Affect
    assessment, 243-245
    definition, 3, 202, 203
Affective Disorder Rating Scale, 300
Affective disorders
    and depression, 3
    DSM-III contributions, 15, 16
    historical observations, 12-14
    nosology, current controversies, 14, 15
Age effects
    controls for, importance, 135, 136
    growth hormone, 160
    HPA function, 169, 170
    MHPG, 132, 133
    personality measurement, 321
Age of melancholia, 17
Age of onset, 102, 103
Aggression, 8
Agitation
    depression assessment, 202
    multivantaged approach construct, 303, 305, 312
    tricyclic antidepressant effect, 309, 314
Alcoholism
    and affective disorders, 25, 28
    dexamethasone test, 177
Alpha-1 receptors, 119-121
Alpha-2 receptors
    and antidepressants, 119, 121
    and growth hormone, clonidine, 158, 159
    supersensitivity, 121
Alzheimer's disease, 23
Amae, 386
Amitriptyline, 305-315
Amphetamines
    depressive reaction, 24
    growth hormone response, 159, 160
    HPA system stimulation, 173, 174
Anatomy of Melancholy, The (Burton), 17
Anhedonia
    definition, 69, 256
    measures, 256
    and the Pleasure Scale, 69
Animal models, 123
Anorexia nervosa, 162
Antecedent-consequent method, 387
Antidepressants, 119-122
Antihypertensive drugs, 23
Antiparkinsonian drugs, 23
Anxiety
    multivantaged approach construct, 303, 305
    physiology, 7
    tricyclic antidepressant effect, 309, 313, 314
Apomorphine, 156-158
Arbitrary inference, 274, 332
Assertion of Autonomy scale, 326, 327
Assertiveness skills, 218, 253
Assortative mating, 94
Attachment bonds, 325, 326
Attributional Style Questionnaire
    characteristics, 248, 282-286, 335, 336
    cognitive function assessment, 246
    internal consistency, 283
    reliability and validity, 283, 284
    research findings, depression, 335, 336
Attributions
    first-order measures, 281
    and learned helplessness, 200
    measures, 248, 249, 282-286
    second-order measures, 281, 282

Atypical antidepressants, 116, 119, 124
Atypical Depression Diagnostic Scale, 59
Atypical Depression Rating Scale, 58, 59
Audiotapes, marital interaction, 226
Automatic thoughts
  Beck's theory, 274, 332-334
  as state characteristic, 332
  and systematic errors, 332
Automatic Thoughts Questionnaire
  characteristics, 275, 276, 332-334
  cognitive style measurement, 332
  and irrational beliefs, 247
  reliability and validity, 275
  research findings, depression, 333, 334
Autoreceptors, 121
Aversive events, 256, 257

Back translation methods, 385, 386
Balanced cyclothymia, 338
Bandura's theory, 272
Base rate, 33
Bech-Rafaelsen Melancholia Scale
  characteristics, 54
  cross-cultural aspects, 391
Beck Depression Inventory
  and behavioral assessment, 207, 208
  behavioral coding measures correlation, 218, 221, 224
  characteristics, 64, 65
  cross-cultural studies, 389, 390
  and Dysfunctional Attitude Scale, 279
  and forms of depression, 10
  and Hamilton Rating Scale for Depression, 65
  and Hopelessness Scale, 290
  inpatient behavior correlation, 224
  reliability and validity, 64
  response mode content, comparison, 211, 212
  symptom coverage comparison, 211, 212
  versus Visual Analogue Scale, 244
Beck's model
  and cognitive measures, 271-281
  cognitive style, 331-334
  overview, 272-275
  verbal behavior, 200, 201
Behavior, 199-235
Behavior coding
  clinical application, 217
  inpatients, 222-225
  observational systems, 216, 217
  reliability, 218
Behavior coding, cont'd
  validity, 208, 218-222
Behavior therapy, 217
Behavioral Assertiveness Test, 254
Behavioral Assessment Grid, 200
Bereavement, 11
Beta-adrenergic receptors
  and antidepressant action, 119, 120, 144
  human leukocytes, 120
  serotonin interaction, 144
Bias (*see also* Response bias)
  clinician ratings, 209
  and response mode content, scales, 211
  state and trait influence, 322
Binswanger disease, 23
Biogenic amines, 7
Bipolar depression
  dexamethasone test specificity, 177
  epinephrine and norepinephrine, 137, 138
  Eysenck Personality Inventory, 330
  nosology, 14
  personality predisposition, 340
  SADS-L test-retest reliability, 99, 100
Bipolar I disorder
  morbid risk, family data, 103
  SADS-L test-retest reliability, 99, 100
Bipolar II disorder
  morbid risk, family data, 103
  SADS-L test-retest reliability, 99, 100
Bleuler, affective disorders classification, 13
Blood measures, shortcomings, 116
Body weight (*see* Weight effects)
Bonding
  measurement, 347, 348
  and normal depression, 4, 5
Bowlby's theory, 4, 5
Brief Psychiatric Rating Scale
  and antidepressant drugs, 56
  characteristics, 55, 56

Canadian study, 391
Cardiovascular disease, 22
Carroll Rating Scale for Depression, 70, 71
Case narrative, 101, 102
Catechol-O-methyltransferase, 130
Catecholamine hypothesis, 110
CATEGO, 40
Causal attributions (*see* Attributions)
Center for Epidemiologic Studies Depression Scale
  characteristics, 75-78
  cross-cultural studies, 389, 390

Center for Epidemiologic Studies Depression Scale, cont'd
- and forms of depression, 10
- point prevalence rates, 76, 77
- response mode content, 212
- sensitivity and specificity, 77
- symptom coverage comparison, 212

Cerebrospinal fluid
- measurement shortcomings, 116
- neurotransmitter measurement, 114, 115, 138

Change measurement, 36, 54, 55
Character-spectrum disorders, 339, 348
Characterological depression, 339
Child Report of Parent Behavior Inventory, 346, 347
Children's Attributional Style Questionnaire, 248, 249, 284, 285
Chinese culture, 390-392, 394
Ching K-S Social Behavior Scale, 300
Cholecystokinin, 143
Choline, depressive effect, 128
Cholinergic agonists, 127, 128
Cholinergic nerves
- adrenergic balance, 144
- HPA function modulation, 173

Circadian rhythm, 167, 168
Clinical Global Impressions instrument
- characteristics, 60, 61
- and Hamilton Rating Scale for Depression, 52

Clinical reappraisal interview, 44
Clinician rating scales, 48-59
Clinician ratings, 209
Clonidine, 158, 159
Clorgyline
- and growth hormone, 159
- receptor subsensitivity, 119

Cocaine, 24
Coding systems (*see* Behavior coding)
Cognition, 267-292 (*see also* Cognitive style)
- assessment, 200, 201, 210, 245-251, 267-292
- methodological problems, 268-271
- and mood, 7, 8

Cognitive Bias Questionnaire
- characteristics, 276-278
- intercorrelations, 246
- range of vignettes, 284
- reliability and validity, 277

Cognitive content, 271
Cognitive distortions, 250, 251
Cognitive Error Questionnaire, 288, 289
Cognitive Events Schedule
- characteristics, 231, 232, 249, 289
- factor analysis, 246

Cognitive impairment
- multivantaged approach construct, 304-315
- tricyclic antidepressant effects, 308-315

Cognitive processes, 271
Cognitive Response Test
- characteristics, 289
- range of vignettes, 284

Cognitive schemas
- Beck's theory, 250, 273, 274, 331
- definition, 331

Cognitive style, 331-336
Cognitive triad, 272-274, 332
Cohen's kappa, 47
Cohort effects, 103
Communication, 6
Communication skills, 255
Community Adaptation Schedule, 355
Community adjustment, 351
Community surveys (*see also* Social adjustment)
- self-report instruments, 75

Complication approach, 320, 340
Comprehensive Psychopathological Rating Scale, 54
Concerns Dimension Questionnaire, 250
Concordance, twin studies, 90
Concurrent validity, 243
Conflict Resolution Inventory, 253
Conflict resolution skills, 255
Consensual validity, 222, 225
Consensus pedigree, 101, 102
Conservation-withdrawal, 7
Construct validity
- Automatic Thoughts Questionnaire, 275, 276
- social skill measures, 254

Constructs
- and cognition, 267
- definition, 298
- multivantaged approach, 298-315

Control groups, genetic studies, 92-94
Convergent validity, 243
Corticosteroids, 23, 24
Corticotropin-releasing factor, 182, 183
Cortisol
- and HPA system, 167-169
- and TSH response to TRH, 162, 163

Costello's theory, 272
Crandall Cognitions Inventory, 290
Criterion drift, 37

Criterion validity
cognitive measures, 246, 258
depression instruments, 243, 258
social skills measures, 254
structured diagnostic interviews, 47
Criterion variance, 30
Cronholm-Ottosson Depression Scale, 54, 212
Cross-cultural studies, 376-395
depression measurement, 389-395
epidemiology, 389
measurement issues and methods, 385-389
structured interview scales, 37
Culture, 376-395
behavioral definition, 376
and biology, 393, 394
concept, 381-384
measurement issues and methods, 385-389
and psychopathology, 379-381
self-report measures, 269, 270
Cyclic AMP, 117-120
Cyclic GMP, 121, 122
Cyclothymia
definition and concept, 336
measures, 336-338
research findings, depression, 337, 338
Cyproheptadine, 160

Daily logs, 230-232
Darwin's theory, 4, 5
Data collection, genetic studies, 95-102
Defense mechanisms, 8
Delusions, 15
Dementia, 23
Demoralization, 69
Denial, 28
Dependency (*see also* Interpersonal dependency)
in Japanese culture, 386,
Deprenyl, 119
Depressed mood
multivantaged approach construct, 303-315
tricyclic antidepressant effect, 308-315
Depressed mood factor, 244
Depression Adjective Check List
characteristics, 73, 244
cross-cultural studies, 390
Depressive neurosis, DSM-III, 16
Depressogenic schemas, 331
Desipramine, 158, 159
Dexamethasone suppression test
age effects, 169
amphetamine effect, 174
dose-response, 178
frequency of sampling, 178, 179
Dexamethasone suppression test, cont'd
healthy controls, importance, 178, 179
and HPA system, 168
sensitivity and specificity, 175-178
treatment outcome prediction, 179-181
TSH response to TRH correlation, 163
weight effects, 170-172
Diagnostic Interview Schedule
characteristics, 39, 42-45
family study use, 97
reliability, 46-48, 98-101
Dichotomous thinking, 274
Differential diagnosis, 63
Dimensionality issues, 242
Discriminant validity, 243, 258
Distortion dimension, 276-278
Distressed emotion, 303-315
Diurnal variation, 225
Dizygotic twins, 90
Domperidone, 157, 158
L-Dopa, 156, 157
Dopamine
in biological fluids, 113-116
depression mechanism, 125
distribution, 125
and growth hormone, 157
interactive systems, 143-145
neuropeptide interactions, 143, 144
and TSH response to TRH, 164, 165
Dopamine receptors, 125
Dopaminergic system, 164, 165
Double depression, 321
Down-regulation, beta-receptors, 120
Drug abuse, and depression, 20-29
DSM-III
contributions of, 15, 16
current controversies, 14
and medical conditions, 25, 26
and operational criteria, 10
self-criticism/guilt, 275
Dyadic interaction, assessment, 254
Dysfunctional Attitude Scale
and Beck Depression Inventory, 279
characteristics, 278-280, 332
clinical improvement sensitivity, 279
cognitive style measurement, 332
irrational beliefs measurement, 247
research findings, depression, 333, 334
test-retest reliability, 269, 278, 279
Dysphoria
assessment, 243-245
definition, 243
and substance abuse, 28

Dysthymic disorder
  cognitive aspects, 268
  definition and concept, 338, 339
  scales, 337, 339

Efficacy index, 60
Ego Control Scale, 329
Ego Resiliency Scale, 329
Electroconvulsive therapy
  growth hormone effect, 157
  Newcastle Scales, 57
Electrodermal response, 394
Electrophysiological techniques, 117, 118
Emic view, 388
Emotion
  definition, 3
  depression relationship, 4-9
Emotional Facial Action Coding System, 244
Emotional Reliance on Another Person Scale, 326, 327
Emotional Stability Scale, 329
Endocrine disorders, 22
Endocrine measures, 153-185
Endogenomorphic depression
  Hamilton subscale, 52, 53
  nosology, 15
Endogenous depression
  Eysenck Personality Inventory, 329, 330
  nosology controversy, 15
Endogenous-reactive depression, 13
Endorphins, 143
Enkephalins, 143
Epidemiologic Catchment Area studies, 42
Epidemiological field surveys, 93
Epidemiology, cross-cultural studies, 389
Epinephrine
  in anxiety-fear, 7
  HPA system activation, infusion, 174
  NIMH Collaborative Study, 130, 133, 137-139
  unipolar versus bipolar depression, 137, 138
  urinary excretion, 115
Ethnic identity, 393
Ethnocultural factors, 376-395
Ethnopsychopharmacological study, 393, 394
Ethological theory, 325, 326
Etic view, 388
Events schedules, 230-232
Evolutionary theory, 4, 5
Existential complaints, 390
Expectancies, 248
Expected BDI, 248
Expressed emotion, 348
Expressive Movement Scale, 300
Extended pedigrees, 90
Extracted Hamilton, 53
Extraversion
  definition and concept, 327, 328
  measures, 328-330
Eye contact, 215, 216
Eysenck Personality Inventory, 327-329

Facial Action Coding System, 244
Facial electromyogram, 201, 245
Facial expression, 244, 245
Factor analysis
  cognitive measures, 246
  rating scales, criticism, 36
False negatives, 33
False positives, 33
Familial factors, measurement, 344-371
Familial markers, 94, 95
Familial pure depressive disorder, 177
Family history method, 87, 88
Family History — Research Diagnostic Criteria
  characteristics, 41, 95-97
  sensitivity and specificity, 89, 96
Family informants, 97-102
Family studies
  data analysis, 102-106
  data collection, 95-102
  design, 88-95
Family study method
  characteristics, 89, 90
  data collection, 97-102
Fawcett Pleasure Scale, 69, 70
Fear, physiology, 7
Feedback, interview-evaluation, 34, 35
Fight or flight, 7
Fixed-choice format, 289
Fluorometric spectroscopy
  history, 111
  NIMH Collaborative Study, 131
Format, test items, 211
Frequency of Self-Reinforcement Attitudes Questionnaire, 249
Freudian theory, 8
Future of an Illusion, The (Freud), 31

GABA
  cerebrospinal fluid, 126
  depression mechanism, 126, 127
  distribution, 126

Gas chromatography-mass spectrometry
  neurotransmitter measurement, 111, 112
  NIMH Collaborative Study, 131
General Behavior Inventory, 336-338
General Health Questionnaire
  characteristics, 74, 75
  and forms of depression, 10
Generalization
  definition, 199, 200
  and levels of inference, 204
  psychometric domains, 204-214
Genetics
  data analysis, 102-106
  data collection, 95-102
  and measurement, 87-107
GHQ-28 (*see* General Health Questionnaire)
Global Assessment Scale
  behavioral coding correlation, 218
  characteristics, 61
Global causal explanations, 334, 335
Global illness ratings, 59-62
Global Ward Behavior Scale, 300
Grief, depression prototype, 11
Growth hormone, 154-161
Growth hormone inhibitory factor, 165
Guilford-Zimmerman Temperament Survey
  depressed women, 330
  introversion-extraversion, 328

Hallucinations, 15
Hamilton Endogenomorphy Subscale, 52, 53
Hamilton Rating Scale for Depression
  versus Beck Depression Inventory, 65
  behavioral coding correlation, 218, 221, 224
  characteristics, 49-52
  and Clinical Global Impressions instrument, 52
  cross-cultural aspects, 391
  derivatives, 52-54
  and Dysfunctional Attitude Scale, 279
  factor analysis, 50, 51
  and forms of depression, 10
  inpatient behavior correlation, 224
  interrater reliability, 51
  response mode content, 211, 212
  and SADS-C, 53
  symptom coverage comparison, 211, 212
Hand movement, 215, 216
Hassles Scale, 256, 257
Health-Sickness Rating Scale, 61
High-pressure liquid chromatography, 111-113
Histofluorescence technique, 111
Home observations, 217
Homogeneous samples, 36
Homovanillic acid
  in biological fluids, 114, 115
  CSF levels, 125
  NIMH Collaborative Study, 130-137
  sex differences, 132, 137
Hopelessness Scale
  Beck's scale correlation, 290
  characteristics, 72, 290, 291
  and expectancy, 248
  suicide attempters, 290, 291
Hopkins Symptom Checklist, 65
Hostility
  antidepressant drug effect, 309, 313, 314
  multivantaged approach construct, 303, 305
5-HT
  in biological fluid, 113-116
  growth hormone release, 160
  interactive systems, 143-145
5-HT-1 receptors, 122
5-HT-2 receptors, 122
Hyman leukocytes, beta-receptors, 120
5-Hydroxyindoleacetic acid
  in biological fluids, 114, 115
  NIMH Collaborative Study, 130-134
  sex differences, 132, 136
5-Hydroxytryptophan, 160
Hyperadrenal cortisolism, 21
Hypercortisolemia, 21
Hypomania, 176
Hypomanic cyclothymia, 338
Hypothalamic-pituitary-adrenal system
  age effects, 169, 170
  amphetamine stimulation, 173, 174
  characteristics, 167-169
  drug effects, 169
  and insulin hypoglycemia, 174, 175
  physostigmine stimulation, 172, 173
  tests of, sensitivity and specificity, 175-178
  and treatment prediction, 179, 180
Hysterical personality, 323-325

Imipramine
  evaluation, multivantaged approach, 305-315
  opiate addicts, 25
Improvement scale, 60
Indian culture, 392
Infants, separation reaction, 6

Informants, 353, 354
Information processing, 258
Inpatients, behavioral assessment, 222-225
Institute for Personality and Ability Testing Depression Scale, 212
Insulin tolerance test
  growth hormone, 155, 156
  and HPA system, 174, 175
Interactional model, 377
Interactive neuroactive systems, 143-145
Internal causal explanations, 334, 335
Internal-External Locus of Control Scale, 248
Interpersonal behavior, 202, 216, 217, 233, 253, 254
Interpersonal dependency
  definition, 325, 326
  measurement, 326, 327
  psychoanalytic theory, 323, 324
Interpersonal Dependency Inventory, 324-327
Interpersonal efficiency ratio, 216
Interpersonal Events Schedule
  characteristics, 230, 231, 252, 253
  and depression outcome, 252, 253
Interpersonal psychotherapy, 25
Interpersonal sensitivity, 303, 305, 314
Interpretation Inventory, 250
Interrater reliability
  family study data, 98-102
  and generalization, 205
  observational scales, 208
  structured diagnostic interviews, 46-48
Interview-evaluation process, 34, 35
Interview Questionnaire, 250
Interview Schedule for Social Interaction, 358, 369, 370
Interviews (*see also* Structured interview schedules)
  cross-cultural aspects, 391, 392
  observational techniques, 215-222
  social adjustment information, 353, 354
Intrapsychic processes, 8
Introversion
  definition and concept, 327, 328
  measures, 328-330
Inventories, 353
Involutional melancholia, 16
Iproniazid, 110
Irrational beliefs
  measures, 247
  and silent assumptions, 280
Irrational Beliefs Test
  characteristics, 247, 280, 281
  reliability and validity, 280
Item format, 311

Japanese culture, 386, 387, 390-392, 394

Kanashi, 387
Katz Adjustment Scale—Relative's Form, 354, 355, 359
KDS-15 Marital Questionnaire, 357, 367, 368
Kraepelinian approach
  affective disorders classification, 13
  versus Meyerian approach, 6

Lack of Social Self-Confidence Scale, 326, 327
Lazare-Klerman-Armor Personality Inventory, 324, 325
LEAD standard, 47, 48
Learned helplessness model
  and cognition, 200, 201
  definitions and formulations, 334, 335
  GABA, 127
  overview, 281, 282, 334, 335
Leeds Scales, 68, 69
Leukocytes, beta-receptors, 120
Levels of inference, 204
Levels of observation, 241, 242
Lewinsohn's model, 230
Lie scale, 329
Life events, 349
  measurement, 256, 257, 349
  reactive depression, 11, 12
Life Experiences Survey, 256
Linkage markers, 94, 95
Living in Familial Environments system, 254
Loss, and normal depression, 5, 6

Magnification, 274, 332
Mania
  cognitive aspects, 268
  dexamethasone test, 176
  epinephrine and norepinephrine, 137, 138
  historical observations, 12-14
  TSH response, 162
Manic-depression (*see also* Bipolar depression)
  historical observations, 12-14
MAO inhibitors, 119
Marital bonding, 348
Marital interaction
  behavioral coding, 225-227
  KDS-15 Marital Questionnaire, 367, 368

Marlowe-Crowne Social Desirability Scale, 249
Marriage (*see* Marital interaction)
Masked depression, 12
Mathematical models, 106
Maudsley Personality Inventory, 328-330
Means-End Problem-Solving Procedure, 253
Mechanical scoring devices, 209
Medical controls, 93
Medical illness, 12, 20-29
Melancholia, 12, 13
Melanchorii, 387
Melatonin, 120
Memory, 201
Menstrual cycle, 155, 156
Metaclopramide, 164, 165
Metanephrine
  NIMH Collaborative Study, 133, 136
  urinary excretion, 115, 136
3-Methoxy-4-hydroxyphenylglycol (*see* MHPG)
Methysergide, 160
Meyerian approach, 6
MHPG
  age effects, 132
  in biological fluids, 114, 115
  NIMH Collaborative Study, 130-139
  and TSH response to TRH, 163
Microcomputer format, 72, 73
Microiontophoresis, 117
Minimization, 274
MMPI
  cultural aspects, 392
  ego control, 328
  introversion, 329
  neuroticism, 328, 329
MMPI Depression scale
  and behavioral assessment, 207
  behavioral coding correlation, 218, 221
  cross-cultural aspects, 390
  response mode content, 212
  symptom coverage comparison, 212
Mobility, behavioral assessment, 216
Molecular biology, 140
Monoamine oxidase inhibitors, 119
Monozygotic twins, 90
Montgomery-Asberg Depression Rating Scale
  change measurement advantage, 36, 54, 55
  characteristics, 54, 55
Mood
  assessment, 243-245
  cultural aspects, 390
  definition, 3, 206
  versus depression, psychometrics, 206
  depression relationship, 3-17
Mood disorders, 3
Morbid risk, family data, 102, 103
Morphine, prolactin response, 166
Motherhood, 366, 367
Motivation, behavioral definition, 203
Motor behavior, 202, 210, 216
Mourning, 11
Movement, 216
Multidimensional, Multiattributional Causality Scale, 249
Multiple-threshold models, 106
Multiscore Depression Inventory, 212
Multivantaged approach, 241, 242, 297-315
Multivariate methods, 10

Naturalistic studies, 11, 208
Negative automatic thoughts (*see* Automatic thoughts)
Negative cognitive traid (*see* Cognitive traid)
Neighborhood method, 93
Neuroendocrine measures, 153-185
Neurological controls, 129-131
Neurological diseases, 20-29
Neuropeptides
  characteristics, 140, 141
  depression mechanism, 140-143
  neurotransmitter coexistence, neurons, 142, 143
Neurotensin, 165
Neurotic depression, 14, 15
Neurotic-psychotic distinction, 13
Neuroticism
  definition and concept, 327, 328
  measures, 328-330
Neurotransmitters, 109-145
New Clinical Drug Evaluation Unit, 49
Newcastle Diagnostic Scale
  characteristics, 57
  cultural aspects, 391
  and dexamethasone test, 177
Newcastle ECT Prediction Scale, 57
Newcastle Scales, 56-58
NIMH Collaborative Program on the Psychobiology of Depression, 128-139, 298-302
NIMH Mood Scale, 300
Nonverbal behavior
  marital interaction, 227
  quantification, 218-234
Norepinephrine
  in biological fluids, 113-116, 136
  interactive systems, 143-145
  NIMH Collaborative Study, 130, 133, 136-138

Normal depression, 4-8
Normetanephrine
  NIMH Collaborative Study, 130, 133, 136
  urinary excretion, 115, 136
NOSIE-30, 222
Nosology
  current controversies, 14, 15
  and medical conditions, 25-27
  and substance abuse, 25-27
Nuclear magnetic resonance, 140
Nurses' Observation Scale for Inpatient Evaluation (*see* NOSIE-30)

Obesity (*see* Weight effects)
Object relations, 325, 326
Observer scales
  and behavior assessment, 208
  and interview, 215-222
  self-report data correlation, 259
Obsessive personality, 323-325
Open-ended format, 289
Operational criteria
  depressive symptoms, 10
  and personality assessment, 321, 322
Opiates, depressive reaction, 24, 25
Opioid peptides
  neurotransmitter interactions, 143
  prolactin response, 166
Oral personality, 323-325
Organic affective disorders, 25
Outcome prediction
  and dexamethasone test, 179
  multivantaged approach, constructs, 303-315
  tricyclic antidepressants, 307-315
Outliers, 36
Overgeneralization, 274, 332
Overt behavior, 202, 210-234

Pain, 12
Paralinguistic codes, 217-234
Parental Bonding Instrument, 347, 348
Parental characteristics, 346-348
Parenting skills, 255
Pathoplasty approach, 320, 340
Pedigrees, 90, 101, 103
Peptides (*see* Neuropeptides)
Personal Beliefs Inventory, 246, 247, 289
Personal Resources Inventory, 358, 368, 369
Personality and Social Network Adjustment Scale, 355, 359, 360
Personality Inventory, 247
Personality measurement, 319-341
  cultural aspects, 392, 393
  methodological issues, 320-322
Personality traits, 322-339
Personalization, 274
Physical Anhedonia Scale, 256
Physostigmine
  depressive effect, 127, 128
  HPA function stimulation, 172, 173
Plasma measures, 116
Pleasant Events Schedule
  activity level assessment, 202
  characteristics, 230, 255, 256
  factor analysis, 255
Pleasure Scale, 69, 70
Point prevalence rates, 76, 77
Population surveys, 93
Positive reinforcement, 331
Positron emission tomography, 139
Postmenopausal women
  monoamine metabolism, 133, 134
  TSH response to TRH, 163
Postmortem studies, 116
Prediction of outcome (*see* Outcome prdiction)
Predictive validity, 243
Predispositional approach, 319
Present State Examination
  characteristics, 38-41
  community survey use, 75
Primary depression
  dexamethasone test specificity, 177
  nosology, 15
  personality predisposition, 340
  SADS-L test-retest reliability, 99-100
  secondary depression distinction, 26, 27
  TSH response to TRH, 162
Private settings, 207
Probability samples, 32
Proband method, 88
Probenecid technique, 114, 131
Problem solving, 253
Prolactin, 165, 166
Pseudodementia, 23
Psychiatric Epidemiology Research Interview, 75
Psychiatric Epidemiology Research Interview life events scale, 256
Psychoanalytic theory
  dependency, 325, 326
  depression origin, 8
  personality patterns, 323-325

Psychogenic depression
  definition, 5
  and medical conditions, 27, 28
Psychological measurement, 240-260
Psychometrics, 10, 11, 204-207, 242, 243
Psychomotor activity (*see* Activity level)
Psychophysiology
  cognition assessment, 250
  cross-cultural studies, 394
  and emotions, assessment, 245, 259
  and self-report measures, 259
Psychosocial factors, 344-371
Psychotherapy, opiate addicts, 25
Psychotic depression
  dexamethasone test specificity, 177
  nosology, controversy, 15
  SADS-L test-retest reliability, 99-100
Psychotic Inpatient Profile, 224
Psychotic Reaction Profile, 224
Public settings, 207

Radioimmunoassay
  drawbacks, 112
  neurotransmitter measurement, 111, 112
Radioligand assays, 117, 118
Radioreceptor assay, 111, 112
Raskin Three-Area Depression Scale
  behavioral coding correlation, 218, 221
  characteristics, 61, 62
Raters (*see* Interrater reliability)
Rating scales (*see also* Clinician rating scales; Structured interview schedules)
  cross-cultural aspects, 389, 391, 392
  and measurement considerations, 34-36
Reactive depression
  definition, 5
  and medical conditions, 27, 28
  nosology, controversy, 14, 15
Receptor supersensitivity, 122, 123
Receptors, and neurotransmitters, 116-124
Recurrent depression, 99, 100
Refusal rate, 93, 94
Rehm's theory, 272, 286-288
Reinforcement Survey Schedule, 255, 256
Rejection, parental, 346
Relapse, and dexamethasone test, 179-181
Relative risk, 104, 105
Relatives, informant data, 97-102
Reliability
  behavioral coding measures, 218-222
  Diagnostic Interview Schedule, 43, 44
  family informant data, 98-102
Reliability, cont'd
  and generalization, 205, 206
  Hamilton Rating Scale for Depression, 51, 52
  multivantaged approach constructs, 302
  overview, 33
  personality measures, 321, 322
  state and trait influence, 322
  statistical issues, 47
  structured diagnostic interviews, 46-48
REM sleep, 201
Research Diagnostic Criteria
  behavioral coding correlation, 218
  family study reliability, 98-101
  as operational criteria, 10
Reserpine, and prolactin release, 165, 166
Reserpine-induced depression, 24, 109
Response bias
  and control data, 93, 94
  self-rating scales, 62
Response-contingent reinforcement, 331
Response mode, 200-210
Response rate, depression assessment, 202
Risk factors, psychosocial, 346-350
Role functioning, 354-368
Role playing, 234
Rosenberg Self-Esteem Scale, 291, 292

SADS
  characteristics, 39, 41, 42
  cultural aspects, 391
  reliability, 46-48
SADS—Affective Disorders supplement, 41
SADS-C
  characteristics, 41, 56
  and Hamilton Rating Scale for Depression, 53
  multivantaged approach, 300
SADS-L
  characteristics, 41, 42
  family study use, 97
  reliability, 98-101
Sampling, problems of, 32
Sampling periods, 205, 206
Scaling devices (*see* Rating scales)
Schedule for Affective Disorders and Schizophrenia (*see* SADS)
Schedule of Recent Experience, 256, 257
Schizoaffective psychoses, 13
SCL-90 (*see* Symptom Checklist—90)
Second messenger systems, 117, 118

Secondary depression
  and drug reactions, 26, 27
  Eysenck Personality Inventory, 330
  and medical illnesses, 26, 27
  nosology, 15
  SADS-L test-retest reliability, 99, 100
  TRH response to TSH, 162
Secondary mania, 15
Segregation analysis, 106
Selective abstraction, 274. 332
Self-Assessment Guide, 356, 362
Self-Concept Test, 291
Self-control, Rehm's model, 286
Self-control program, 218
Self-Control Questionnaire, 286, 287
Self-Control Scale, 253
Self-Control Schedule, 287, 288
Self-criticism/guilt, 275
Self-disclosure
  dyadic interactions, 254
  and social skill, 252
Self-esteem
  learned helplessness measures, 334, 335
  measures, 247
  and mood, 7
Self-medication, 25, 28
Self-monitoring, 230-232
Self-Rating Questionnaire for Depression, 212
Self-rating scales
  characteristics, 62-78
  criticism, 35, 62, 63
  and differential diagnosis, 63
Self-references, 218
Self-reinforcement, 249, 250
Self-report instruments
  and behavioral assessment, 207, 208, 213, 214
  cognitive assessment, 268, 269
  cross-cultural studies, 389-391
  cultural factors, 269, 270
  observational measure correlation, 259
  and psychophysiologic measures, 259
  social skills assessment, 252, 253
  state and trait influence, 322
  symptom coverage comparison, 211
  validity and reliability, 269, 322
Seligman's theory
  cognitive measures, 281-286
  overview, 281, 282, 334-336
  and response mode, 200, 201
Senile dementia, 23
Sensitivity
  family history method, 89
Sensitivity, cont'd
  and reliability, 33, 34
Separation, 4-6
Serotinergic system, 160
Serotonin (*see* 5-HT)
Severity, 35, 36
  Beck Depression Inventory, 65
  Leeds Scales, 69
Severity Scale, 60
Sex effects
  controls for, importance, 135, 136
  monoamine metabolites, 132
  personality measurement, 321
Significant others, 354
Silent assumptions, 279, 332
Situational depression (*see* Reactive depression)
Situational factors
  and assessment generalization, 206, 207
  and behavioral assessment, 233
Sleep disorder
  multivantaged approach construct, 304
  and tricyclic drug evaluation, 309
Sociability scale, 329, 330
Social adjustment, 350-371
  controversies, 352, 353
  definition and components, 352
  historical overview, 351
  measurement, 350-371
  operational approaches, assessment, 353
  and symptoms, 352, 353
Social Adjustment Scale, 356
Social Adjustment Scale — Self-Report
  characteristics, 356, 361, 362
  and Social Support Network Inventory, 370
Social Anhedonia Scale, 256
Social Behavior Assessment Schedule, 357, 364, 365
Social communication, 6
Social factors, 344-371
Social Functioning Schedule, 357, 365, 366
Social Interaction Self-Statement Test, 253
Social learning theory, 325, 326
Social Maladjustment Schedule, 356, 363
Social Problem Questionnaire, 356, 363, 364
Social Readjustment Rating Scale, 256, 257
Social Role Adjustment Instrument, 357, 366, 367
Social role functioning, 354-368
Social skills
  assessment, 251-255
  behavioral measures, 228, 229, 253, 254, 259; validity, 254
  definition, 251

Social skills, cont'd
  self-report measures, 259
Social support
  definition, 349, 350
  measurement, 349, 350, 368-370
Social Support Network Inventory
  characteristics, 358, 370
  and Hamilton Rating Scale for Depression, 370
Somatization
  multivantaged approach construct, 303
  tricyclic antidepressant evalution, 309, 314
Somatostatin, 165
Specificity
  family history method, 89
  and reliability, 33, 34
Spectrometric technique, 111
Speech behavior, 201, 215-217
Speech pause time, 216
Speech rate, 215-217
Stable causal explanations, 334, 335
Staff-Residents Interaction Chronograph, 225
State dependency
  multivantaged approach constructs, 302-304
  personality measures, 322
  and psychometrics, 205, 206
  and self-report, 269, 322
Steroids, 23, 24
Story completion test, 288
Stress, 11, 12
Stressful life events (*see* Life events)
Structured and Scaled Interview to Assess Maladjustment
  characteristics, 355, 360, 361
  correlation with Personality and Social Network Adjustment Scale, 360
Structured Clinical Interview for DSM-III, 39, 45, 46
Structured interview schedules, 37-48
  characteristics, 37-48
  criticism, 35
  cross-cultural aspects, 391, 392
  generalization, 209
  reliability, 46-48, 409
  social adjustment, 361
Subaffective dysthymia, 339
Subclinical approach, 320, 340
Subcortical dementias, 23
Subjective awareness, 7, 8
Subjective Probability Questionnaire, 246, 248, 289
Substance abuse, 20-29
Suicidal Ideation Scale, 269
Suicidal Intent Scale, 290, 291
Supersensitivity, receptors, 122, 123
Surveys (*see* Social adjustment)
Switzerland study, 391
Symptom Checklist—90
  and behavioral assessment, 207
  characteristics, 65, 66
  multivantaged approach, 300
  response mode content, 212
  symptom coverage comparison, 212
Symptomatic depression, 9-17
Symptoms
  behavioral definition, 203
  coverage of, scales, 211
  and social adjustment, 352, 353
Syndrome, measurement problems, 32

Test-retest reliability
  and generalization, 205, 206
  SADS-L, 98-101
  self-report scales, 269
Therapeutic community, 359, 360
Threshold models, genetic studies, 106
Thyroid-stimulating hormone, 161-165
Thyrotropin-releasing hormone, 161-165
Time, and generalization, psychometrics, 205, 206
Time-Sample Behavior Checklist, 225
Token economy, 224, 225
Trait factors
  cyclothymia, 337, 338
  and personality assessment, 322
  and psychometrics, 205, 206
Trait markers, genetic studies, 94, 95
Trauma, reactive depression, 11, 12
Tricyclic antidepressants
  evaluation, multivantaged approach, 305-315
  mechanism of action, receptors, 119-122
Twin studies, 90
Two-threshold model, 106

Unipolar depression
  dexamethasone test specificity, 177
  morbid risk, family data, 103
  norepinephrine and epinephrine, 137, 138
  nosology, controversy, 14
  personality predisposition, 340
  TSH response to TRH, 162, 163

Unpleasant Events Schedule, 230, 231, 257
Up-regulation, alpha-receptors, 120
Urinary measures
monoamine metabolites, 138
shortcomings, 116

Validity
behavioral coding measures, 218-222
and depression measurement, 31, 32
and generalization, 205, 213, 214
Hamilton Rating Scale for Depression, 51, 52
multivantaged approach constructs, 302
overview, 31-33, 243
self-report scales, 269
structured diagnostic interviews, 46-48
Vanillylmandelic acid
NIMH Collaborative Study, 130-133, 136
urinary excretion, 115, 136
Vasopressin, 155
Verbal behavior
assessment, 200, 201, 210, 227, 229
marital interaction, 227
sequential characteristics, 229
Video Interview Behavior and Symptom Scale, 300
Visual Analogue Scale
versus Beck Depression Inventory, 244
characteristics, 73, 74, 244
Vitamin disorders, 22
Vulnerability factors, 270

Wakefield Self-Assessment Depression Inventory, 68
Wakefield scale, 212
Ward Behavior Checklist, 254
Ward Behavior Inventory, 224
Ward observations, 222-225
Wechsler scale, 212
Weight effects
dexamethasone test, 171, 172
HPA system, 170-172
Western culture, 380-394
Williamsburg Conference on Depression, 129
Wolpe-Lazarus Assertiveness Scale, 253
Women
and marriage, depression, 225, 226
social role assessment, 366, 367
World Health Organization study, 391, 393

Yuutsu, 386

Zimmerman's Inventory to Diagnose Depression, 78
Zung's Depression Status Inventory, 67, 68
Zung Self-Rating Depression Scale
and behavioral assessment, 207
characteristics, 66, 67
cross-cultural studies, 389, 390
and forms of depression, 10
response mode content, 212
symptom coverage comparison, 212

DATE DUE

DEC 15 2009			
GAYLORD			PRINTED IN U.S.A.